NEUROLOGICAL SYMPTOMS IN
BLOOD DISEASES

NEUROLOGICAL SYMPTOMS IN BLOOD DISEASES

Nello d'Eramo   and   Mario Levi

Translated by John Iliffe

UNIVERSITY PARK PRESS

Baltimore • London • Tokyo

UNIVERSITY PARK PRESS
International Publishers in Science and Medicine
Chamber of Commerce Building
Baltimore, Maryland 21202

A revised and updated translation of the Italian work *I sintomi neurologici nelle emopatie*, published by "Leonardo" Edizioni Scientifiche, Rome.

LIBRARY OF CONGRESS CATALOGING IN PUBLICATION DATA

D'Eramo, Nello.
  Neurological symptoms in blood diseases.

  Translation of I sintomi neurologici nelle emopatie.
  Bibliography: p.
  1. Neurologic manifestations of general diseases. 2. Blood—Diseases. I. Levi, Mario, joint author. II. Title.
RC343.D3913   616.8'04'71   72-1871
ISBN 0-8391-0703-X

*In honored memory
of Professor Giovanni Di Guglielmo,
for many years our revered teacher
of hematology*

CONTENTS

FOREWORD

In association with the various disorders of the hematopoietic system, neurologic manifestations of all kinds have been observed. Some no doubt have been coincidental and quite unrelated to the hematologic disorder. Others have been minor and inconsequential. Still others have been important though not necessarily directly related to the hematologic disease. Then there are some which are intimately related to the hematologic condition, as for example, the combined system disease which is encountered in pernicious anemia. Moreover, neurologic manifestations may seriously complicate therapy, as for example, the meningeal manifestations of acute leukemia which may develop in spite of an otherwise apparently complete remission of the disease with chemotherapy.

Reports regarding neurologic manifestations associated with hematologic disorders are widely scattered throughout the world literature. Some are single case reports; others are systematic studies of series of cases. Professors d'Eramo and Levi have undertaken the very laborious task of assembling this literature in a form which makes it available to us all. For this, scientific medicine owes them a debt of gratitude. The Italian edition of their monograph has been published in elegant form with excellent typography, good illustrations, and a full bibliography. The English translation does no less and also brings the literature up to date to the time of publication. It is a welcome addition to the hematologic literature.

Maxwell M. Wintrobe, M.D., PH.D.
*Professor and Head, Department of Medicine,
and Director, Laboratory for Study of
Hereditary and Metabolic Disorders,
University of Utah College of Medicine,
Salt Lake City*

FOREWORD TO THE ITALIAN EDITION

In the broadest sense of the term, diseases of the blood, that is diseases involving the constituents of the circulating blood and the hematopoietic tissues, must be regarded as truly general diseases, for they are clearly capable of causing modifications and alterations in the most disparate parts and organs of the body. Thus the study of blood diseases provides an instance of the reconstitution, on the phenomenological plane, of the unity of pathology, today obscured by the multiplicity of specializations characteristic of modern medicine.

The value of monographs such as this lies primarily in the contributions they make toward a deeper and more unified knowledge of diseases. Here the complex subject of hemopathies is thoroughly explored and analyzed in detail. Copious references are made to the literature, to personal communications, and to the authors' own numerous cases.

Since the involvement of the nervous system during the course of blood diseases is not infrequent and can lead to serious problems in diagnosis and treatment, my former pupils, Nello d'Eramo and Mario Levi, have performed a most useful service by assembling from the world literature the most valuable contributions dealing with the diagnosis and treatment of hemopathies, and by offering their conclusions to the medical profession in a single, broad, exhaustive treatise.

The authors accurately report and critically evaluate specific cases of blood diseases not only to analyze them but also to supply clinical data to support their analysis. These cases are supplemented by numerous references to the authors' own case series.

It gives me great satisfaction to know that this work was begun at the Medical Center of Rome under my direction. It was continued there under my successors, and was completed only after several more years of work and study by d'Eramo, while he was Head Physician at the City Hospital of Avezzano, and by Levi, while he was Head Physician at the City Hospital of Rieti. Their work was finally completed in the course of their professional practice in Rome.

The present monograph consists of descriptions of neurological complications in the broadest sense, including both functional and anatomical complications. As may readily be expected, such complications are frequently related to central nervous system hemorrhage or to infiltrative invasion, either of which may be secondary expressions of an underlying blood disease.

The medical practitioner will be particularly interested in the systematic and comprehensive exposition of the numerous syndromes and particular symptoms of nervous distress which demonstrate that central and peripheral neurological suffering in clinically encountered blood diseases is far-reaching and complex, indeed. This complexity is emphasized by the tendency of neurological signs to precede symptoms of underlying diseases and often to be forerunners of their clinical manifestations. With this knowledge the practitioner not only can avoid errors in diagnosis, but also will be more apt to follow a correct diagnostic course from the beginning.

Awareness of the possibility that neurological complications may be encountered in cases of polycythemia vera, erythroblastosis fetalis, or sarcoidosis could be significantly important to the clinician.

The authors devote special attention to the various forms of anemia, notably pernicious anemia (Biermer's disease). Leukemia and reticulosis are also treated at considerable length. The section dealing with porphyria is indeed excellent. A rich and fully up-to-date bibliography is provided with each chapter.

Of greater importance is the completeness, the modernity, and clarity of the text, and the fact that the work is based on a sound foundation of personal case experience, resulting in a monograph of highest clinical interest, on both the theoretical and practical levels; a work, indeed, that I take great pleasure in presenting to the medical profession, particularly to those whose concern lies with hematology and neurology.

Cesare Frugoni, M.D.
Professor Emeritus
Formerly Head, Department of Medicine
University of Rome, Italy

PREFACE

Changes in the nervous system that appear in the course of blood diseases are primarily referable to five factors:

1. metabolic disturbances
2. hypoxemia
3. ischemia (caused by compression or occlusion of vessels supplying the nerves), leading to hemodynamic disturbances and stasis
4. proliferation of infiltration of blood or reticulo-histiocyte cells
5. hemorrhage.

Neurological complications of this kind may be of particular importance as the first clinical sign of the underlying disease and hence a possible cause of erroneous diagnosis. Furthermore, the particular physiological features of the nervous system may sometimes result in their raising special therapeutic problems. Nerve involvement in blood diseases would seem to be fairly common, though clinical symptoms are not always present. No exact data are available, since statistical evidence based on systematic neurological and postmortem examinations is lacking. In the case of some diseases, however, such as leukemia, the published statistics give, on the whole, data on which a sufficiently documented judgment can be formed.

Occasionally, assessment of a correlation between hemopathy and neurological picture is difficult; the two conditions may, indeed, be completely independent of each other.

Both the central nervous system, with its various subdivisions, and the peripheral system may be involved. Therefore a great variety of clinical pictures may be observed, some of which may be particularly complex.

Chapter I

NEUROLOGICAL SYMPTOMS
IN ANEMIA

Decreased hemoglobin levels may result in neurological changes secondary to anemic anoxia. Such changes appear as various forms of nervous
pain, often cerebral. These are readily differentiated both anatomically
and clinically and are classified as "anemic anoxia neuropathies" (*Magri
and Fasano*). Hypoxic changes in the nervous system are, in any event,
rare and usually of slight extent in anemia.

In chronic anemia, particularly in serious cases, tissue nutrition may
reach a critical stage because of hypoxemia. Total blood quantity is not
diminished, however, and a regulatory mechanism, in the form of a
hyperkinetic circulatory syndrome (*d'Eramo et al.*), sometimes results in
outstanding increases in blood supply to the organs and nervous system.
Thus an anemia picture with 4.6 g% Hb may present brain venous O_2
pressure values around 25 mm Hg, i.e. well above the critical limit of
approximately 19 mm Hg (*Opitz and Schneider*). This explains the fact
that some intensely anemic subjects can continue to work and, in some
cases, can walk to the hospital for treatment (as in the case of a patient
suffering from pernicious anemia, with a red blood cell count of
1,100,000/mm³ and a hemoglobin level of 26%, reported by *Borchers and
Mittelbach*).

Of course, chronic anemia may nevertheless sometimes be accompanied by reversible neurological signs, particularly psychological disturbances.

General hypoxemia and decreased blood volume are factors of great
importance in anemia caused by hemorrhage and may lead to shock and
collapse in severe cases. Patients commonly complain of muscular
weakness, headache, dizziness, tinnitus, nausea, vomiting, transient or
permanent loss of vision, and they present pyramidal or extrapyramidal
symptoms (the latter may even constitute a form of parkinsonism:
necrosis of the globus pallidus after serious blood loss has been
observed). Heavy hemorrhage can also lead to atrophy of the optic

1

nerves. Other signs observed include decreased comprehension, disturbed sleep, and psychological changes.

The more serious disturbances attributable to hemorrhage occur at the height of the episode in only about 25% of cases; in the remainder they are observed from two to three days to two weeks later. Neurological symptoms are more commonly associated with bleeding from the digestive tract (35–40% of cases) and the uterus (20–30%) than with traumatic hemorrhage.

Borchers and Mittelbach report the case of a 53-year-old man who initially presented asthenia and dark stools caused by bleeding from an ulcer. These symptoms were ignored for six days, in spite of pronounced circulatory collapse on the sixth evening. Total bilateral amaurosis was observed on waking on the seventh morning and did not respond to emergency transfusion treatment.

Serious aplastic anemia may lead to psychological and sensory disturbances, sometimes even to coma (*De Renzi*); remissions, however, are not uncommon.

Anemia may, on the other hand, be accompanied by forms of neurological impairment that are clearly of a primary nature as far as the anemia is concerned, both conditions being mutually independent and of separate pathological origin (*Legramante and Zilli*). Such associations, first described by *Lichtheim* in 1887, were given the name "neuroanemic syndromes" by *Mathieu* in 1925. They are particularly common in pernicious anemia—originally they were thought to be confined to this form—and are occasionally observed in other megaloblastic perniciosiform types, in sideropenic anemia, and in both congenital and acquired hemolytic anemias (so-called neurohemolytic syndromes).

I. Pernicious Anemia (Biermer's Disease)

Neurological impairment in pernicious anemia is attributable to lack of vitamin B_{12} (fig. 1), *i.e.* to the cause of the primary disease. This, in turn, is caused by atrophic gastritis (a typical feature of the disease) and by a corresponding failure to secrete Castle's intrinsic factor, followed by nonabsorption of vitamin B_{12} by the intestinal mucosa. About 40% of cases present serum anti-intrinsic factor autoantibodies (*Schwartz; Taylor; Najean and Bernardy; Glass*). These autoantibodies inhibit the absorption of vitamin B_{12} by preventing its union with the intrinsic factor or by causing the precipitation of such a union (*Glass*). It must also be noted that about 70–90% of patients present cytoplasm autoantibodies

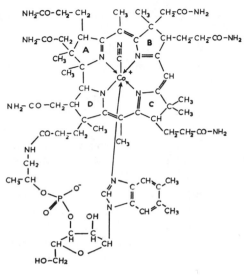

a

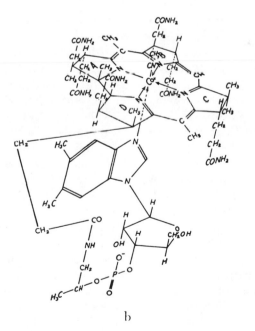

b

Fig. 1. Vitamin B12: (*a*) formula; (*b*) spatial arrangement (Figs. 1 and 2 in *Smith*).

antagonistic to gastric wall cells (*Dameshek et al.; De Boer et al.; Irvine; Kravetz et al.*).

The part played by vitamin B_{12} in the metabolic processes responsible for the functional efficiency and anatomical integrity of the myelin sheaths of nerve fiber is well known.

Several explanations have been advanced for the damage caused to these formations by a lack of vitamin B_{12}. Both in pernicious anemia and in simple vitamin B_{12} deficiency, increased p-hydroxyphenylpyruvic acid values are observed (*Bussi et al.; Wekes et al.*) and *Sinclair* has suggested that this acid combines with lipoic acid, resulting in inhibition of the conversion of the pyruvate to acetylcoenzyme A and ultimately causing nerve tissue damage. Support for this view may be seen in reports (*Earl et al.*) of increased blood pyruvic acid levels in some cases of funicular myelosis (combined system disease).

Other investigators (*Ling and Chow; Register*) maintain that vitamin B_{12} deficiency is followed by decreased levels of the nonprotein sulfhydryl groups (reduced glutathione) required for the oxidation of pyruvic aldehyde; this substance is thus free to combine with lipoic acid and cause nerve damage.

The most widely-held view, however, is that vitamin B_{12} deficiency is followed by depressed nucleoprotein synthesis, since the vitamin is indispensable for this process because of its activity in the metabolism of both DNA and RNA (*Nieweg et al.*). DNA is found only in the cell nucleus. During mitosis, the cell must double its chromosome component. This necessarily involves increased synthesis and it is here that vitamin B_{12} is indispensable. If it is lacking, cell reproduction is depressed and this is of particular consequence in tissues where cell turnover is rapid (hematopoietic tissue and the digestive tract epithelia); cytogenetic anomalies referable to DNA metabolic disorders have, in fact, been observed in the bone marrow of patients with pernicious anemia (*Kahn and Martin*). RNA, on the other hand, is found in the cytoplasm and nucleoli and is particularly abundant in nerve tissue, where cell multiplication is very low. Depressed RNA formation caused by vitamin B_{12} deficiency will thus result in damage to the nervous system. Such damage is not necessarily associated with anemia, since the two conditions are mutually independent (*Birkett-Smith*).

Folic acid is also important in nucleoprotein synthesis but is involved solely in the metabolism of DNA. Its lack of influence on RNA synthesis has been seen as an explanation for the fact that folic acid deficiency, while provoking perniciosiform changes in the hematopoietic system and digestive apparatus, does not result in damage to the nervous system (*Baldwin and Dalessio*). It should be noted, moreover, that the administration of massive doses of folic acid in megaloblastosis accompanied by neurological signs may, while improving the anemia picture, aggravate the nervous disturbances or even be responsible for their onset. Since the active forms of folic acid are converted as a result of the action of vitamin B$_{12}$ (*Bethell et al.*), such massive administration leads to increased vitamin B$_{12}$ consumption and hence to its depletion (*Vilter et al.*). Nervous system involvement therefore becomes likely.

Evidence of the particular sensitivity of the nervous system to vitamin B$_{12}$ deficiency has been given by *Begemann*. He found congenital hydrocephalus and crystalline changes in 28% and 54% respectively of rats born of mothers kept on a vitamin B$_{12}$-free diet. He also refers to the useful results obtained from the massive administration of this vitamin in the treatment of many forms of peripheral nerve degeneration.

Evident neurological involvement is a feature of about 20–30% of pernicious anemia cases (*Bensançon;Wintrobe; Villa and Bussi*), while 10% present signs of serious damage (*Grinker and Kandel*). If patients with only minimal signs are taken into account, however, the percentage rises to 90% (*Smithburn and Zerfas; Goldhamer et al.; Davidson*).

Nerve tissue changes in pernicious anemia were extensively studied before the introduction of replacement treatment, since the inevitably fatal outcome of the disease at that time ensured an abundant supply of necropsy material.

Neuroanemic syndromes in pernicious anemia may involve any part of the nervous system, from the brain to the peripheral nerves. The spinal cord, however, is the most commonly observed site, the funiculi posteriores being the first to be involved, followed by the laterales, particularly the spino-cerebellar and pyramidal tracts (fig. 2). This picture, known as "subacute combined sclerosis of the spinal cord," "combined system disease," or "funicular myelosis," forms the basis of the most typical example of neurological involvement encountered in the disease, *i.e.* Lichtheim's syndrome.

At a later stage, transverse fusion of the affected areas may lead to the creation of a characteristic ring-shaped appearance of the spinal cord; in exceptional cases, involvement is solely or primarily confined to the lateral white columns (Rieser-Russell syndrome, or "pure spastic paraplegia").

In other rare forms the typical impairment of white matter includes the ventral roots; sometimes the dorsal roots are involved, though only in advanced cases.

Damage to the spinal cord originates in the lower cervical and upper dorsal areas. Later in an ever-decreasing number of cases it spreads

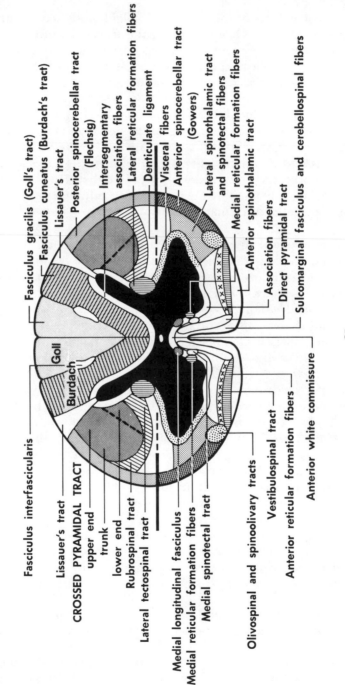

Fasciculus interfascicularis

Lissauer's tract

CROSSED PYRAMIDAL TRACT
upper end
trunk
lower end
Rubrospinal tract
Lateral tectospinal tract

Medial longitudinal fasciculus
Medial reticular formation fibers
Medial spinotectal tract

Olivospinal and spinoolivary tracts

Vestibulospinal tract

Anterior reticular formation fibers

Anterior white commissure

Fasciculus gracilis (Goll's tract)
Fasciculus cuneatus (Burdach's tract)
Lissauer's tract
Posterior spinocerebellar tract
(Flechsig)
Intersegmentary
association fibers
Lateral reticular formation fibers
Denticulate ligament
Visceral fibers
Anterior spinocerebellar tract
(Gowers)
Lateral spinothalamic tract
and spinotectal fibers
Medial reticular formation fibers
Anterior spinothalamic tract

Association fibers
Direct pyramidal tract
Sulcomarginal fasciculus and cerebellospinal fibers

Goll
Burdach

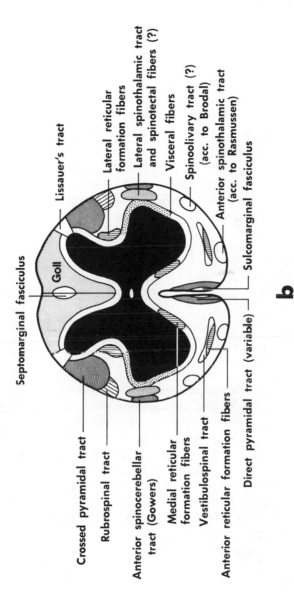

Septomarginal fasciculus

Goll

Lissauer's tract

Lateral reticular formation fibers

Lateral spinothalamic tract and spinotectal fibers (?)

Visceral fibers

Spinoolivary tract (?) (acc. to Brodal)

Anterior spinothalamic tract (acc. to Rasmussen)

Sulcomarginal fasciculus

b

Crossed pyramidal tract

Rubrospinal tract

Anterior spinocerebellar tract (Gowers)

Medial reticular formation fibers

Vestibulospinal tract

Anterior reticular formation fibers

Direct pyramidal tract (variable)

Fig. 2. Arrangement of the posterior funiculi of the spinal cord: (*a*) in the upper cervical segment; (*b*) in the lumbosacral segment (from Figs. 32*A* and 32*B* in *Masquin and Trelles*).

upwards and downwards, but rarely goes beyond the cervical marrow. In fact, changes in the elongated cord and the subcortical cones of the cerebral motor areas are uncommon. Equally rare is degeneration of the spinal ganglia, peripheral nerves, and of the celiac, mysenteric, and submucosal plexuses.

Macroscopic examination of the cord generally reveals little more than a slight decrease in size (*Bardeci*), together with edema (*Whitby and Britton*), changes in consistency, and, in chronic cases, slight decoloration resulting from sclerosis (*Trelles and Escalante*).

Histologically, the noninflammatory nature of the changes in the spinal tracts will be apparent. Usually only the myelin sheaths are affected, exhibiting distinct sites of dissolution, whereas the axons remain unimpaired for long periods. Simultaneous involvement of both will be observed only in extremely acute cases. Demyelinization is followed by partial cicatricial gliosis. This gives the spinal cord a so-called perforated field (*Peters*) or "beehive" appearance, marked by the presence of vacuolar spaces of various size filled with colliquated material and surrounded by connective tissue. In acute cases, small perivasal lymphocytic infiltrates may be observed. Punctiform hemorrhages, probably caused by capillary damage induced by hypoxemia, have also been reported.

As previously stated, cerebral lesions are not common. A distinction is drawn between specific and aspecific lesions. The former are histologically identical with lesions of the spinal cord and are found primarily in the parietal and frontal lobes, though they have also been observed in the corpus callosum, the internal capsule, and the white matter. Aspecific lesions appear when the hemoglobin level falls below 40% (*Ulbricht*). They are also present in other forms of anemia and appear to be related to tissue hypoxia: they include small perivasal hemorrhages attributable to diapedesis, the less common major intracerebral and meningeal hemorrhages, and parenchymal softening and necrosis.

Peripheral nerve involvement is even less common, especially as far as the cranium is concerned. Lesions consist of degeneration of the myelin sheaths—usually the largest (*Greenfield and Carmichael*)—though the axons may also be affected. Connective tissue repair reaction is poor (*Foster*). The anterior tibial nerves would seem to be the site of choice (*von Noorden*).

Neurological symptoms often appear well before hematological signs in pernicious anemia (in 25% of cases, *Wintrobe*), and may often be misinterpreted.

Lichtheim's syndrome is the most typical picture. This is observed mainly in subjects aged from 40 to 55 years and presents a fundamentally sensory symptom pattern in most cases: distal paresthesia (often permanent) involving first the lower and then the upper extremities. These signs are commonly misdiagnosed at first and may even be interpreted as cervical arthrosis; in a case reported by *Labauge et al.*, incessant reciprocal rubbing together of the fingers had led to an initial diagnosis of Parkinson's disease. Such paresthesias run a gradual course over periods of months or years and appear well in advance of more explicit pictures of nerve involvement. They rarely occur suddenly or run a rapid course. Though normally painless, they may occasionally cause lancinating pains, but never to the degree of those of tabes dorsalis (*Begemann*). Paresthesias of the trunk, with sensations of chest and abdominal constriction, have also been reported (*Thompson*).

Some workers attribute these paresthesias to involvement of the posterior funiculi, others (*Greenfield and Carmichael*) to damage to the peripheral nerves.

Motility disturbances follow, giving a picture similar to that of spastic paraplegia. The patient is usually able to walk. The organic character of the involvement will be demonstrated by changes in the reflexes. These are commonly depressed or even absent, particularly in the lower limbs. Here either posterior funicular or peripheral damage may be responsible; where such damage is limited in extent, however, exaggerated reflexes may be observed. Babinski's reflex (a sign of involvement of the lateral white columns) is often present.

Abdominal and cremasteric reflex behavior is not constant and either normal or nil responses may be obtained.

The motor symptoms are accompanied by a particular sensory syndrome. This includes subjective features (little or no pain, psychro-esthesia, sensation of walking on cotton, *etc.*) and well-defined objective signs: total retention of skin tactile, thermal, and pain sensitivity, marked changes in deep sensibility (loss of sense of position—first noticeable in the big toe—astereognosis and, more particularly, complete lack of response to tuning-fork vibrations first noticeable at 256 Hz) and static and dynamic cerebellar syndrome (ataxospastic gait, Romberg's sign).

The cerebrospinal fluid is usually normal, though slight changes in albumin content and weakly positive Nonne-Apelt and Pandy reactions may be observed. Increased phospholipid and, to a lesser extent, cholesterol values have been reported (*Carrega Cassafonth et al.*); *Introzzi* observed one case with increased glucose values.

The spontaneous evolution of the disease, which takes 12–18 months, is expressed as total flaccid paraplegia, with spinal automatism, sphincter disturbances, and trophic changes (edema and eschar). In two untreated cases, *Pant et al.* observed signs of a partial transection of the spinal cord, including a sensory level on the trunk. Massive transection, with spastic tetraplegia and neck sensory level, has since been reported by *Sollberg*.

In some cases, a few or even only one of the symptoms of the neuroanemic syndrome will be present. In Dejerine's "long radicular fiber syndrome," the posterior column nerve damage appears as paresthesia and deep anesthesia; in "pure spastic paraplegia" (Rieser-Russell syndrome, see above), too, a lateral column neurological picture develops.

Versé has reported funicular myelosis with psychological changes in a pernicious anemia patient aged two years and five months.

Brain symptoms in pernicious anemia are essentially psychological or psychotic. *Wintrobe* considers that minor disturbances (irritability and some depression) are present in two out of every three cases. However, true psychoses (*P. Emile-Weill* and *De Morsier* encephaloanemic syndromes) are both rare and protean. *Emile-Weill* distinguished between depressive, hypersthenic, and mixed types. Furthermore, such mixed types may be observed in a diphasic or recurrent version in which melancholic depression alternates with periods of neurohypersthenia.

Psychotic complications in pernicious anemia may appear as: a simple slowing down of ideation; states of anxiety or maniac agitation; stuporous depression; euphoria; visual or auditory hallucinations, which may assume characteristics of delirious melancholia; dementia or schizophrenic changes in behavior.

Besides the work of Emile-Weill and De Morsier, mention should also be made of the contributions of *Olmer; Columbo; Frià; Sarrouy and Portier; Gottwald; Roger; and Sollberg* to the study of psychological changes in pernicious anemia.

When marked cerebral signs are present, the cause may well lie in the patient's predisposition, quite apart from vitamin B$_{12}$ deficiency.

Psychological changes often appear long before the abnormal blood picture and may even be so striking as to mask it completely, with the result that it remains both undiagnosed and hence untreated. Irreversible brain lesions may occur in the form of widespread demyelinization of the white substance of uneven severity, most pronounced at the cortex-subcortex transition zone and unaccompanied by glial proliferation (*Adams and Kubik*).

In a personal case (reported by *Di Guglielmo*), a woman of 51 years with anemia of seven years' standing presented funicular myelosis and, more recently, psychological disturbance comprising depression, mental confusion, and loss of memory. Apathy and lack of interest in her surroundings were particularly noticeable in this subject. Occasionally, prolonged intractable anorexia was also observed.

Electroencephalographic evidence of a slowing down of electrical activity frequently points to widespread cerebral involvement in pernicious anemia (*Samson et al.; Walton et al.*). These signs are present in about two out of three untreated cases (*Thompson*) and appear to be unrelated to the degree of anemia, the extent of nerve involvement, or the patient's age.

Polyneuritis is sometimes reported as the initial or as the most outstanding clinical symptom (*Mathieu; van Bogaert; Alajouanine; Sollberg; etc.*). *Kampmeier and Jones* have observed retrobulbar neuritis, while *Enoksson and Norden* have collected 29 published examples of this lesion, in nine of which it was the initial symptom of vitamin B12 deficiency. In such forms, this includes fogging and loss of vision, central or paracentral scotoma, and disturbances of color vision. Partial regression is obtained with vitamin therapy, though color vision remains impaired, together with temporal paleness of the optic disk. Atrophy of the optic nerve, however, is rarely observed in pernicious anemia (*Castle and Minot; Amyot*).

Papillar edema is an equally uncommon finding (*Reid and Harris; Murphy and Costanzi*). Examination of the fundus oculi may reveal widespread retinal paleness and small roundish hemorrhagic patches scattered over the whole of the retina (*Stirpe*). A case of thrombosis of the central vein of the retina has been reported by *Stirpe*. In another case, homonymous hemianopsia regressed with improvement of the blood picture. Hemorrhagic retinitis responds to treatment more quickly than the anemia. Examination of the fundus may thus be of assistance in prognosis (*Storti*).

Neuro-ophthalmological associations are more commonly observed in males (*Hamilton et al.*). It has therefore been suggested that, apart from vitamin B12 deficiency, another etiopathogenetic factor—identified by *Freeman and Heaton* in tabagism—is also operative in these cases.

Very exceptionally, upward or downward gaze paralysis (Parinaud's syndrome) has been reported (*Kissel et al.*).

Nystagmus was observed by *Erbslöh* in 1% of his series. Involvement of the auditory nerve, changes in the sense of taste and smell, dysarthria, and pharyngeal and laryngeal paralysis have also been reported.

Lockner et al. observed electroneurographic signs of median nerve impairment in 33% of a series of 34 cases of pernicious anemia. Subjective symptoms, however, were present in only 7%. Neuropathy would seem to be an early sign rather than a late complication.

A Parkinson-type picture was present in a case observed by *Portuonod y de Castro*; this improved considerably with hepatotherapy.

The diagnosis of these neurological signs may sometimes present difficulty and may not be recognized for some time (*Wieck*), particularly since—as has been stated—the symptom picture may be free of hematological signs of pernicious anemia; *Boudin and Barbizet* report a case in which signs of nerve damage appeared at least five years before the hematological symptoms.

It should, of course, be remembered that pernicious anemia is one of the leading causes of spinal marrow change. *D'Eshougues* places it immediately after multiple sclerosis and tumors, and ahead of syphilis.

In addition to the purely hematological studies that must be made of peripheral blood and bone marrow and to biochemical investigation of the gastric juice for achylia, early detection of pernicious anemia will depend on the determination of serum vitamin B_{12} levels (*Birkett-Smith*), urinary and stool excretion of the vitamin, liver scanning after ingestion of labeled vitamin B_{12}, and evaluation of the gastric juice intrinsic factor content. Schilling's test (1954) is also useful (*Cossa*): when ordinary vitamin B_{12} is injected into the pernicious anemia or gastrectomized patient, urinary excretion of labeled vitamin derived from absorption pools in the liver is extremely low, but will return to normal after administration of intrinsic factor.

Lichtheim's syndrome may be confused with multiple sclerosis. In addition to causing spastic paralysis of the lower extremities, multiple sclerosis may also be responsible for paresthesia and deep sensitivity changes; differential diagnosis, however, is made possible by the fact that the neuroanemic syndrome runs a subacute course, whereas multiple sclerosis is punctuated by periods of regression.

Other points of difference from multiple sclerosis are: absence of nystagmus (noted by *Erbslöh* in only 1% of his pernicious anemia series), absence of intention tremor, the possible persistence of abdominal wall reflexes, and the predominant involvement of the lower limbs (*Bodechtel and Schrader*).

The association of spastic paraplegia and deep sensibility disturbances must also be differentiated from intramedullary tumors and posterior spinal compression caused by a prolapsed disk. Dejerin's "long radicular fiber syndrome" can be distinguished from tabes dorsalis both by syphilis-negative serum and liquor findings and by the presence of unimpaired superficial sensibility. "Pure spastic paraplegia" must also be distinguished from Erb's myelitis.

A useful diagnostic aid in pernicious anemia polyneuritis is constituted by the fact that there is no predominance of superficial sensibility impairment in the overall pattern of sensibility changes.

It should not be forgotten that funicular myelosis is not the sole prerogative of pernicious anemia. As well as in other blood diseases (perniciosiform, sideropenic, and hemolytic anemia, leukemia, and reticulosis), it may be observed in: avitaminosis (beriberi and scurvy), poisoning (alcoholism, ergotism, and lathyrism), Addison's and Basedow's diseases, diabetes mellitus, acute yellow atrophy of the liver, nephritis, carcinosis, diseases of the pancreas, long-standing infections (*Begemann*). Idiopathic forms have also been reported. About 30% of all cases of funicular myelosis are not attributable to pernicious anemia (*Bodechtel and Schrader*).

In diagnosing psychological symptoms, the possible simulation of Korsakoff's syndrome in the absence of evidence of anemia should be borne in mind.

Immediate administration of vitamin B_{12} is the basic therapy for the nerve lesions of pernicious anemia, since they are reversible only in the early stages. Later, involvement of the axons leads to permanent damage, since these formations are totally incapable of regenerative activity. There are greater chances of success in young subjects.

Treatment with vitamin B_{12} has now completely replaced raw liver, liver, and gastric extracts. Since it achieves total regression, it has reversed the former extremely poor prognosis for nerve lesions in pernicious anemia.

Early diagnosis of the nature of the neurological signs is essential, particularly where symptoms of anemia are delayed or masked. Pernicious anemia can cause more damage in its early stages when its clinical picture is not fully clear.

Some workers (*Lereboullet and Pluvinage, etc.*) advise massive doses of vitamin B_{12} to overcome the slight but real danger of vitamin resistance. Daily intramuscular administration of 4,000 µg for two weeks is followed by consolidation and then by maintenance doses.

Others (*Creyssel et al.*), however, dispute the validity of this method and point out that vitamin B_{12} treatment is equally effective at minimal doses. Moreover, it has been shown that urinary excretion of this vitamin is directly proportional to the dose administered.

Labauge et al. recommend 100 µg per day until the peak of the reticulocyte crisis, followed by the same dose per week until correction of the anemia and 100 µg thereafter per month for life. They state that a period of two months is usually enough for correction of the symptoms of anemia, whereas resolution of the neurological picture is a much longer process and depends on how early treatment is begun.

As examples, we may cite two cases reported by *Garcin* in which four years and nine years passed before the total regression of a bilateral

Babinski's reflex and paresthesia respectively; paresthesia is, in any event, much slower to disappear than disturbances in gait and deep sensibility.

In some cases, the reappearance of osteotendinous reflexes under therapy may be expressed by their presentation in exaggerated form. This has been attributed to rapid regression of the peripheral component, cord changes being poorly responsive to treatment (*Thompson*). In successfully treated cases, the onset of electroencephalographic regression is usually noted within seven days (*Thompson*).

Suspension of vitamin B$_{12}$ administration may lead to relapse of both the blood and the neurological picture. The recurrence of nerve lesions, indeed, may well progress to paraplegia, though its course is usually insidious and gradual over a period of several months; sudden relapses are very occasionally observed.

Some workers (*Heinrich and Gabbe*) advise intraspinal administration of vitamin B$_{12}$ in advanced cases of funicular myelosis.

Reasons have already been given for the total contraindication of folic acid in neuroanemic syndromes and in megaloblastosis in general. In any event, this substance should be used with extreme caution and should not be administered in the commonly encountered forms of anemia with ill-defined pictures and uncertain diagnosis. An instructive example may be seen in the history of four patients reported by *Conley and Krevans.* These subjects presented cord sclerosis and achylia unaccompanied by anemia or megaloblastosis. Since they had made extensive use of reconstituent tablets containing folic acid, this substance had probably been responsible for preventing the onset of frank pernicious anemia, but may have encouraged the neurological disturbances.

Pearson et al. report the case of a 32-month-old boy who presented severe involvement of the nervous system, including ataxia and coma, following several treatments with folic acid for megaloblastic anemia (later diagnosed as pernicious). Rapid and dramatic improvement of the neurological picture was obtained with vitamin B$_{12}$, though the patient was left with partial deafness and retarded mental development, probably the result of prolonged B$_{12}$ deficiency. In reporting the neurological picture observed on the administration of folic acid, the writers stress the necessity of determining the etiology of megaloblastic anemia beyond all doubt so that proper treatment can be prescribed. They offer a combined therapeutic-diagnostic criterion: the administration of daily physiological doses (25–100 μg) of folic acid will lead to the prompt remission of folic acid deficiency anemia, but unlike massive folic acid doses, they will have no effect on vitamin B$_{12}$-deficiency forms.

Collateral treatment of pernicious neuroanemic syndromes includes 100 mg/day vitamin B₁ and blood transfusions.

II. *Perniciosiform Anemia*

Neurological symptoms are observed in other forms of megaloblastosis, though much less frequently than in pernicious anemia.

Funicular myelosis, usually expressed in the form of paresthesia, is occasionally observed in the **gastrectomized patient** (agastric anemia) (*Pawlovsky, Tomoda*) and may, indeed, occur many years after surgery (*Henning; Stöhr*) as a result of the exhaustion of vitamin B₁₂ deposits. Paraparesis, unaccompanied by sensibility impairment, was observed seven years after gastrectomy by *Cacudi* in one case; regression was obtained with vitamin B₁₂. Funicular myelosis following partial gastrectomy has been reported by *Williams et al.*, and others.

Nerve involvement is also rare in **sprue**, though damage attributable to funicular myelosis is occasionally reported (*Woltman and Heck; Kant and Lubing*). However, psychological disturbances (depression and irritability) are relatively common.

Bothriocephalus anemias display only rare (*Björkenheim*) and rather slight forms of nerve involvement (mild paresthesia and slight ataxia).

In megaloblastic anemias considered to be folic acid deficiency states, the administration of this substance is not usually followed by the appearance of neurological complications; funicular signs are not normally observed.

When such anemia is the result of **pregnancy**, spinal damage is unusual; slight involvement was reported in one of eight cases by *Strauss and Castle*. *Di Guglielmo* has suggested that the rarity of neurological signs may be an aid in distinguishing this form from pernicious anemia. Aphonia, unaccompanied by other signs of nerve involvement and cured with anemia therapy, was observed in only two of a series of 335 pregnancy anemia patients collected by *Giles*. Cases of retinal hemorrhage have been reported (*Thompson and Ungley; Lowenstein et al.*).

Babinski's reflex, sluggish patellar reflexes, and depressed sensibility to vibration have been observed as symptoms of spinal cord involvement in megaloblastic anemia attributable to **anticonvulsant drugs** (*Silber*): diphenylhydantoin, primidone, phenobarbitone, and methophenobarbitone have been incriminated in this respect. The first case of megaloblastic anemia referable to anticonvulsants was reported by *Mannheimer et al.* in 1952.

III. Iron Deficiency Anemia

To judge by the very small number of cases reported in the literature, neuroanemic syndromes are rarely encountered in iron deficiency anemia. Iron treatment brings rapid relief. Little is therefore known of the particular anatomical and pathological features of neurological damage associated with this form of anemia.

Such deficiencies may vary considerably in etiology (diet, idiopathic hypochromic anemia, chlorosis, intestinal parasitosis, pregnancy, partial gastroresection, and gastroenterostomy). The rarely encountered neuroanemic syndromes are attributable to idiopathic hypochromic anemia or, where psychoanemic forms are concerned, to chlorosis.

Evidence for the association of the neurological lesion with the anemia may be seen in the effectiveness of the administration of iron. It has, however, been suggested that iron deficiency has an indirect effect on nerve tissue by interfering with intestinal absorption of vitamin B$_{12}$ and hence a fall in levels. This view is supported by reports of cases in which hypochromic iron deficiency anemia has given way to a typically megaloblastic form (*Gram; Lenhartz; Greppi*). Subnormal blood levels of vitamin B$_{12}$ in iron deficiency anemia have also been observed to become normal after the administration of iron.

On some occasions, however, secondary iron deficiency may mask megaloblastic anemia, which may appear subsequently and will undoubtedly be the source of any neurological symptoms that are observed.

Both hemicrania (in chlorosis) (*Daniels and Roelofs*) and funicular myelosis (*Chevallier et al.*) have been described. Brain damage, with predominantly psychological symptoms, is a notable feature of chlorosis and includes irritability, emotivity, restlessness, a tendency towards sadness and melancholia, and loss of ability to concentrate; peripheral nerve involvement primarily consists of neuritic symptoms (paresthesia, sluggishness of the extremities, depression or loss of reflexes) (*Worster-Drought and Shafar; Whitby and Britton*). Associations of cranial and peripheral nerve damage may result in the appearance of a particularly serious picture ("encephalic and polyneuritic forms," *Mathieu*). *Scuro et al.* have reported a case of iron deficiency anemia in which an extremely serious polyneuritic picture was accompanied by the involvement of some of the cranial nerves (right 6th, both sides of the 7th, and the 9th and 10th), together with signs of damage to the spinal cord and brain. Total remission was obtained with iron therapy.

Cases of papillitis caused by congestion were observed by *Watkins*. He attributed them to local tissue reaction to hypoxemia. Mention may also be made of the observations made by *Capriles* with reference to intracranial hypertension in an iron-deficiency series. Two female subjects (aged 19 and 27 years) with an anemia picture similar to classic chlorosis complained of headaches followed by disturbed vision. Apart from a slight degree of stiffness of the neck, there were no objective neurological signs; frank edema of the papilla was observed, however, together with increased cerebrospinal fluid pressure, though fluid albumin values were normal. There were no ventriculographic or gas encephalographic signs. Rapid and lasting regression was obtained with blood transfusions and iron gluconate. *Capriles* points out that early treatment is essential if further deterioration of vision is to be prevented. Thus, in another case, a 37-year-old woman with a one year history of headaches progressed to complete blindness in spite of iron treatment with decompressive trepanation of the skull and repeated spinal punctures. In yet another case, on the other hand, endocranial hypertension was not accompanied by papillitis. It is suggested that such hypertension is the result of cerebral edema, this in turn caused by tissue and capillary anoxia induced by anemia. Decreased iron-bearing enzyme levels probably aggravate the anoxia.

Papillary edema has also been observed in various states of anemia by *Reid and Harris; Murphy and Costanzi* (see above under pernicious anemia); *Lubeck; and Schwaber and Blumberg*. This was attributed to changes in the relationship between retinal artery and vein pressure or between cerebrospinal and intraocular fluid pressure (*Aita*). A clinical picture of cerebral pseudotumor was present in the case observed by *Murphy* and *Costanzi*. An example of severe bilateral papillitis, with small flame-like peripapillary hemorrhagic radiations, has been reported by *Stirpe* in a case of Lederer's anemia.

Iron deficiency may also produce neurological symptoms without causing anemia (*Hittmair*).

IV. Hemolytic Anemia

Cases of neurohemolytic syndromes began to appear in the literature well over half a century ago. A case reported by *Salomon* (1914) was followed by those of *Curshmann; Lemaire et al.; Cassano and Benedetti; Michelazzi;* and others.

In a critical review of these cases, *Sarrouy and Portier* (1951) stressed that they could not be regarded simply as coincidences and made a considerable advance towards their nosographical classification. Up to that time, reported cases had dealt only with congenital forms; since then, neuroanemic syndromes have also been observed in acquired hemolytic anemia.

The hemolytic crises of **constitutional hemolytic icterus** may be accompanied by severe headache, vertigo, vasomotor reactions, or generalized cramp-like symptoms. Such disturbances are undoubtedly secondary manifestations of the state of anemia which occurs during the crisis. The literature also contains reports of individual cases of spastic paraplegia, Strümpell-Lorrain paraplegia, funicular changes, Friedreich's disease, P. Marie's ataxia, myoclonic epilepsy with amyostatic syndrome and cerebellar disturbances, muscle atrophy, and tabes-like syndromes (*Salomon; Curshmann; Lemaire et al.; Dumolard et al.; Michelazzi; Pecorella; Portier et al., and others*).

Heavy demands on vitamin B_{12} reserves caused by enormously increased erythropoiesis in response to the hemolytic crisis are considered to constitute the pathogenesis of funicular changes. Strong support for this view comes from the clear signs of megaloblastosis observed during the crisis.

There is, however, also a possibility that neurological damage owes its origin to the same hereditary defect as the primary disease; this agrees with the classification "neuroanemic syndrome."

Nerve damage is frequently observed in **sickle-cell or drepanocytic anemia.** *Rowland* reported serious neurological complications in 29% of a 92 patient series collected over a period of ten years.

The term sickle-cell anemia includes a group of systemic blood diseases in which the red cells display a sickle-like appearance in anoxia (sickling test) caused by the presence of typical pathological hemoglobin (S). Electrophoretic studies have revealed associations of hemoglobin S with other forms. The homozygous S disease (SS) must thus be distinguished from various heterozygous forms including: SA, the simple heterozygous form consisting of the association of the abnormal hemoglobin S with the normal A; SC, a double heterozygous form (two abnormal hemoglobins); SF (more correctly SAF), in which the presence of the F hemoglobin typical of thalassemia ("microcytemia" of *Silvestroni and Bianco*) has given rise to the term thalassodrepanocytosis (*i.e.,* the "anemia microdrepanocitica" first described by *Silvestroni and Bianco* in 1945).

Neurological involvement in sickle-cell anemia is more common in America (*Hugues et al.; Patterson et al.; Wintrobe*) than in Africa (*Raper; Lambotte-Legrand and Lambotte-Legrand*). This may be attributable to the higher frequency of heterozygotism in the African continent or to the more rapid course of the disease, which does not allow the neurological lesions time to establish themselves.

Signs of nerve involvement are rather uncommon in thalassodrepanocytosis.

Damage to the nervous system primarily involves the brain and is essentially vascular. Massive and single softening (case reported by *Connel*) or small, bilateral, multiple, and variously developed softening (*Thompson et al.*) may be observed in the cortex and, less frequently, in the white substance. Necrosis of the pons (*Wertham et al.*) or the cerebellum (*Tori*) is rare. Cerebral, cerebromeningeal, or subarachnoid hemorrhage is occasionally reported. In cerebromeningeal forms, the hemorrhage site is sometimes of considerable extent and may involve the ventricular cavities (*Fadell and Crone*). In other cases, however, small, multiple hemorrhagic sites are observed (*Thompson et al.*). Subdural hematoma is not unknown (*Bauer and Fischer*). Associations of hemorrhage and softening of the brain have been reported (*Walker and Murphy; Thompson et al.*).

Thrombosis of the lumen of the different vessels because of the accumulation of red cells is a typical finding; aggregates of this kind have a site of choice in the capillaries. Involvement of the arteries, particularly the superficial branches of the internal carotid (*Connel*), is reported occasionally. Reports of damage to the cortical veins have been given by *Thompson et al.*, while *Penna de Azevedo and Ford* have described lesions of the venous sinuses.

Fatty thrombi may be found in the lumen of the vessels and are a characteristic feature of sickle-cell anemia (*Vance and Fisher; Wade and Stevenson; Brittingham and Phinizzi; and others*). Fat emboli are usually disseminated and often associated with red cell accumulation thrombi and, more frequently, with bone necrosis of vascular origin.

Endothelial proliferation and thickening of the arteriolar media have been described; the anatomical picture in such cases may recall that of thromboangiitis obliterans.

Damage to the spinal cord was observed by *Wertham et al.* This included multiple (cervical and lumbar) degeneration, with zonal demyelinization of the posterior and (less frequently) the lateral column and gliosis of the anterior cornua.

Low concentrations of O_2 are held responsible for the formation of intravasal red cell clumps. The abnormal hemoglobin S (less soluble than the normal type) tends to take the form of crystallized birefracting tactoids under these conditions, giving the cell its characteristic sickle shape. Decreased circulation rate caused by sickle cell rigidity is followed by increased blood viscosity and hence by congestion and risk of thrombosis. These changes lead to anoxia and this further enhances sickle-cell formation (*Harris*'s vicious circle).

In sickle cell anemia, in fact, the onset of anoxia, however caused (infection, acute infantile dehydration, or puerperalism), may encourage neurological involvement.

Fatty embolism of the cerebral vessels is assumed to be the result of bone marrow necrosis caused by skeletal tissue infarct. *Wertham et al.,* on the other hand, stress that the fat corpuscles are formed of lipoids and not neutral fats, this being a sign of disturbed red cell fat metabolism and not of marrow damage.

A complicated pathogenesis must undoubtedly be postulated for the intracranial hemorrhage observed in sickle cell anemia and no clear explanation can be offered for its frequent occurrence during transfusion treatment, after correction of the basic disease.

Little anatomical data are available on thalassodrepanocytosis. *Silvestroni and Fontana* studied the spleens of three splenectomized patients and *Romeo* and *Ascenzi and Silvestroni* have each presented an anatomical and histological study of one case. In that of *Ascenzi and Silvestroni,* increased dura mater tension and small hemorrhages were noted on both sides of the falx cerebri. Brain weight was 1,460 g. The cerebral circumvolutions were rather flat, while the meninges were finely injected and the veins congested with slight hemorrhagic suffusions at the upper end of the border between the frontal and the right parietal lobes. Slight overall loss of nerve substance consistency was observed, with a gelatinous appearance at some points of the cerebellum: the arbor vitae was virtually indistinguishable. Histological examination of the cortex and subcortical layers showed signs of edema and capillary and venular engorgement on the part of continuous clumps of conglutinated sickle cells. Edema, hemorrhage, and capillary engorgement caused primarily by sickle cells were also observed in the cerebellum.

Cerebral vascular accidents and epileptic crises are also observed, especially in homozygous forms of the disease; these occur most frequently during acute hemolytic attacks, whether in second infancy, adolescence, or early adulthood. On some occasions, the neurological signs are the first symptoms of the primary disease. Their presence in heterozygous forms is by no means impossible (*McCormick*).

Sudden onset, mild symptoms, rapid regression, and ready recurrence form the general pattern of these cerebral accidents. Headache is common (*Hugues et al.; Patterson et al.*) and is often relieved by epistaxis or spinal puncture (*Margolies*). Migraine, vertigo, tinnitus, deafness, transient blindness, and diplopia have all been reported.

Epileptic crises are relatively frequent (*Hugues et al.; Hill et al.*), usually during anemic episodes. *Languillon* reports the case of a Guadeloupe native in which the diagnosis of idiopathic epilepsy, made in infancy, had eventually to be replaced by that of sickle-cell anemia because of the association of the convulsive episodes with the recrudescence of hemolysis. Signs of epilepsy might also be interspersed with periods of coma. The reason for such episodes is not clear, though they may be considered as being the equivalent of epilepsy. In a case of this type reported by *Kampmeier,* the later course included meningeal hemorrhage and right hemiplegia.

Cortical hemiplegia, usually partial and sometimes accompanied by aphasia, must be considered a major cerebral accident and is very often part of a particularly serious neurological picture, whose first symptoms include vegetative disturbances and coma. Hemiplegia will be less serious when related to softening of the cerebral tissue, whereas cerebral or ventricular hemorrhage will be responsible for more drastic episodes. The possibility of softening accompanied by hemorrhage must not be overlooked (*Cook; Kampmeier*).

Clinical pictures dependent on massive cerebral necrosis (*Connel*) or fat embolism are particularly serious; in the latter case, the typical picture has two stages: first, violent dorsal and lumbar pain resulting from the vertebral infarct; second (after 2–3 days), deep and commonly irreversible coma (*Wade and Stevenson*).

Isolated aphasia is very exceptional (*Bosselman and Kraines*). Subarachnoidal hemorrhage has been reported (*Sydenstricker et al.; Arena; Ballard and Bondar*). Ophthalmological changes are an important feature of sickle cell. anemia. Vitreous hemorrhages are common and the most usual cause of blindness. Disturbances of the fundus result in proliferating retinitis, with occlusion of the central artery of the retina, and vitreous hemorrhage. Cases of hemianopsia have also been reported.

Lastly, psychological changes (confusion, agitation, drowsiness, etc.) have been described (*Ribstein et al*).

Occasionally, the symptom picture of brain involvement may be unusually protean, as in cerebral malaria (*Thompson*).

Damage to the spinal cord seems to be extremely rare. The literature contains very few cases and only one anatomical study (*Wertham et al.*). Combined medullary sclerosis has been reported (*Cassano and Benedetti; Trincao and Madeira*), as well as progressive spasmodic paraplegia with deep sensibility disturbances (*Charmot and Reynaud*). Partial regression was obtained in the latter case when the number of blood cells rose.

The clinical picture of funicular myelosis in the case reported by *Cassano and Benedetti* did not change when vitamin B_{12} was administered, but proved responsive to vitamin B_1.

Cord changes of this type are considered to be an expression of systemic degeneration of the marrow or the result of anoxia induced by stasis and vascular obliteration.

Wintrobe has reported a case in which the initial neurological picture was interpreted as poliomyelitis. A radiculomedullary syndrome in a case presented by *Ford* was caused by crushing of the vertebrae following a succession of bone infarcts. Sciatic neuralgia with signs of 4th and 5th lumbar infarct was observed in a case reported by *Legant and Ball.* Polyneuritis has also been described.

Neurological signs have been observed by *Silvestroni and Bianco* in thalassodrepanocytosis: convulsions, violent headache followed by fatal coma; occipital headache (case studied anatomically and histologically by *Ascenzi and Silvestroni*) followed by mental confusion and loss of consciousness with tonic-clonic contractions of the right arm and semiface. A desire to eat small pieces of plaster ("geophagist's anemia," *Caminopetros*) is often observed.

The liquoral changes in sickle-cell anemia include increased pressure, xanthochromia, and increased protein and cell levels (*Wintrobe; Ribstein et al.*). Sickle cells are also found.

Both localized and diffuse electroencephalographic abnormalities have been reported. These may at times be more impressive than might have been expected from the clinical picture (*Hill et al.; Portier et al.*). Examination of the fundus oculi will often reveal tortuous retinal vessels (*Smith and Conley*).

Some neurological episodes (hemorrhage, softening of the brain) are always potentially fatal. Regression, with or without sequelae, is possible, however, though recurrence must usually be expected. This may occur several times (*Cowley-Chavez et al.*), either mirroring the first episode or with a different symptom picture (*Bridgers; Ford*).

The sequelae of these episodes may include chronic encephalopathy, marked by the presence of long-standing epilepsy, or infantile cerebral hemiplegia, or various degrees of delayed mental development. Associations of these signs are common (*Anastasopoulos et al.*). Unilateral or widespread cerebral atrophy may be observed radiologically.

Sickle-cell anemia may be heralded by neurological symptoms and these are commonly misinterpreted.

Kampmeier has reported the case of a young patient who was admitted five times for convulsion complicated by variously diagnosed coma and fever. Sickle-cell anemia was not identified until the fourth admission. *Yoyo et al.* observed a case in which a patient was admitted in what was thought to be a state of alcoholic excitement but was later identified as sickle-cell anemia psychosis.

Pictures of this kind are more common in the heterozygous forms of drepanocytosis, which are often hematologically silent. On the other hand, cerebral accident in a young African or American Negro, or in an inhabitant of the Mediterranean basin should always be thought of in terms of an association with sickle-cell anemia. Careful screening of other possibilities will, of course, be required in the course of differential diagnosis. Focal epilepsy, for example, will raise the suspicion of intracranial tumor, whereas meningocerebral hemorrhage in a Caucasian child must be considered as a possible expression of cerebrovascular deformity. In a case reported by *Wertham,* meningocerebral hemorrhage attributed to sickle-cell anemia was found on necropsy to be the result of the rupture of a congenital aneurysm of the middle cerebral artery. Cerebral angiography will also give the diagnostician useful data concerning obliteration of the large arterial vessels, a condition that rarely forms part of the sickle-cell picture (*De Mello et al.*). In the adult, thought must always be given to the possibility of hypertension or atherosclerosis. Lastly, it must not be forgotten that a meningeal infection caused by ordinary pyogens or tuberculosis may easily arise in the course of drepanocytosis and simulate a hemorrhage attributable to the primary disease: here lumbar puncture will prevent a false diagnosis.

Sickle-cell anemia has no specific remedy. Prophylactic measures designed to prevent incomplete blood O_2 saturation offer the best chance of avoiding the consequences of circulation blocks. Methylene blue has proved useful in the treatment of the psychotic symptoms (*Yoyo et al.; Ribstein et al.*).

Systemic damage to the nervous system (cretinism) has been observed in **ovalocytary** (elliptocytary) **anemia;** divergent squint (*Gerrits and De Vries*) and mental deficiency have also been reported (*Fernandez Ithurrat e Silvestre*).

Psychoasthenia would seem to be the most common sign (*Greppi and Di Guglielmo*) in **thalassemia minor** (Rietti-Greppi-Micheli disease). This may be the result of congenital diencephalic disturbance. Electroencephalography and gas encephalography have shown serious brain changes and a tendency to develop diffuse cerebral atrophy (*Greppi and Di Guglielmo*). *Cabibbo et al.* and *Pompili and Sinibaldi* have each reported a case of funicular myelosis in this disease.

In **Cooley's anemia** (thalassemia major), extrapyramidal symptoms were observed by *Davison and Wechsler* in a 10-year-old Italian boy. These workers compared the neurological picture in their case with that of hepatolenticular degeneration. Werdnig-Hoffmann type amyotrophy was noted by *Colarizi and Mengoli* in a 9-month-old boy with "hemolytic icterus with increased globular resistance."

It has been suggested that the neurological lesions of thalassemia major follow the same hereditary pattern as the principal disease.

Examination of the brain will very often reveal widespread edema of the nervous substance, which may be so marked as to give a sieve-like appearance to the parenchyma (*Frongia*). Anemic pallor is commonly observed in the cerebral tissue, together with hemorrhagic sites and thickening of the leptomeninges or the dura, sometimes with the appearance of fibrino-hemorrhagic pachymeningitis (*Maggioni and Ascenzi; Frongia*).

In **methemoglobinemia,** there is an accumulation of a trivalent ferric-iron that cannot combine in respiratory exchanges and involvement of the nervous system may be observed. In congenital enzymopenic methemoglobinemia, according to *Finch,* mild headache, under stress or depression, vertigo, and other similar disturbances are occasionally reported. Retarded mental development (9 of 58 cases in the series of *Fialkow et al.*) is attributed to potentiation of genetic tendencies to oligophrenia by the primary disease (*Tönz*). Other neurological symptoms include hypotonia, areflexia, athetosis, squint, etc. Pathological electroencephalographic pictures may also be observed.

In **paroxysmal nocturnal hemoglobinuria** (Marchiafava-Micheli syndrome), venous thrombosis of the brain or portal vein system is the most frequent cause of death (*Dacie*); the spinal cord is never involved. Thrombophilia is here attributable to blood cell instability in the face of the action of plasma hemolytic factors, now considered to form part of the complement: platelet lysis leads to the release of thromboplastin, which is then converted to prothrombin and thrombin. In a case reported by *Perreau et al.,* thrombosis of the upper longitudinal sinus of the dura mater in a 37-year-old man had given rise to bilateral papillary edema. Thrombosis of the hepatic veins was also observed in this subject. *Atamer* reports an example of hemiplegia observed by *Pierce and Aldrich.* Left hemiplegia with swallowing and behavior disturbances was reported by *Reynes et al.* Necropsy showed venous thromboses and serious hemorrhagic softening sites in the brain.

Coma and meningeal manifestations (*Lederer, etc.*), paresis, delirium, and agitation—attributed to purpura and brain edema—have been reported in **acquired hemolytic anemia caused by autoantibodies** in children. A 60-year-old patient described by *Lesbros and Bigonnet,* with signs of atherosclerosis, presented signs of disturbed vision and hearing simultaneously with cold-induced hemoglobinuric accidents with jaundice (icterus). In a case reported by *Milliez et al.,* an apparently acquired hemolytic icterus was complicated by combined medullary sclerosis. Splenectomy was followed by rapid regression of the hemolytic symptoms (Coombs test negative) and clinical cure occurred within one year of the appearance of the neurological signs. Reference may also be made to a 40-year-old patient observed by *Cattan et al.*, who presented extrapyramidal symptoms and brain and sensory disturbances (recurrent confusion and delirium, hypersomnia) in chronic hemolytic anemia attributable to cold agglutinins. The cerebral lesions simulated those described for nuclear icterus and the patient also presented atrophic cirrhosis of the liver and Sjögren's syndrome. Unusually serious chronic cold agglutinin disease was observed by *Borchers and Mittelbach* in a 60-year-old man. The symptom picture had developed over a period of 15 months, starting with typical cyanosis of the extremities, which passed from the hands to the face and, more particularly, to the ears, nose, and cheeks, and had reached a point where even the slightest exposure to cold was followed by circulatory disturbances (dizziness, headache). Hemolysis was virtually absent and both the icterus and the anemia were mild. A particularly serious episode of intravasal red cell agglutination could not be resolved even by intense heating of the patient and led to deep cyanosis and fatal coma. The terminal cold agglutinin titer was 1:262,000 and the agglutinates could not be dissolved below 45°C *in vitro*. Necropsy revealed cord pallor, whereas the cerebral cortex was deep red-blue in color. Histological examination of the vessels showed that clumped, homogenized red cell fragments were present at only a few points, whereas a partly granular amorphous blood deposit was observed elsewhere; the vessels were surrounded by edema and signs of glial and mesenchymal proliferation.

These data show that a hemolysis leads to the impregnation of the brain with bilirubin and this, coupled with intravasal cold agglutination of the red cells, is to be regarded as a fundamental factor in the causation of damage to the nervous tissue in these types of anemia. When funicular myelosis is present, however, and the primary anemia is of syphilitic origin, there may well be a relationship between the two conditions.

Pasero and Muratorio observed a 56-year-old patient suffering from chronic autoantibody hemolytic anemia, with high titer cold agglutinins (complete and incomplete) and Raynaud's phenomenon, who presented a multi-site neurological picture. This included: slowly increasing motility disturbances (flaccid tetraplegia), muscle hypotrophy, deep sensibility disturbances of the lower limbs, osteotendinous areflexia and erection deficit; slight signs of cerebellar compression and facial tics were also present. Facial herpes zoster had been observed some months prior to admission. The clinical picture became slightly worse over the subsequent two years and pathological deterioration and atrophy of the brain became evident; the cerebrospinal fluid was normal. These workers suggest that massive red cell lysis gives rise to toxic products interfering with nerve activity and causing nerve damage. In autoantibody forms of the disease, nerve changes may be attributable to the same cause as the primary disease. In this respect, it may be pointed out that a structural link between red cells and the myelin sheaths may be seen in the globular membrane lipoproteins, these being particularly involved in hemolysis (*Crosby*).

A more recent report (*Bodechtel et al.*) concerns a patient with cold agglutinin anemia showing a clinical picture with a substantial neurological component. Necropsy revealed extensive lesions of the gray substance and degeneration of the dentate nuclei.

Anemia caused by marrow aplasia may be encountered in *chronic benzolism:* acute erythemia or leukemic myelosis have also been observed. In addition to the pathological blood picture, spinal complications may also be noted. These recall the combined sclerosis picture of neuro-anemic syndromes (*Pennacchietti*).

Erythroblastosis fetalis is a form of hemolytic anemia caused by isoantibodies, most commonly attributable to mother-fetus Rh incompatibility and much less frequently to ABO or other blood group incompatibility.

As is well known, neonatal hemolytic pictures may occasionally be attributable to autoantibody anemia in the mother, to the administration of high doses of vitamin K (particularly in the premature infant), to hemoglobin diseases (sickle-cell anemia, thalassemia), to hereditary spherocytosis or congenital nonspherocytic anemias, especially that caused by erythrocyte glucose 6-phosphate dehydrogenase (G6PD) deficit (*Di Toro*).

Particularly **grave signs of nervous** involvement are observed in this disease and the sequelae are equally serious. Nervous system damage is the result of toxic brain bilirubin concentrations (see also above in acquired hemolytic anemia).

When indirect bilirubin values in the serum exceed 18–20 mg%, diapedesis of the substance, which is released particularly in the area of the cerebral gray nuclei (*Schmorl's* "Kernicterus") may occur. Bilirubin deposits in the brain are an expression of the liposolubility of the indirect form; the direct form is water-soluble and is excreted in the urine. The neonatal brain may contain a lipoid with a special affinity for indirect bilirubin. Increased permeability of the hemato-encephalic barrier, a still obscure feature of the first eight days of life, is clearly a fundamental factor in the bilirubinic impregnation of nerve tissue, since jaundice (icterus) no longer leads to nervous system involvement after this period. Impregnation is also related to decreased glycuronyl-transferase activity in the neonatal liver, since insufficient glycurone-conjugation of indirect to water-soluble direct bilirubin takes place. It may be noted that nuclear jaundice brought on by such liver enzymatic insufficiency may be observed in the premature infant, quite apart from any question of immunological abnormality. Here the bilirubin liberated in the course of physiological hemolysis is not conjugated.

Bilirubin impedes cell metabolism (*Zetterström and Ernster*) and its action on brain tissue is shown in the form of abnormal phosphorylation and depressed tissue respiration (*Di Cagno et al.*).

Orth (1875) reported the first anatomical observation of erythroblastosis fetalis. Yellow staining is macroscopically evident in the wet brain; this is sometimes widespread, but is more commonly limited, the gray nuclei of the base being the site of choice. Such staining usually appears on the third day of life and disappears on the 15th–20th, occasionally as late as the third, fifth, or sixth month; it is poorly light- and formalin-fast. From the end of the first year the brain is macroscopically normal. In some cases, its size is reduced, the cortex is abnormally thin, and the ventricles are distended.

Apart from rare examples of yellowish granulation within the cell, histological examination will reveal no trace of bilirubin, even in the initial stage of the disease, since the pigment is destroyed during preparation of the sections; frozen sections may permit its visualization. Silver impregnation in this first stage (confined to the first week of life) reveals considerable changes in the nerve fibrils, including their dislocation and replacement by granulous masses. Nissl-stained nerve tissue often has a rarefied appearance, caused both by decreased cell content and by serious and unusual changes (edematous degeneration, acute swelling, and Nissl's serious degeneration) in the remaining cells. *Bertrand et al.* hold that edematous degeneration, with swelling and gradual vacuolization of the cytoplasm, is the most common lesion. Stain affinity is lost, the nucleus becomes pyknotic or loses its chromatin, and only the nucleolus remains. Acute tumefaction is thought to be very rare. Here the nucleus is swollen and globular and dendron and neurite alterations are observed.

Nissl degeneration has been closely studied by *Alzheimer* and consists of extensive tigrolysis, with the concentration of coarse lumps of chromophil substance on the periphery of the notably changed cell. Both elongations and indentations of the cell border may be observed or even frank shrinkage, with the crowding of irregularly shaped strips of cytoplasm around the nucleus so as to give a picture of total atrophy. Glial reaction is virtually nonexistent. Vasal congestion is intense, though hemorrhage sites are rare. Only one case of thrombosis has been reported (*Wiener and Brody*). Topographically speaking, the histological lesions are much more extensive than the areas of bilirubin staining (*Bertrand et al.; Sansone and Brusa*). No firm parallel between the two parameters can be shown (*Sansone and Brusa*).

As already stated, nuclear jaundice (kernicterus) is most commonly attributable to maternal isoimmunization in response to mother-fetus Rh incompatibility. Other causes have been assigned, though it should be noted that many observations date from the period before the discovery of the Rh factor by Landsteiner and Wiener (1940) and must therefore be treated with reserve (*Bertrand et al.*). These same workers also point out that the type of nerve changes found in nuclear jaundice may also be seen in diseases where neither hemolysis nor jaundice is present.

In erythroblastosis fetalis, a nuclear jaundice episode is required to produce a clear neurological picture and its so-called sequelae in the later stages. This means that nerve involvement frequency is linked to that of nuclear jaundice. The latter, however, has been variously assessed, values of from 90% to 12% having been proposed. This discrepancy is primarily explained by the fact that the term "kernicterus" (nuclear jaundice) is sometimes extended to include the mild nervous disturbances that may be observed during the course of any form of hemolytic disorder in the neonate.

Muscle hypotonia is the most common sign of the clinical picture, particularly in the terminal stage. The physiological hypertonia of the neonate is completely absent. The patient lies heavily in his cot, limbs completely distended. The normal flexion of the thighs on the pelvis and legs on the thighs and that of the elbows and fingers are absent and the hands are occasionally laid flat, this being totally abnormal in the neonate. Symptomatological demonstration of hypotonia is obtained by the methods of Kernig (complete extension of the legs on the thighs while the latter are flexed on the pelvis) and André-Thomas (bringing of the hand and forearm to the contralateral shoulder).

Hypertonia is a less common sign. This is distinguished from the physiological pattern by the abnormal distribution of tension as displayed by the adoption of typical attitudes. The picture is more correctly stated as an association of hypertonia and hypotonia. Enhanced tension in one muscle group may be combined with depressed tension in another group (e.g., in its antagonist); alternatively, hypertonia suddenly gives way to hypotonia, either spontaneously or as a result of a symptom-eliciting manipulation.

With respect to the nucha, backward flexion of the head is a typical sign. Hypertonia of the vertebral muscles will be revealed by the ease with which the hand can be passed under the back when the patient is placed on a table in dorsal decubitus. There will also be a notable readiness to shift from dorsal to lateral decubitus. In hypertonic forms, the infant finds anterior flexion of the trunk difficult. In the normal subject, this is easier than posterior flexion (André-Thomas). Vertebral muscle hypertonia may reach the point of frank opisthotonos, with horizontal dorsal and lumbar skin folds.

Limb hypertonia is expressed in a great variety of attitudes, such as extension and adduction of the lower limbs (as in the Egyptian mummy), "boxer on guard" pose of the upper limbs, hyperextension of the elbow with antepulsion of the arm and forced pronation of the forearm.

Simultaneous presentation of these attitudes gives what is known as the "hunting horn" appearance, though this is rarely observed in its entirety. This attitude is often accompanied by an upward and backward flexion of the tip of the tongue, making feeding a considerable problem.

Upward or downward rotation of the eyes, whether permanent or intermittent, is common. Fixed gaze or hypertonia of the levator palpebrae may be observed. Stridor is very common. This is apparently linked to hyperextension of the head and may be the cause of swallowing disturbances.

Muscle hypertonia tends to adopt a paroxysmal pattern and simulation of convulsive pictures is not uncommon.

In serious cases, osteotendinous reflexes disappear. If the child is brusquely lifted by the feet so that its head touches the examination table, a symmetrical complex of upper limb movements will be observed: extension of the forearm on the arm, followed by forward adduction of the arms (clutching movement or Moro's reflex). This cannot be elicited in the terminal stage and may be transiently absent at the conclusion of blood transfusion.

Somnolence, usually of slow onset, is a common companion of hypotonia: *Péhu and Dollet,* however, observed a case marked by the sudden onset of lethargy and consider this a pathognomic sign. Initially, vagitus is relatively rare and is often replaced by a more or less suppressed groan. Where hypertonia predominates, however, somnolence is not present and the patient will cry and react vigorously, albeit abnormally, to various stimuli; Moro's reflex is often exaggerated and states of agitation are not rare.

Respiration may be rapid and irregular. Acute pulmonary edema was observed in the terminal stage in a case reported by *Bertrand et al.* Temperature regulation disturbances are very common and both increased and decreased values are observed (mainly the former). A central origin is presumed for both these and respiratory disturbances, including the pulmonary edema just mentioned.

Other symptoms include: convulsion (not to be confused with parox-ysmal deterioration of hypertonia), myoclonia, nystagmus-like move-ment of the eyeballs, athetosis (absent, however, from the large series presented by *Bertrand et al.*), and paralysis of the cranial nerves (6th and 7th in the same series).

Anorexia is an early sign and vomiting may also be observed.

The prognosis for untreated cases is always fatal. There are three stages: first, icterus, pallor, spleen enlargement; second, more intense icterus, hepatomegaly (general condition still good, however); third, hemorrhage, nerve involvement as described above, this being the most constant and the most outstanding feature of the picture. The transition between stages is usually gradual, though the onset of the terminal stage (2nd–5th day of life) may be sudden and is always rapid (a few hours). Its duration may be equally short, though 24–36 hour periods are more common.

Terminal stage signs may be present at birth with a picture recalling that of fetoplacental anasarca. The skin is pale and dirty yellow (often cyanotic), with signs of edema, purpura, and ecchymosis; the spleen and liver are swollen and enlarged. Respiration is shallow and irregular and resuscitation is necessary; the vagitus is feeble. There is frank hypotonia and normal reflexes cannot be elicited.

Repeated transfusions may, if done at an early stage, lead to regression. A steady state is reached and lasts for 12, 24, or 48 hours, followed by the onset of a usually rapid recovery. Total clinical cure, *i.e.* the attainment of apparently normal health, may be achieved within six months or one year. Other patients, however, display noticeably retarded psychomotor development; yet this, however grave, will always lack the extrapyramidal element typical of the classic kernicterus sequel pattern (see later). The three cases of oligophrenia in the series of *Bertrand et al.* contrast strongly with the hypertonia and idiocy that are regularly part of the post-kernicterus neurological picture.

In addition to these "comprehensive" (*Bertrand et al.*) forms of nuclear jaundice, in which both the blood and the neurological picture are markedly abnormal, other forms with less drastic hemolysis and a different neurological picture are observed. Here jaundice is noted 3–12 hours after birth in an apparently healthy infant and is clearly defined by the 24th hour. Anemia is mild (red cell count usually above 2,500,000/mm³) and spleen but not liver enlargement is present. The general condition remains good and hemorrhage does not occur. Neurological symptoms appear in a minority of cases, usually on the

third day of life. The syndrome is indicative of extrapyramidal involvement but may also be observed in the course of the "comprehensive"
forms.

The main features include muscle hypertonia (nucha, back, lower
extremities), which may be intermittent and localized. When the
symptoms are slight, they may be difficult to interpret. Abnormal
movement (myoclonia) is less common. Agitation (not inconsistent with
the adoption of fixed attitudes) is more frequent than somnolence. The
vagitus is typically superacute in about one out of three cases. Convulsions are infrequent. Hyperthermia (of central nervous system origin) is
not unusual and paralysis of the oculomotor muscles may be observed.

Osteotendinous reflexes can be elicited but their discovery is impeded
by hypertonia. Moro's reflex is obtainable, often in an exaggerated form.
Deep respiratory disturbances are rare, except in the terminal stage,
though irregular rhythm and inconstant hiccuping may be more often
observed.

Larval extrapyramidal forms (*Dereymaeker*) and isolated symptoms are
known, including abnormal attitude, slight hypertonia, a distressing
vagitus, or abnormal eye movements.

By comparison with the particularly high mortality of nuclear jaundice, survival is the most frequent prognosis for these extrapyramidal
forms. Neurological and psychological sequelae may remain, however.
These are often extremely serious and at times appear disproportionate
to the acute symptom picture. Progress to a "comprehensive" form is not
unknown. In extrapyramidal forms, a symptom such as a certain degree
of somnolence, usually present in the "comprehensive" form, may be
virtually deprived of significance by reason of its detachment from its
normal framework.

As far as differential diagnosis is concerned, neurological signs of
nuclear jaundice must be distinguished from neonatal anoxia (rapid
regression without hemolysis), meningeal or cerebromeningeal hemorrhage (effusion into the posterior cranial fossa or upper cervical region
may give rise to opisthotonos or tonic contracture of the dorsum) and
from disturbances subsequent to blood transfusion (apnea crisis, tonic
and clonic convulsions, muscle hypertonia). Serum examination is
essential in the diagnosis of kernicterus: mother and child antigen
incompatibility is investigated and the maternal serum is examined for
immune antibodies; a positive Coombs test offers valuable confirmation.

The clinical picture of the sequelae is dominated by signs of
extrapyramidal involvement. Muscle hypertonia is typically the first to
appear and primarily affects the posterior musculature: the nucha is
thrown backwards, making opisthotonos (fig. 3a) a typical attitude (care

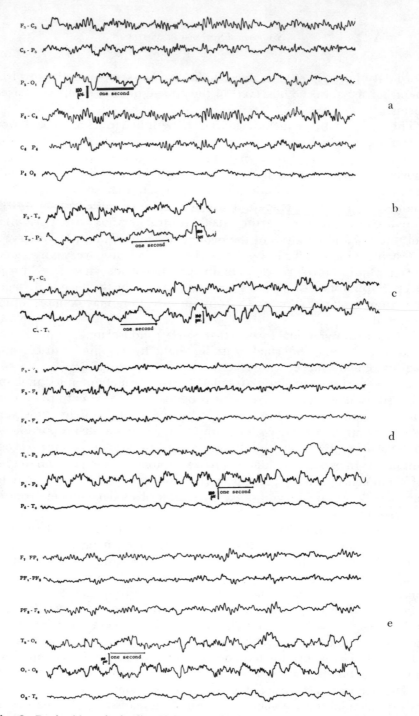

Fig. 3. Erythroblastosis fetalis: EEG traces in five patients with neuro-psychological sequelae (*a–e*). Decreased δ-wave frequency and amplitude, including plateaus, may be observed in some leads (Figs. 1–14 in *Bertrand et al.*)

must be taken to avoid confusion between this sign and precocious control of the head). The upper extremities are usually in hyperextension, abduction, and pronation and the hand is closed to form a fist. The lower limbs are in adduction and extension, or in semiflexion (fig. 3b), with talipes equinovarus. The face lacks expression. Paroxysmal attacks of increased hypertonia may be such as to throw the infant from the arms of the person holding him (*Fitzgerald et al.*).

Hypertonia may also be associated with hypotonia. The patient cannot hold an object in his hand for long and his legs may suddenly collapse under him.

Abnormal movements form the second fundamental aspect of the extrapyramidal sequelae picture and appear during a central nervous system maturation stage (*Coquet, Dereymaeker*), in which hypertonia tends to regress. Athetosic or choreoathetoid movements (fig. 3 c, d), particularly of the face, tongue, and jaws, are most common, the limbs being rarely involved (*Coquet*). Such abnormal movements are principally demonstrated in association with voluntary actions (speaking, mastication). Myoclonia and spasms have also been observed.

Pyramidal involvement is less common, though hemiplegia (*Spiller*) and Babinski's reflex in association with reflex exaggeration (*Brock and Wolf; etc.*) have been reported. A cerebellar syndrome, with ataxia and dysmetria, has also been described. Deglutition disturbances (*Vaughan*) may result in severe bronchopneumonia. *Deschamps and van Bogaert* observed a case of cord involvement, with amyotrophy areflexia, and lesions of the anterior and posterior gray columns. Various examples of cranial nerve impairment have been reported: facial paralysis (*Segarra-Obiol*); trismus (*Hoffer and Hausmann*); 8th, 9th, and 10th pair damage (*Spiller; Boucomont; etc.*).

Epilepsy, oculogyric crisis, optical atrophy, decreased sharpness of vision, blindness (in a case described by *Cappell*, this was histologically attributed to cortex lesions), and hearing disturbances have all been observed. Some workers (*Lightwood and Colver; Docter*) have reported nonvestibular nystagmus, interpreted as secondary to fundus changes.

Other signs include increased salivation, intense sweating crises, hyperthermia episodes not attributable to infection, and increased susceptibility to infection. Hydrocephalus was observed in a case reported by *Dereymaeker*, though this may have been a purely coincidental association.

Brain changes are a virtually constant feature of the clinical picture: impaired intelligence, retarded speech, with poor vocabulary and difficulty of expression, and disturbed affect.

Electroencephalographic findings included decreased δ-wave frequency and plateaus (*Bertrand et al.*).

The diagnosis of erythroblastosis fetalis sequelae may be particularly difficult. As the neonatal period recedes the maternal serum antibody values gradually fall, at a rate that is characteristic of the individual subject. On the other hand, a record of early neonatal jaundice (*i.e.*, with onset during the first day of life), classified as intense and persistent (duration of at least 12 days), with anemization and the appearance of neurological signs, coupled with evidence of nonidentical mother and child blood group classification, will add up to a significantly demonstrative picture. A familial history of neonatal or fetal accidents, generally increasing in seriousness, from anemia to premature delivery of a stillborn child, may also form a basis for reaching a diagnosis.

The differential diagnosis of neurocerebral sequelae may require the investigation of possible meningitis (the fontanelle not stretched, normal liquor finding), the uncommon neurological consequences of trauma during partus maneuvers, and other conditions giving rise to an extrapyramidal picture (Ramsay-Hunt's pallidoprogressive degeneration, Hallervorden-Spatz syndrome, Vogt's cerebromacular degeneration, Wilson's disease, *etc.*).

By contrast with the acute stage, during which nervous tissue lesions are widespread and bear no relation to the clinical picture, neurocerebral sequelae in subjects who survive tend to present localized anatomically and histologically demonstrable changes that conform to the clinical picture to a certain extent. The anatomical finding is essentially cicatricial. Areas of brain porosity may be observed. Yellowish staining of the nuclear formations is rare. Microscopic evidence of cerebral gliosis may be found; there will be signs of nerve ganglion rarefaction, caused by irreversible nerve lesions. These are expressions of changes that occurred during the acute stage and have resulted in complete disappearance of the parts involved. Myelin changes are infrequent (demyelinization, for example, is rare). In exceptional cases, vascular lesions may be found: congestion, areas of softening with hemorrhagic suffusion, perivascularities, *etc.*

No constant topographical arrangement of such changes has been established. The impression gained is that localization is essentially a function of the intensity of the initial process. Extensive, symmetric degeneration of the central auditory pathways is sometimes reported (*Dublin*).

The prognosis for patients with neurocerebral sequelae is very uncertain because of their hypersensitivity to infection; death attributable to intercurrent disease may well occur before puberty.

The treatment of erythroblastosis fetalis is essentially based on early, copious and, if necessary, repeated exchange transfusion, the aim being to maintain blood bilirubin values below 18 mg%. In recent years, prenatal therapy has been introduced (injection of O Rh-negative blood into the fetal peritoneal cavity (*Liley*); fetal exchange blood transfusion following hysterotomy (*Adamsons et al.*). Prenatal diagnosis can be obtained by means of spectrophotometric examination of an amniocentesis specimen; this will be found to contain pathological pigments (bilirubinoids). In addition to preventing the onset of nuclear jaundice, timely transfusion may halt the further development of bilirubin-induced brain disease. It is well known that the neurological sequelae are less frequent and less serious in proportion to the timeliness of the transfusion (*Di Giacomo and Dardi; etc.*).

Additional therapy includes the routine use of cortisones. Prednisolone must be administered for several days after transfusion until blood bilirubin levels show a clear fall. *Kellner and Stoermer* report good results with an association of prednisolone and Periston N. *Murano* has emphasized that cortisone treatment, by stimulating hepatic transglycurone-conjugation, potentiates bilirubin elimination. This worker studied chromatographic traces of serum biliary pigment diazoderivatives and found that cortisones led to the appearance of a band referable to diglycuronide alongside the free bilirubin band. The latter, of much greater intensity, represented the sole pretreatment blood bilirubin quota.

Kitchen et al. have suggested the employment of hyperalbuminous blood during the first half of the blood transfusion. Alternatively, and perhaps with greater reason, they recommend the injection of concentrated albumin 30–60 minutes before commencing the transfusion. Albumin recalls tissue bilirubin into the circulation. *Diamond and Schmid*, moreover, have demonstrated experimentally that human plasma albumin, by forming a bond with bilirubin, prevents the latter from crossing the hemato-encephalic barrier.

Prevention of erythroblastosis fetalis arising from Rh incompatibility has been attempted in a number of countries by injecting the Rh-negative mother with an anti-D immunoglobulin. The results have been very satisfactory.

REFERENCES

Anemia in general

BORCHERS, H. G. and MITTELBACH, F.: Neurologische Störungen bei Blutkrankheiten. Internist, Berl. 2:105–117 (1961).

ERAMO, N. D'; GAETANO, G. DE; CANDELORO, A. and VINCENZONI, M.: Il cuore nelle
    emopatie (contributo clinico). Nota I: nelle anemie (cuore da anemia). Gaz. int. Med.
    Chir. 69:1001–1016 (1964).
LEGRAMANTE, A. and ZILLI, E.: Le sindromi neuro-anemiche. Policlinico, Sez. prat.
    70:637–656 (1963).
LICHTHEIM, H.: Zur Kenntnis der perniciösen Anämie. Verh. Cong. inn. Med. 6:84–99
    (1887).
MAGRÌ, G. and FASANO, V. A.: Vascolopatie cerebrali (Ediz. Minerva Medica, Turin 1959).
MATHIEU, P.: Les syndromes neuro-anémiques (Doin, Paris 1925).
OPITZ, E. and SCHNEIDER, M.: Über die Sauerstoffversorgung des Gehirns und den
    Mechanismus von Mangelwirkungen. Ergebn. Physiol. 46:126–260 (1950).
RENZI, S. DE: Le anemie aplastiche. Il sangue (Atti IX Settim. Med. Osped.), Rome 1964,
    140 (Il Pensiero Scientifico, Rome 1964).

Pernicious anemia (Biermer's disease)

ADAMS, R. D. and KUBIK, C. S.: Subacute degeneration of brain in the pernicious anemia.
    New Engl. J. Med. 231:1–9 (1944).
ALAJOUANINE, T.: Sur les syndromes neuro-anémiques; in Questions médicales d'actualité
    (Masson, Paris 1937).
AMYOT, R.: Les syndromes neuro-hématologiques. Union méd. Canada 90:1118–1126
    (1961).
BALDWIN, J. N. and DALESSIO, D. J.: Folic acid therapy and spinal cord degeneration in
    pernicious anemia. New Engl. J. Med. 264:1339–1342 (1961).
BARDECI, C. A.: Encéfaloneuropatías anémicas. Acta neurol. lat. amer. 7:103–131 (1961).
BEGEMANN, H.: Die perniziöse Anämie; in Heilmeyer and Hittmair, Handbuch der
    gesamten Hämatologie, vol. III, 395–418 (Urban & Schwarzenberg, Munich-Berlin
    1960).
BESANÇON, F.: Études cliniques et biologiques sur l'anémie pernicieuse; Thése Paris (1955).
BETHELL, F. H.; MEYERS, M. C. and NELEIGH, R. B.: Vitamin B12 in pernicious anemia and
    puerperal macrocytic anemia. J. Lab. clin. Med. 33:477 (1948).
BIRKETT-SMITH, E.: Neurological disorders in vitamin B12 deficiency with normal B12
    absorption. Danish med. Bull. 12:158–162 (1965).
BODECHTEL, G.: in Heilmeyer and Begemann, Blut and Blutkrankheiten, p. 264 (Springer,
    Berlin-Göttingen-Heidelberg 1951).
BODECHTEL, G. and SCHRADER, A.: Die Mangelkrankheiten des Nervensystems; in Klinik
    d. Gegenwart, vol. III (Urban & Schwarzenberg, Munich-Berlin 1956).
BOER, W. G. R. M. DE; NAIRN, R. C. and MAXWELL, A: Pernicious anaemia autoantibody to
    gastric parietal cells. Immunofluorescence test with rat stomach. J. clin. Path.
    18:456–459 (1965).
BOGAERT, L. VAN: La polynévrite anémique. Ann. Med. 22:321–329 (1927).
BOUDIN, G. and BARBIZET, J.: Neuropathie achylique biermérienne isolée pendant 5 ans
    avant l'apparition du syndrome hématologique. Bull. Soc. méd. Hôp., Paris
    72:964–966 (1956).
BUSSI, L.; POZZA, G.; ERIDANI, S.; FAVA, P. L. and MICHELI, E. DE: Studio sulle
    megaloblastosi in midolli normali allevati in vitro: influenza dell'acido fenilpiruvico e
    paraidrossifenilpiruvico. Biol. lat. 6:28 (1953).
CÁRREGA CASSAFONTH, C. F.; BRAGE, D. and RIVAS, L.: La lipidorraquia en las anemias
    perniciosas; la lipemia; el componente neural, la secreción gástrica y sus interrela-
    ciones. Sem. méd., B. Aires 55:403 (1948).
CASTLE AND MINOT: in Amyot.
COLOMBO, P.: Sindrome psico-anemica a tipo delirante-allucinatorio in corso di anemia
    perniciosa. Guarigione rapida dopo trasfusione di sangue ed epatoterapia d'urto.
    Med. int. 59:1–3 (1951).

CONLEY, C. L. and KREVANS J. R.: New developments in diagnosis and treatment of pernicious anaemia. Ann. intern. Med. 43:758–766 (1955).

COSSA, P.: Diagnostic des syndromes neuro-anémiques par le test de Schilling. Acad. de Méd. (December 1964). J. Méd., Bordeaux 142:1978 (1965).

CREYSSEL, R.; BONDOT, M.; PAYEN, G.; CHIPPAUX, C.; MOREL, P. and CROIZAT, P.: Données statistiques sur l'évolution hématologique de la maladie de Biermer. L'inutilité des doses massives de vitamine B₁₂. Rev. lyonn. Méd. 4:219–227 (1955).

DAMESHEK, W.: Theories of autoimmunity; in Conceptual advances in immunology and oncology (Harper & Row, New York 1963).

DAMESHEK, W.; SCHWARTZ, R. and OLINER, H.: Current concepts of autoimmunization: an interpretative review. Blood 17:775–783 (1961).

DAVIDSON, S.: Clinical picture of pernicious anemia prior to introduction of liver therapy in 1926 and in Edinburgh subsequent to 1944. Brit. med. J. i:241 (1957).

EARL *et al.*: in Legramante and Zilli.

EMILE-WEILL, P.: in Labauge *et al.*

ENOKSSON, P. and NORDEN, A.: Vitamin B₁₂ deficiency affecting the nerve optic. Acta med. scand. 167:199–208 (1960).

ERBSLÖH, F.: Das Zentralnervensystem bei Krankeiten des Blutes; in Lubarsch and Henke, Handbuch der speziellen pathologischen Anatomie und Histologie, vol. XIII/2: 1468–1525 (Springer, Berlin-Göttingen-Heidelberg 1958).

ESHOUGUES, J. R. D': Les syndromes neurologiques des anemies hyperchromes. Algérie méd. 64:1041–1044 (1960).

FOSTER, D. B.: Degeneration of peripheral nerves in pernicious anemia. Arch. Neurol., Chicago 54:102–109 (1945).

FREEMAN A. G. and HEATON, J. M.: The aethiology of retrobulbar neuritis in Addisonian pernicious anemia. Lancet i:908–911 (1961).

FUÀ, C.: Osservazioni clinico-terapeutiche sulle sindromi neuroanemiche. Rass. clin.-scient. 27:147–150 (1951).

GARCIN: in Besançon.

GLASS, G. B.: Recent status of the physiology and immunology of intrinsic factor and its clinical significance. Simp. Int. Fattori Eritropoicsi, Pavia 1968.

GOLDHAMER, S. M.; BETHELL, F. H.; ISAACS S. and STURGIS C. C.: The occurrence and treatment of neurologic changes in pernicious anemia. J. amer. med. Ass. 103:1663 (1934).

GOTTWALD, W.: Die neurologischen und psychotischen Syndrome der perniziösen Anämie. Medizinische 3:85–88 (1953).

GREENFIELD J. G. and CARMICHAEL, E. A.: The peripheral nerves in cases of subacute combined degeneration of the cord. Brain 58:483–491 (1935).

GRINKER, R. R. and KANDEL, E.: Pernicious anemia: results of treatment of the neurologic complications. Arch. intern. Med. 54:851–871 (1934).

GUGLIELMO, G. DI: Le anemie megaloblastiche (D'Agostino, Naples 1955).

HAMILTON, H. E.; ELLIS, P. P. and SHEETS, R. F.: Visual impairment due to optic neuropathy in pernicious anemia: report of a case and review of the literature. Blood 14:378–385 (1959).

HEINRICH, H. C. and GABBE, E. E.: Intravitale Retention und Exkretion des Aquocobamids, einer für die Therapie geeigneten natürlichen Vitamin B₁₂-Depotform. Klin. Wschr. 39:689–691 (1961).

INTROZZI: in Ferrata and Storti, Le malattie del sangue, vol. I, p. 727 (Fr. Vallardi, Milan 1958).

IRVINE, W. J.: Immunological aspects of pernicious anaemia; in Baldwin and Humphrey, Autoimmunity (Blackwell Scient. Publ., Oxford 1965). Clinical and pathological significance of parietal cell antibodies. Proc. roy. Soc. Med. 59:695–698 (1966).

KAMPMEIER, R. H. and JONES, E.: Optic atrophy in pernicious anemia. Amer. J. med. Sci. 195:633–638 (1938).

KAHN, M. H. and MARTIN, H.: Zytogentische Untersuchungen bei perniziöser Anämie. Blut 18:129–141 (1968).

KISSEL *et al.*: in Labauge *et al.*

KRAVETZ, R. E.; NOORDEN, S. VAN and SPIRO, H. M.: Parietal cell antibodies in patients with duodenal ulcer and gastric cancer. Lancet i:235–237 (1967).

LABAUGE, R.; IZARN, P. and CASTAN, P.: Les manifestations nerveuses des hémopathies. Rapport LXI Congr. Franç. de Psychiatrie et de Neurologie, Nancy 1963 (Masson, Paris 1963).

LING, C. T. and CHOW, B. F.: The influence of vitamin B_{12} on carbohydrate and lipide metabolism. J. biol. Chem. 206:705–709 (1954).

LOCKNER, D.; REIZENSTEIN, P.; WENNBERG, A. and WIDÉN, L.: Peripheral nerve function in pernicious anemia before and after treatment. Acta haemat., Basel 41:257–263 (1969).

MORSIER DE: in Labauge *et al.*

MASQUIN, P. and TRELLES, J. O.: Precis d'anatomo-physiologie normale et pathologique du système nerveux central (Doin, Paris 1966).

MURPHY, T. E. and COSTANZI, Y. Y.: Pseudo-tumor cerebri associated with pernicious anemia. Ann. intern. Med. 70:777–782 (1969).

NAJEAN, Y. and BERNARD, J.: Anémie pernicieuse et vitamine B_{12}. Evolution des idées concepts physio-pathologiques. Rev. Prat., Paris 16:1887–1901 (1966).

NIEWEG, H. O.; FABER, J. G.; VRIES, J. A. DE and STENFERT KROESE W. F.: Relationship of vitamin B_{12} and folic acid in megaloblastic anemia. J. Lab. clin. Med. 44:118–132 (1954).

NORDEN, C. VON: Untersuchungen über schwere Anämien. Char. Ann. 16:217–266 (1891).

OLMER, J.: L'épatothérapie dans les syndromes neuroanémiques. Nutrition, Paris 7:103–111 (1937).

PANT, S. S.; ASBURY, A. K. and RICHARDSON, E. P. JR.: Myelopathy of pernicious anemia. A neuropathological reappraisal. Acta neurol. scand. 44(supplem. 35):7–36 (1968).

PEARSON, H. A.; VINSON, R. and SMITH, R. T.: Pernicious anemia with neurologic involvement in childhood. Report of a case with emphasis on dangers of folic acid therapy. J. Pediat. 65:334–339 (1961).

PETERS, G.: Patologia del sistema nervoso (Sansoni, Florence 1955).

PORTUONDO Y CASTRO, J. M. DE: Anemia macrocítica (estudio de 40 casos) (Seoane, Fernandez y Cía, Havana 1950).

REGISTER, U. D.: Effect of vitamin B_{12} on liver and blood non-protein sulphydryl compounds. J. biol. Chem. 206:705–709 (1954).

REID, H. A. and HARRIS, W.: Reversible papilloedema in pernicious anemia. Brit. med. J. i:20 (1951).

ROGER, H.: Les syndromes neuroanémiques. Marseille méd. 91:473–490 (1954).

SAMSON D. C. *et al.*: Cerebral metabolic disturbances and delirium in pernicious anemia. Arch. intern. Med. 90:4–14 (1952).

SARROUY, C. and PORTIER, A.: Les syndromes neurohémolytiques. Presse méd. 59:1062 (1951).

SCHWARTZ: in Dausset, Immuno-hématologie (Flammarion, Paris 1956). In editorial (Autoimmune and autoallergic hemolytic anemias) in New Engl. J. Med. 169:1381–1383 (1963).

SINCLAIR, H. M.: Vitamine e sistema nervoso (Il Pensiero Scientifico, Rome 1956).

SMITH, E. L.: Vitamin B_{12} (Methuen, London 1963).

SMITHBURN, K. C. and ZERFAS, L. G.: The neural symptoms and signs in pernicious anemia: effects of liver extract. Arch. Neurol., Chicago 25:1100–1110 (1931).

SOLLBERG, G.: Seltenere neurologische Syndrome und Verlaufsformen der B_{12}-Avitaminose. Med. Welt, Stg. 7:341–348 (1969).

STIRPE, M.: Il fondo oculare nelle anemie ed emoblastosi. Osservazioni sulla casistica esaminata nel Policlinico di Roma durante il decennio 1955–1964. Boll. Ocul. 44:577–591 (1965).

STORTI, E.: Diagnostic des maladies du sang (Doin, Paris 1959).

TAYLOR, K. B.: Inhibition of intrinsic factor by pernicious anaemia sera. Lancet ii:106 (1959).

TERZANI, A.: Le sindromi neurologiche dell'anemia di Biermer. Riv. Clin. med. 39:574–621 (1939).
THOMPSON, R. B.: A short textbook of haematology (Pitman Medical, London 1961).
TRELLES, J. O. and ESCALANTE, S.: Sobre dos casos anatomoclínicos de mielosis funicular de Lichtheim. Rev. Neuropsiquiat. 22:541–584 (1959).
ULBRIGHT: in Peters, Patologia del sistema nervoso (Sansoni, Florence 1955).—And in Pintus, G.; Muratorio, A. and Giannini, A.: Le sindromi neuropsichiche da carenza alimentare (Omnia Medica, Pisa 1959).
VERSÉ, H.: Perniziöse Anämie mit funikulären Symptomen im Kleinkindesalter Z. Kinderheilk. 99:325–337 (1967).
VILLA, L. and BUSSI, L.: L'anemia perniciosa. Relaz. LX Congr. Soc. Ital. Med. Intern., Rome 1959 (Pozzi, Rome 1959).
VILTER, R. W.; HONIGAN, D.; MUELLER, J. F.; JANOLD, T.; VILTER, C. F.; HAWKINS, V. and SEAMAN, A.: Studies on the relationships of vitamin B12, folic acid, thymine, uracil and methyl group donors in persons with pernicious anemia and related megaloblastic anemias. Blood 5:695–717 (1950).
WALTON, J. N. *et al.*: The EEG in pernicious anemia and subacute combined degeneration of the cord. Electroenceph. clin. Neurophysiol. 6:45–64 (1954).
WHITBY, L. E. H. and BRITTON, C. J. C.: Disorders of the blood (Churchill, London 1963).
WIECK, H. H.: Funikuläre Spinalerkrankung, die über Jahre nicht erkannt wurde. Med. Welt, Stg. 4:197–198 (1964).
WINTROBE, M. M.: Clinical hematology (Lea & Febiger, Philadelphia 1961).
WOKES *et al.*: in Legramante and Zilli.

Perniciosiform anemia

BJÖRKENHEIM, G.: Neurological changes in pernicious tapeworm anemia. Acta med. scand. 260 (suppl.) : 1–125 (1951).
CACUDI, G.: A proposito delle sequele neurologiche nei gastroresecati (neuropatia periferica con anemia macrocitica ipercromica). G. Clin. med 66:189–198 (1965).
GILES, C.: An account of 335 cases of megaloblastic anaemia of pregnancy and the puerperium. J. clin. Path. 19:1–11 (1966).
GUGLIELMO, G. DI: *loc. cit.*
HENNING: in Stöhr.
KANT, F. and LUBING, H. N.: Syndrome of non tropical sprue with unusual neurologic and psychiatric picture. Wisconsin med. J. 46:1095–1097 (1947).
LOWENSTEIN, L.; PICK, C. and PHILPOTT, N.: Megaloblastic anemia of pregnancy and the puerperium. Amer. J. Obstet. Gynec. 70:1309–1337 (1955).
MANNHEIMER, E.; PAKESCH, F.; REIMER, E. E. and VETTER, H.: Die hämatologischen Komplikationen bei der Epilepsiebehandlung mit Hydantoinkörpern. Med. Klin. 47:1397–1401 (1952).
PAWLOVSKY, A.: Alteraciones de los elementos figurados de la sangre en los gastrectomizados. Medicina, Madr. 13:301–316 (1953).
SILBER, R.: Recenti acquisizioni in tema di anemie megaloblastiche non addisoniane. Aggiornamenti Emat., Rome 1:237–259 (1964).
STÖHR, O.: Die totale Magenresektion und der Wert des Vitamin B12 in der Behandlung der Folgezustände. Arch. klin. Chir. 272:326–344 (1952).
STRAUSS, M. B. and CASTLE, W. B.: Studies of anemia in pregnancy; etiologic relationship of gastric secretion defects and dietary deficiency to hypochromic and macrocytic (pernicious) anemias of pregnancy and treatment of these conditions. Amer. J. med. Sci. 185:539–551 (1933).
THOMPSON, R. B. and UNGLEY, C. C.: Megaloblastic anemia of pregnancy and the puerperium. Quart. J. Med. 20:187–204 (1951).
TOMODA, M.: Agastrische perniziöse Anämie. Chirurg, Berl. 25:49–58 (1954).
WILLIAMS, J. A.; HALL, G. S.; THOMPSON, A. G. and COOKE, W. T.: Neurological disorders after partial gastrectomy. Brit. med. J. iii:210–212 (1969).

WOLTMAN, H. N. and HECK, F. J.: Funicular degeneration of the spinal cord without pernicious anemia: neurologic aspects of sprue, nontropical sprue and idiopathic steatorrhea. Arch. intern. Med. 60:272–300 (1937).

Iron deficiency anemia

AITA, J. A.: Neurologic manifestations of general diseases (C. Thomas, Springfield, Ill. 1964).

CAPRILES, L. F.: Intracranial hypertension and iron-deficiency anemia; report of four cases. Arch. Neurol., Chicago 9:147–153 (1963).

CHEVALLIER, P.; ALAJOUANINE, T. and STEWART, A.: in Mathieu.

DANIELS, A. P. and ROELOFS, C. O.: Hypochromic anemia with symptoms of ocular fundus. Ned. T. Geneesk. 79:3835–3848 (1935).

GRAM, H. G.: Further observations on a family showing many cases of pernicious anemia. Acta med. scand. 34 (suppl.): 107–113 (1930).

GREPPI, E.: Sulle anemie ipocromiche da microcitosi e sulla loro evoluzione in anemia perniciosa. Haematologica 15:573–592 (1934).

HITTMAIR, A.: Eisenmangel. Med. Klin. 55:677–683 (1960).

LENHARTZ, H.: Diagnostische und therapeutische Erwägungen bei perniziöser Anämie. Münch. med. Wschr. 77:669–675 (1930).

LUBECK, M. J.: Papilledema caused by iron deficiency anemia. Trans. amer. Acad. Ophthal. Otolaryng. 63:306–310 (1959).

MATHIEU, P.: *loc. cit.*

MURPHY, T. E. and COSTANZI, J. J.: *loc. cit.*

PENNACCHIETTI, M.: Alterazioni sistemiche del midollo spinale nella patologia internistica (patologia del midollo spinale nelle intossicazioni professionali). Atti delle Giornate Mediche Triestine, Trieste 1962, 161–175 (Ediz. Scuola Med. Osped. Trieste).

REID, H. A. and HARRIS, W.: *loc. cit.*

SCHWABER, J. R. and BLUMBERG, A. G.: Papilledema associated with blood loss in anemia. Ann. intern. Med. 55:1004–1007 (1961).

SCURO, L. A.; MOROCUTTI, C. and NACCARATO, R.: Grave sindrome neuroanemica in anemia ipocromica sideropenica (Esito di guarigione). Riv. Neurol. 32:463–476 (1962).

STIRPE, M.: *loc. cit.*

WATKINS: in Freeman and Heaton (*loc. cit.*).

WHITBY, L. E. H. and BRITTON, C. J. C.: *loc. cit.*

WORSTER-DROUGHT, C. and SHAFAR, J.: Achlorhydric hypochromic anaemia associated with peripheral neuritis with report of two cases. Brit. med. J. ii:273–276 (1939).

Hemolytic anemia

ADAMSONS, K.; FREDA, V. J.; JAMES, L. S. *et al.*: Prenatal treatment of erythroblastosis fetalis following hysterotomy. J. Pediat. 35:848–855 (1965).

ALZHEIMER: in Bertrand *et al.*

ANASTASOPOULOS, G.; DIAKOGHIANNIS, A. and RUTSONIS, K.: Emiplegia con epilessia in un caso di anemia drepanocitica. Minerva med. 47/I:843–844 (1956).

ARENA, J. M.: Cerebral vascular lesions accompanying SCA. J. Pediat. 14:745–751 (1939).

ASCENZI, A. and SILVESTRONI, E.: Étude anatomo-clinique d'un cas de maladie microdré-panocytique. Acta haemat., Basel 18:205–218 (1957).

ATAMER, M. A.: Blood diseases (Grune & Stratton, New York-London 1963).

BALLARD, M. S. and BONDAR, H.: Spontaneous subarachnoid hemorrhage in sickle cell anemia. Neurology, Minneap. 7:443–444 (1957).

BAUER, J. and FISCHER, J. L.: SCA with special regard to its nonanemic variety. Arch. Surg., Chicago 6:553–563 (1943).

BERTRAND, I.; BESSIS, M. and SEGARRA-OBIOL, J. M. (with the collaboration of BUHOT, S. and KOUPERNIK, C.): L'ictére nucléaire. Séquelle de la maladie hémolytique du nouveau-né. Étude clinique et anatomique (Masson, Paris 1952).

BESSIS, M.: Transfusion sanguine et actualités hématologiques (Masson, Paris 1954).

BODECHTEL, G.; BORCHERS, H. G. and KOLLMANNSBERGER, A.: Enzephalopathie bei Blutkrankheiten. Dtsch. med. Wschr. 91:673–682 (1966).

BOSSELMAN, B. and KRAINES, H.: Mental changes including aphasia in a patient with SCA. Amer. J. Psychiat. 94:709–712 (1937).

BOUCOMONT, J.: Hépatonéphrite infectieuse et ictère nucléaire. Arch. franç. Pédiat. 1:7 (1944).

BRIDGERS, W. H.: Cerebral vascular disease accompanying sickle cell anemia. Amer. J. Path. 15:353–362 (1939).

BRITTINGHAM and PHINIZZI: in Labauge *et al.* (*loc. cit.*).

BROCK, S. and WOLF, A.: Cerebral complications of icterus gravis neonatorum. Arch. Neurol., Chicago 36:1368 (1936).

CABIBBO, S.; CANNATA, D.; BRUNETTI, M. and MIRALDI, C.: Mielosi funiculare in corso di emopatia mediterranea. Progr. med., Naples 17:833–839 (1961).

CAGNO, L. DI; LANGE, M. M. and CASTELLO, D.: Esiti immediati e tardivi della malattia emolitica del neonato da Rh ed ABO. Conv. Sez. Piemontese Soc. Ital. Pediat., Turin 1963. Minerva pediat. 15:1207–1235 (1963).

CAMINOPETROS, J.: Recherches sur l'anémie érythroblastique infantile des peuples de la Méditerranée orientale: étude nosologique. Ann. Méd. 43:27–61 (1938). Étude anthropologique, étiologique et pathogénique: la transmission héréditaire de la maladie. Ann. Méd. 43:104–125 (1938).

CAPPELL, D. F.: Mother child incompatibility problem in relation to nervous sequelae of haemolytic disease of newborn. Brain 78:486-494 (1947).

CASSANO, C. and BENEDETTI, G.: Neuroanemia emolitica costituzionale con drepanocitosi. Boll. Soc. Med. Chir., Pisa 7:303–316 (1939).

CATTAN, R.; AJURIAGUERRA, J. DE; CARASSO, R.; DAUSSET, J.; HOPPELER, A. and ZERAH, CH.: Anémie hémolytique acquise de l'adulte avec cirrhose atrophique, syndrome nerveux complexe et syndrome de Gougerot-Sjögren. Sem. Hôp., Paris 26:801–810 (1952).

CHARMOT, C. and REYNAUD, R.: Anémie drépanocytaire avec paraplégie spasmodique, lésions hépatiques et altérations osseuses. Méd. trop., Marseille 17:826–829 (1957).

COLARIZI, A. and MENGOLI: Ittero emolitico a resistenze eritrocitarie aumentate e amiotrofia tipo Werdnig-Hoffmann. Proc. 6th Congr. Int. Pediat. (Zürich 1950).

CONNEL, J. M. C.: Cerebral necrosis in sickle cell disease. J. amer. med. Ass. 118:893–895 (1942).

COOK, W. C.: A case of SCA with associated subarachnoid hemorrhage. J. Med. 11:541–542 (1930).

COQUET, K.: Les séquelles neurologiques tardives de l'ictère nucléaire. Ann. paediat., Basel 163:83 (1944).

COWLEY-CHAVEZ, O.; ALONSO FRONTAO, J. and DUENAS, H.: Las manifestaciones neurologicas en la anemia sickle cells. Reporte de un caso. Arch. Hosp. Universit., Cuba 6:550–560 (1953).

CROSBY, W. H.: Pathogenesis of spherocytes and leptocytes (target cells). Blood 7: 261–274 (1952).

CURSHMANN: Über funikuläre Myelose bei hämolytischem Ikterus. Dtsch. Z. Nervenheilk. 122:119–125 (1931).

DACIE, J. V.: The haemolytic anaemias congenital and acquired; 2nd ed., part IV, p. 1134 (Churchill, London 1967). Editoriale: le più recenti acquisizioni in tema di anemie emolitiche. Aggiornamenti Emat., Rome 6:157–165 (1969).

DAVISON, C. and WECHSLER, I. S.: Erythroblastic (Cooley's) anemia and neurologic complications (status dysmyelinatus). Amer. J. Dis. Child. 58:362–370 (1939).

DEREYMAEKER, A.: L'ictère nucléaire; Thèse Louvain (1948).

DESCHAMPS, A. and BOGAERT, L. VAN: Idiotie, épilepsie, choreo-athétose double avec un syndrome médullaire, séquelles tardives de l'ictère nucléaire. Acta neurol. belg. 48:480 (1948).

DIAMOND, I. and SCHMID, R.: Experimental bilirubin encephalopathy. The mode of entry of bilirubin ^{14}C into the central nervous system. J. clin. Invest. 45:678–689 (1966).

DOCTER, J.: Kernicterus neurological sequelae of erythroblastosis fetalis. J. Pediat. 27:327–334 (1945).

DUBLIN: in Labauge *et al.* (*loc. cit.*).

DUMOLARD, C.; SARROUY, C. and PORTIER, A.: Ataxie cérébelleuse associée à un syndrome de splénomégalie chronique avec anémie. Bull. Soc. méd. Hôp., Paris (meeting 14 January 1938) 54:71–76.

FADELL, E. and CRONE, R. I.: Cerebral hemorrhage as a manifestation of the sickle cell phenomenon; case report with autopsy finding. Amer. J. Obstet. Gynec. 73:212–214 (1957).

FERNANDEZ ITHURRAT and SILVESTRE: in Di Guglielmo, G.; Pontoni, L. and Silvestroni, E., Emopatie familiari. Relaz. L. Congr. Soc. Ital. Med. Intern., Rome 1949 (Pozzi, Rome 1949).

FIALKOW, P. J.; BROWDER, J. A.; SPARKES, R. S. and MOTULSKY, A. G.: Mental retardation in methemoglobinemia due to diaphorase deficiency. New Engl. J. Med. 273:840–845 (1965).

FINCH, C. A.: Medical progress: methemoglobinemia and sulfhemoglobinemia. New Engl. J. Med. 239:470–478 (1948).

FITZGERALD, G. M.; GREENFIELD, J. C. and KOUNINE, B.: Neurological sequelae of 'Kernicterus'. Brain 62: 292–310 (1939).

FORD, F. R.: Diseases of the nervous system in infancy, childhood and adolescence; 4th ed., 890–891 and 909 (C. Thomas, Springfield, Ill. 1960).

FRONGIA, N.: Il morbo di Cooley e le eritroblastosi subcroniche al tavolo anatomico (collana monografie Rass. Med. sarda) (Soc. Editor. Ital., Cagliari 1955).

GERRITS and VRIES DE: in Di Guglielmo *et al.* (*loc. cit.*).

GIACOMO, B. E. DI and DARDI, G.: Esiti immediati e tardivi della malattia emolitica del neonato da Rh ed ABO. Conv. Sez. Piemontese Soc. Ital. Pediat., Turin 1963. Minerva pediat. 15:1248–1250 (1963).

GREPPI, E. and GUGLIELMO, R. DI: Die Thalässamien; in Heilmeyer und Hittmair, Handbuch der gesamten Hämatologie, vol. III, 520–557 (Urban & Schwarzenberg, Munich-Berlin 1960).

HARRIS: in Labauge *et al.* (*loc. cit.*).

HILL, F. S.; HUGUES, J. G. and DAVIS, C. B.: Electroencephalographic findings in sickle cell anemia. J. Pediat. 6:277–285 (1950).

HILL, F. S. and DAVIS, C. B.: Further electroencephalographic studies in sickle cell anemia. Amer. J. Dis. Child. 84:214–217 (1952).

HOFFER, W. and HAUSMANN, M.: Ikterus neonatorum gravis: Folgezustaende und Pathogenese. Mschr. Kinderheilk. 33:193 (1926).

HUGUES, J. G.; DIGGS, L. W. and GILLESPIE, C. E.: Involvement of nervous system in sickle cell anemia. J. Pediat. 17:166–184 (1940).

KAMPMEIER, R. H.: Sickle cell anemia as cause of cerebral vascular disease. Arch. Neurol., Chicago 36:1323–1329 (1936).

KELLNER, H. and STOERMER, J.: Der Kernikterus; seine Pathogenese und Therapie unter Berücksichtigung neuer Erkenntnisse über das direkte und das indirekte Bilirubin. Dtsch. med. Wschr. 83:1983–1987 (1958).

KITCHEN, W. H. *et al.*: Human albumin in exchange transfusion. A quantitative study of the influence of added human albumin on bilirubin removal. J. Pediat. 57:876–883 (1960).

LAMBOTTE-LEGRAND, J. and LAMBOTTE-LEGRAND, C.: L'anémie à hématies falciformes en Afrique noire. Sang 23:560–568 (1952).

LANGUILLON, J.: L'anémie à hématies falciformes. À propos de 6 observations personnelles chez des noirs de la Guadeloupe. Sang 22:565–580 (1951).

LEDERER, M.: Three additional cases of acute hemolytic (infectious) anemia. Amer. J. med. Sci. 179:228–236 (1930).

LEGANT, O. and BALL, R. P.: Sickle cell anemia in adults: roentgenographic findings. Radiology 51:665–675 (1948).

LEMAIRE, A.; DUMOLARD, A. and PORTICI, A.: Deux cas familiaux de maladie de Friedreich avec maladie hémolytique chez des indigènes algériens. Bull. Soc. méd. Hôp., Paris (meeting 9 July 1937) 53:1084–1087.

LESBROS, A. and BIGONNET, J.: Manifestations neurologiques, ophtalmologiques et otologiques chez un sujet présentant des crises d'hémoglobinurie paroxystique a frigore et le phénomène de la grande auto-agglutination des hématies. Rev. Oto-Neuro-Ophtal. 21:331–349 (1949).

LIGHTWOOD, E. and COLVER, T.: A boy exhibiting nervous symptoms ascribed to Kernicterus with septic neonatal jaundice as cause. Proc. roy. Soc. Med. 31:559 (1937).

LILEY, A. W.: The use of amniocentesis and fetal transfusion in erythroblastosis fetalis. Pediatrics 35:836–847 (1965).

MEGRAITH, B.: Pathological anatomy of Mediterranean and tropical diseases; in Doerr and Uehlinger, Spezielle pathologische Anatomie, vol. V, 379–541 (Springer, Berlin-Heidelberg-New York 1966).

MAGGIONI, G. and ASCENZI, A.: Morbo di Cooley (Abruzzini, Rome 1948).

MARGOLIES, M. P.: Sickle cell anemia; composite study and survey. Medicine, Balt. 30:357–443 (1951).

McCORMICK, W. F.: The pathology of sickle cell trait. Amer. J. med. Sci. 241:329–335 (1961).

MELLO, A. DE; GUIMARAES, E. L. and GUARINO, D.: Manifestações nervosas da eritrofalcemia. Arq. brasil. Med. 46:409–426 (1956).

MICHELAZZI, A. M.: Anemia emolitica familiare con sintomatologia nervosa. Rass. Fisiopat. clin. ter. 12:145–162 (1940).

MILLIEZ, P.; LAROCHE, CL.; DUBOST, CH.; DREYFUS, B. and DAUSSET, J.: Maladie neuro-hémolytique apparemment acquise. Présence d'anticorps circulants du type incomplet. Influence des exsanguino-transfusions. Remarquables résultats de la splénectomie sur l'hémolyse et sur les troubles neurologiques. Bull. Soc. méd. Hôp., Paris 67:771–779 (1951).

MURANO, G.: Rilievi sulla profilassi dell'ittero nucleare; in Scritti in onore del Prof. G. Tesauro (XXV anno di insegnamento), vol. II, 1480–1512 (Montanino, Naples 1962).

ORTH, J.: Ueber das Vorkommen von Bilirubinkrystallen bei neugeborenen Kindern. Virchows Arch. path. Anat. 63:447 (1875).

PASERO, G. and MURATORIO, A.: Le sindromi neuroemolitiche. A proposito di una osservazione di anemia emolitica acquisita da autoimmunizzazione associata a sindrome neurologica plurifocale. Sist. nerv. 12:458–484 (1960).

PATTERSON, R. H.; WILSON, H. and DIGGS, L. W.: Sickle cell anemia: surgical problem; further observation on surgical implications of sickle cell anemia. Surgery 28:393–403 (1950).

PECORELLA, F.: Sindrome neuroanemica in soggetto con ittero emolitico familiare. Riv. Clin. pediat. 44:690–701 (1946).

PÉHU, M. and DOLLET, M.: L'ictère nucléaire du nouveau-né. Rev. franç. Pédiat. 15:349–390 (1939).

PENNA DE AZEVEDO, A.: Sobre o diagnostico histologico da anemia drepanocytica. Mém. Inst. Oswaldo Cruz 32:517–520 (1937).

PERREAU, P.; GUNTZ, M. and SIMARD, C.: Thrombose des veines sus-hépatiques, thrombose des veines crâniennes et hémoglobinurie paroxistique nocturne. Arch. Mal. Appar. digest. 55:919 (1966).

PIERCE, P. P. and ALDRICH, C. A.: Chronic hemolytic anemia with paroxysmal nocturnal hemoglobinuria (Marchiafava-Micheli syndrome); report of a case with marked thrombocytopenia in 5-year-old child. J. Pediat. 22:30–42 (1943).

POMPILI, A. and SINIBALDI, L.: La sindrome neuroemolitica. Considerazioni a proposito di un caso. Riv. Neurol. 39: 265–274 (1969).

PORTIER, A.; NATTER, S.; GARRE, H. and MASSONAT, J.: Thalassémie et syndromes neuro-hémolytiques. Presse méd. 60:725–728 (1952).

PORTIER, A.; MASSONAT, J.; GARRE, H. and NATTER, S.: Nouvelles contributions à l'étude des syndromes neuro-hémolytiques. Sem. Hôp., Paris 30:1632–1644 (1954).

RAPER, A. B.: Sickle cell disease in Africa and America. A comparison. J. trop. Med. Hyg. 53:49–53 (1950).

REYNES, M.; DIEBOLD, J.; COULET, T.; CAMILLERI, J. P. and DELARUE, J.: Les lésions anatomiques de l'hémoglobinurie paroxystique nocturne. Arch. Anat. path. 17:79–86 (1969).

RIBSTEIN; YOYO and LEVIGNERON: Complications nerveuses et complications mentales de l'hémoglobinose hétérozygote AS. J. Méd., Bordeaux 142:955–961 (1965).

ROMEO, F.: Anemia microdrepanocitica (studio clinico ed emato-istologico). Haematologica 39:1–34 (1955).

ROWLAND, L. P.: Neurologic manifestations in sickle cell disease. J. nerv. ment. Dis. 115:456–457 (1952).

SALOMON, H.: Hämolytischen Ikterus und Degeneration der Hinterstränge. Med. Klin. 10:438 (1914).

SANSONE, G.: Le malattie del feto e del neonato da incompatibilità di sangue (Ediz. Minerva Medica, Turin 1950).

SANSONE, G. and BRUSA, A.: Studio anatomo-istologico di un caso di malattia emolitica neonatale con particolare riguardo alle lesioni del sistema nervoso. Minerva pediat. 6:64–68 (1954).

SARROUY, C. and PORTIER, A.: *loc. cit.*

SCHMORL, G.: Zur Kenntniss des Ikterus neonatorum, insbesondere der dabei auftretenden Gehirnveränderung. Verh. dtsch. orthop. Ges. 6:109 (1903).

SEGARRA-OBIOL, J. M.: La ictericia nuclear; Disert. Madrid (1951).

SILVESTRONI, E.: Anemia drepanocitica e drepanocitosi; in Introzzi Trattato italiano di medicina interna, part III, vol. II. 1339–1343 (Abruzzini, Rome 1961).

SILVESTRONI, E. and BIANCO, I.: Una nuova entità nosologica: la malattia microdrepanocitica. Haematologica 29:445–488 (1946). La malattia microdrepanocitica (II Pensiero Scientifico, Rome 1955).

SILVESTRONI, E. and FONTANA, M.: Studio anatomo-istologico della milza in alcune emopatie familiari. Arch. ital. Anat. Istol. pat. 26: 293–314 (1953).

SMITH, E. W. and CONLEY, C. L.: Clinical features of genetic variants of sickle cell disease. Bull. Johns Hopk. Hosp. 94:289–318 (1954).

SPILLER, W. G.: Severe jaundice in the newborn child; a cause of spastic cerebral diplegia. Amer. J. med. Sci. 149:345 (1915).

SYDENSTRICKER, V. P.; MULHERIN, W. A. and HOUSEAL, R. W.: SCA. Two cases in children with necropsy in one case. Amer. J. Dis. Child. 26: 132–154 (1923).

THOMPSON, R. B.: *loc. cit.*

THOMPSON, R. K.; WAGNER, J. A. and McLEOD, C. E.: Sickle cell disease; report of a case with cerebral manifestations in absence of anemia. Ann. intern. Med. 29:921–928 (1948).

TÖNZ, O.: The congenital methemoglobinemias. Bibl. Haematologica, No. 28 (Karger, Basel-New York 1968).

TORI, G.: Clinical and radiological observations in 102 cases of sickle cell anemia. Radiol. Clin. 23:87–108 (1954).

TORO, R. DI: La malattia emolitica del neonato (Ediz. Minerva Medica, Turin 1966).

TRINCAO, C. and MADEIRA: Un caso de células falciformes com invulgares alterações neurológicas e ósseas num Portugués branco. Gaz. méd. portug. 2:851–869 (1949).

VANCE, B. M. and FISHER, R. C.: Sickle cell disease; two cases, one presenting fat embolism as fatal complication. Arch. Path. 32:378–386 (1941).

VAUGHAN, V. C.: Kernicterus in erythroblastosis fetalis. J. Pediat. 29:462–473 (1946).

WADE, L. J. and STEVENSON, L. D.: Necrosis of the bone marrow with fat embolism in sickle cell anemia. Amer. J. Path. 17:47–54 (1941).

WALKER, D. W. and MURPHY, J. P.: Sickle cell anemia complicated by acute rheumatic heart disease and massive cerebral hemorrhage; report of a case. J. Pediat. 19:28–37 (1941).

WERTHAM, F.; MITCHELL, N. and ANGRIST, A.: The brain in sickle cell anemia. Arch. Neurol., Chicago 47:752–767 (1942).

WIENER AND BRODY: in Labauge *et al.* (*loc. cit.*).

WINTROBE, M. M.: *loc. cit.*

YOYO, M.; RIBSTEIN, M. and CASSIUS LINVAL, J. DE: Drépanocytose et hemoglobinopathies à la Martinique. Leur traitement. Presse méd. 70:2197–2200 (1962).

ZETTERSTRÖM, R. and ERNSTER, L.: Bilirubin, an uncoupler of oxidative phosphorylation in isolated mitochondria. Nature, Lond. 178:1335–1337 (1956).

Chapter II

NEUROLOGICAL SYMPTOMS
IN POLYCYTHEMIA VERA

Erbslöh lists polycythemia vera (formerly Vaquez' disease) third after pernicious anemia and leukemia as a hematopathic source of neurological complications in a high percentage of cases. The original case described by *Vaquez* (1892) presented a 40-year-old male with severe vertigo, buzzing in the right ear, and vomiting episodes. Eight of the nine cases of polycythemia vera reported by *Osler* (1903) were accompanied by nervous symptoms, and involvement of the nervous system has frequently been featured in the later literature relating to this disease (*E. Levi* (1905); *Müller* (1910); *Christian* (1916); *Sloan* (1933); *DuVoir et al.* (1935); *Johnson and Chalgren* (1951); *etc.*).

In polycythemia vera, various physical and chemical changes in the blood picture (*Alajouanine et al.*) are responsible for neurological accidents with a vasculohematic substrate, and cerebral sites are primarily involved.

Nearly every internal organ in cases of polycythemia vera will show signs of capillary stasis and congestion. These are an expression of circulatory deceleration, resulting from increased red cell mass and platelet number, as well as from high blood viscosity. This high viscosity is proportional to increases in the number of figured cells. Diminished cerebral blood flow has been shown experimentally (*Nelson and Fazekas; etc.*): a rate of 20–25 cm³/min/100 g in polycythemia patients was observed in contrast to a normal value of 56–60 cm³. Increased cerebrovascular resistance (4.3 instead of 1.6) has also been shown.

Stasis is aggravated by the fact that the jugular foramina (where the internal jugular veins begin) cannot be enlarged. Thus vasal dilatation and the resultant improved drainage of the encephalic circulation cannot be secured (*Lengsfeld*). The cerebrovascular system must therefore undergo changes analogous to the adaptation of a container to its content. Such changes may be transient or permanent. Considerable passive dilatation of the venous capillary bed can be demonstrated by the presence of distention of the retinal veins (*Wintrobe; Stirpe*) on examination of the fundus oculi, or, at necropsy, by the observation of notable increases in cerebral vein caliber. *Courville* has reported a necropsy picture of exceptionally severe congestion of the meningeal veins. These were broad and tortuous and covered almost the entire cerebral cortex, which was slightly atrophic. Histological examination of the brain revealed frank enlargement of the veins, with angular and corkscrew patterns, thinning of the vessel walls, and small aneurysms. However, the arteries showed fewer signs of adaptation. Corkscrew formation of the extracranial segment of the carotid artery has been shown arteriographically, together with an absence of opacification of the ipsilateral anterior cerebral artery (*Lafon et al.*).

Active vasomotor mechanisms may result in temporary changes in passive cerebral congestion (*Alajouanine et al.*). Increased histaminemia and CO_2 levels and the beneficial effect of warmth may be responsible.

Polycythemia patients are predisposed to cerebral ischemia resulting from diminished blood flow and increased O_2 consumption: there is abnormal venous blood O_2 desaturation but normal arterial saturation. Depressed circulation and its determining factors, particularly increased platelet number and adhesivity (*Shield and Pearn*), and high blood viscosity, together with decreased clotting times, encourage the formation of red cell thrombi in various sites. Venous or arteriocapillary thrombosis, rather than arterial thrombosis, is observed in the brain. The thrombi lack fibrin and are formed of clumped cells that adhere only weakly to the vessel and can be readily detached. Adhesion to arterial walls is facilitated by the presence of atheromas, which are common in patients with this disease.

Coagulation studies have shown that clot formation in polycythemia vera is incomplete. The clots themselves are usually fragile and imperfectly formed (*Rosenthal*). This is a result of increased red cell mass and many cells are not caught within the fibrin mesh, but remain free (so-called "falling out" phenomenon). Poor adhesion and clot friability in thrombosis of the brain and other organs in polycythemics give rise therefore to delayed organization and hence to longer periods of reversibility than in other diseases (*Goldstein*).

It is also true that hemorrhage may occur in polycythemia and may reach serious proportions or even be fatal when the brain is involved.

This fact appears to conflict with the marked tendency toward thrombosis associated with the disease, but is attributable to considerable vasodilatation:the tourniquet test is frequently slightly positive. In addition to clot fragility, the pathogenic significance of which has recently been emphasized by *Cocconi et al.*, relative fibrinogenopenia resulting from a decrease in plasma mass has been suggested by

Stefanini and Dameshek as a factor involved. *Fiehrer,* however, suggests that increased fibrinogen consumption—hence transient hypo-fibrinogenemia or afibrinogenemia—is the result of occasional massive platelet lysis, followed by the release of thromboplastic substances, the production of thrombin, and the formation of numerous small thrombotic sites in parenchymal tissue.

The anatomic picture of the brain in polycythemia vera is marked by intense vascular congestion, particularly in the venous trunks, which gives the color of cyanotic hyperemia to the nerve formations. This picture, which has been studied by *Courville, Kotner and Tritt,* and *Erbslöh,* may on rare occasions be associated with meningeal edema (*Hutchison and Miller*). In spite of chronic distention, the vessel wall may often appear normal, though signs of thinning and fragility, sometimes leading to aneurysms (*Courville*), are by no means uncommon. Frank thickening of all the cerebral vessel walls is less frequent. It has already been noted that atherosclerosis is common. The surface of the incised brain displays a contrast between the dark red cortical matter and the paler white matter (*Erbslöh*). The latter may have a marbled appearance, as a result of irregular blood distribution in the terminal pathways.

Local softening, usually in circumscribed, multiple disseminated sites of varying age, is commonly observed. The patient reported by *Hutchison and Miller* presented necrosis of the two occipital, left temporal, and cerebellar lobes, the left lenticular nucleus, and the right thalamus. The formation of such sites is encouraged by the circulatory deceleration and anoxia already referred to, and they are an expression of vascular obliteration attributable to such causes as thrombosis, atherosclerosis, and arterial stenosis; angiospasms have also been cited as causes (*Winther*).

Hemorrhage is very common and is widely held to be one of the main causes of death. Massive cerebral hemorrhages, however, are rare (*Erbslöh*), those of slight or average severity being far more frequent. These are usually multiple and disseminated (*Erbslöh*), though zonal patterns are sometimes observed, as in the case reported by *Duvoir et al.* Meningeal hemorrhage is not exceptional. Subdural hematoma, reported by *Drew and Grant,* is still a unique finding (*Labauge et al.*). Softening of the brain and hemorrhage may be concomitant.

Neurological and psychological symptoms in polycythemia vera may both precede and overshadow strictly hematological signs, and exact diagnosis may thus be extremely difficult. Nineteen out of sixty-two cases presented by *Croizat et al.* were of this kind, and 78% of the 163 patients reported by *Tinney et al.* displayed neurological signs; in 38%, these signs had been the reason for consulting the physician.

Physical and mental asthenia is one of the more common features of the protean neuropsychological symptom picture of polycythemia (55% of the 541 cases presented by *Calabresi and Meyer*). The mental signs include ready brain fatigue, poor memory, and inability to concentrate. Mental confusion and somnolence are sometimes reported, and irritability and depression to the point of weeping may also be observed. Diminished libido and sexual potential are other signs.

Headache is a frequent and, indeed, virtually constant symptom (51% and 45% of the series of *Lawrence* and of *Calabresi and Meyer*, respectively). It is an expression of endocranial hypertension, primarily venous in nature, and is most commonly present as a simple but persistent sensation of fullness or heaviness, of hot flashes, or of an oppressive feeling of a flow of blood to the head. Patients may, however, complain of active head pain of a pulsating type, and true hemicrania crises are not unknown. *Parkes Weber* reports the interesting case of a 43-year-old man who had suffered from ophthalmic migraine episodes for ten years, often with diplopia or even vertigo. Diagnosis was guided by the appearance of erythrosis, the observation of splenomegaly, and a red cell count of 9,500,000 cells per mm³. Migraine crises were observed in 4 out of 56 and 9 out of 163 of the cases reported by *Brockbank* and *Tinney et al.*

Vertigo is also common (44% of the series of *Calabresi and Meyer*). It usually takes the form of a vague sense of malaise, coupled with a feeling of instability, which may occur simultaneously with headache crises.

Although Menière's disease was observed in the initial case of polycythemia vera reported by Vaquez, the typical picture of this disease (buzzing in the ears, copious, often recurrent, vomiting episodes that follow a critical course and may last several minutes or several hours) is not commonly reported. *Magni* observed five such cases and suggested that vestibular signs were attributable to vascular disturbances in the inner ear, with involvement of the peripheral receptors, whereas irritative symptoms were caused by vasomotor disturbances of the labyrinth. This relationship to circulatory changes of the inner ear had been previously noted by *Bieling*. When serious damage to these formations or particularly frequent recurrences of the disturbances occur, irreversible changes may result. In the case reported by *Boucher et al.* vestibular symptoms, with onset antedating the frank appearance of polycythemia vera by a number of years, were later associated with an alternative syndrome involving the pons. This may be seen as proof of the central rather than the peripheral origin of vertigo. In any event, it may be (following *Labauge et al.*) that the discrepancies among the reported cases are only apparent, since both the arteria labyrinthi and the pons arterial branches have a common origin in the basilar artery.

Disturbances of vision are reported by polycythemia patients also. These include ready eye fatigue, photophobia, blurred vision, scotoma, and transient amaurosis. There are also signs of pain affecting the extremities, often the great toe, as well as other parts of the body (precordial region and abdomen). Such pain is usually severe, with cramp-like seizures, paresthesia, or deep tension (*Lhermitte*). The picture may recall pain caused by torsion or crushing and may mimic that of an erythromelalgia crisis (11 cases reported by *Croizat et al.*). Onset is more common at night and is encouraged by decubitus. Insomnia follows, though the pain may be eased by walking. Concomitant features include joint swelling, true intra-articular effusion, ecchymoses, and purpuric extravasation.

Cerebromeningeal hemorrhage is of particular importance in polycythemia vera. Its onset may be acute and striking. Death from such a hemorrhage is not uncommon, and it can be said that such episodes, with their accompanying symptomatic picture, are often the terminal neurological event in polycythemia, following a history of minor disturbances.

Cerebral ischemia in polycythemia finds its most common clinical expression in hemiplegia due to softening. Aphasia, hemianopsia, and decreased sensibility may also be observed. *Johnson and Chalgren* stress the frequency of hemianesthesia, sometimes as an isolated sign; deep sensibility would seem to be primarily involved (*Alajouanine et al.*).

Hemorrhagic and thrombotic cerebrovascular accidents (or their associations) are a fairly frequent component of all the reported case series: 24% *Friedberg*; 20% *Videbaek*; 17% *Garrett*; 14% *Beal*; 9% *Calabresi and Meyer*; 7% *Norman and Allen*; *Burris and Arrowsmith*. However, *Labauge et al.* hold that these percentages, based on clinical observation, do not give a true picture. They submit that only by close anatomical and clinical comparison can the exact frequency of cerebrovascular accidents be ascertained and the incidences of hemorrhagic and ischemic episodes, which are associated in many cases, be distinguished.

We have stated that cerebral hemorrhage is often the terminal neurological event in polycythemia after a history of minor disturbances. This applies to ischemia also. Occasionally the presentation or recurrence of a minor disturbance may be the direct prelude to a serious cerebral accident. *Lafon* reported the case of a 63-year-old man whose first episode consisted of sudden, severe dizziness that caused him to fall in the street, but regressed rapidly. A second attack, accompanied by vomiting, occurred the same evening and lasted for 48 hours. A few days later, a third episode progressed to severe right hemiplegia.

Meningeal hemorrhage may be a recurrent sign, as in a case presented by *Tizianello*. Here, however, consideration must be given to the possibility of cerebrovascular deformity associated with polycythemia. Reference may usefully be made to the symptom picture in a case of meningeal hemorrhage reported by *Sloan*.

A 40-year-old man presented sudden subarachnoid hemorrhage, right brachiofacial paralysis, and aphasia. Examination revealed erythrosis, liver and spleen enlargement, and dilatation of the retinal veins. Successive red cell counts of 6,160,000 and 7,250,000 cells/mm^3 were observed.

The clinical onset of ischemia is rarely sudden. In most cases, the picture unfolds slowly and gradually and may simulate that of cerebral neoplasia (papillary changes may be observed in the fundus oculi). Note the two cases of polycythemia reported by *Christian* (1916) and two others presented by *Burris and Arrowsmith* (1953) in which cerebral thrombosis was diagnosed as cerebral tumor.

Ischemic complications display a notably protean symptomatology. Their natural history may include rapid regression (even within the space of one day) to the point of complete disappearance of the clinical picture, followed by recurrence after an interval of a few days.

In a case observed by *Levi* (1905) a complex neurological picture was attributed to slight, diffuse hemorrhage of the nervous structures. Rapid and almost total regression followed. The neurological signs were preceded by intense vertigo and consisted of right hemiparesis, serious contralateral superficial sensory deficiency, speech disturbances, and paralysis of the pharyngeal muscles, with bilateral Babinski's reflex. Hemiparesis of slow onset regressed totally within a few days in a case reported by *Andrews*.

The case reported by *Lafon et al.* is important. In a 57-year-old male with polycythemia and left hemiparesis, an electroencephalogram (EEG) revealed an abnormal right frontocentral area, and thrombosis of the ipsilateral anterior cerebral artery was demonstrated arteriographically. After one year of venesection and oral ^{32}P, the hemiparesis disappeared completely. Thrombosis was still evident in the arteriogram, but the examination showed that treatment had favored the establishment of an efficient compensatory circulation via the right middle cerebral artery and thus prevented the formation of new vasal occlusions.

The varying patterns of the ischemic picture, with their regressions and recurrences, bring to mind the now well-understood picture of incomplete stenosis of the greater vessels of the neck (*Labauge et al.*). By way of explanation, *Millikan et al.* rightly postulate basilar or carotid artery insufficiency; the latter possibility is clearly documented by the arteriographic findings of *Lafon et al.*

Cerebrovascular changes in polycythemia may give rise to isolated pathological signs without paresis, and apraxia has been reported (*Schoen and Doering*).

Slight apraxia of the right arm and leg, attributable to circumscribed cerebral thrombosis, was observed by *Wick* in a 12-year-old girl. Treatment brought about the regression of these symptoms, though slight spastic hemiplegia remained.

Involvement of the cerebellum was described by *Dammert and Kaipanen* (one case of hemorrhage) and *Videbaek* (two cases of thrombosis).

To complete the picture, pseudobulbar syndrome (*Bredemann*) and Wallenberg's syndrome (*Videbaek*: two cases) have been reported in polycythemia.

Less commonly, changes in the central gray nuclei may be responsible for abnormal body movements (usually chorea or choreoathetosis), a parkinsonian association of chorea and tremor (*Alajouanine et al.*), or torsion spasms (*De Secondi*). The chorea of polycythemia is marked by acute onset (gradual onset in a case observed by *Gautier-Smith and Prankerd*) and a tendency to regress, particularly under treatment, though recurrences are common. In a typical case described by *Harvier et al.*, regression coincided with the onset of warm weather, while the numerous and annually worsening recurrences occurred during cold periods.

An interesting case of chorea in polycythemia, accompanied by gangrene of the fingers of one hand, is reported by *Bogolepov*.

A 70-year-old male had suffered from polycythemia for ten years. Four years before admission, an episode of nocturnal loss of consciousness had been followed by chorea. This had regressed after ^{32}P, venesection, and oxygen therapy, only to reappear three years later accompanied by speech disturbances and trophic changes involving the fingers of the right hand. The patient also complained of occasional headache and dizziness.

On admission, the clinical and hematological signs of polycythemia were accompanied by a choreic picture involving mainly the muscles of the face and tongue, though the trunk and extremities were also affected.

The patient's speech was hindered and indistinct. The chorea symptoms became worse during speaking. Writing was difficult and untidy. Facial and limb electromyograms showed asymmetrical oscillations (fig. 4). Dry gangrene of the nail and half of the second phalanx of the right

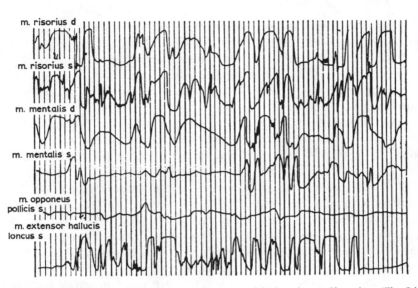

Fig. 4. Polycythemia vera: electromyogram in a case with choreic manifestations (Fig. 2 in *Bogolepov*).

index finger was still present and sores with areas of necrosis were visible on the first, third, and fourth fingers.

Chorea was attributed to circulation changes involving the basal ganglia, and the dystrophy of the right hand was ascribed to circulation disturbances in the extremities, polycythemia being incriminated in both instances. Hereditary chorea was excluded, as was Raynaud's syndrome —reported as a complication of polycythemia by *Patrassi and Jona*—and attention was drawn to an earlier case with gangrene of the toes presented by *Borisova*.

Parkinsonian symptoms were present in a 60-year-old male with polycythemia studied clinically and necroptically by *Courville*. This patient displayed decreased comprehension also and died from cardio-respiratory insufficiency following bronchopneumonia. Necropsy revealed intense venous congestion of the brain, as already described, the basal ganglia being also involved.

Parkinsonian symptoms as a complication of polycythemia are cited from the literature and from personal data by *Kramer* and by *Shoen and Doering*.

Convulsions are thought to be uncommon in polycythemia and have, in fact, been reported only by *Tinney el al., Alajouanine et al., Forsberg,* and *Schoen and Doering*. In one case described by *Alajouanine et al.,* the picture was complicated by serious speech disturbance, dysesthesia (paresthesia and transient anesthesia) in one foot, and disturbed balance. These signs were observed for 26 years before polycythemia was diagnosed, and they disappeared with the administration of ^{32}P. In the case reported by *Schoen and Doering,* convulsion episodes were accompanied by short periods of unconsciousness and occurred over a number of years.

Fainting and mental depression have been observed occasionally (5% of the series of *Calabresi and Meyer*). Silent polycythemia with a red cell count of 8,800,000 cells mm^3 was revealed by the onset of narcocataplexy in a case described by *Lhermitte and Peyre*.

Slight psychological disturbances may occur in polycythemia and, less commonly, true symptoms of psychosis—usually in predisposed subjects. Transient or paroxysmal mental confusion is the most frequent sign (*Müller*), though confusion may also be protracted to a true confusion and dementia syndrome (*Haber*). Depressive psychosis with melancholia has been noted also. Yet such dysthymiac psychoses always appear as organic forms and are often preceded or accompanied by headache, vertigo, or hemiparesis (*Levin*). Such signs are generally attended by a confusion syndrome resulting in prolonged stupor, as observed by *Levin*. The organic nature of these psychological changes is demonstrated by the anatomical evidence collected by *Winkelmann and Burns* (frank dilatation of the cerebral vessels, blood stasis, and anoxia-induced cell change).

Olfactory and optical hallucinations and Korsakoff-type syndromes have also been reported (*Hiller*).

In a personal case of polycythemia in a 38-year-old man admitted for cardiac decompensation we noted decreased intellectual capacity (slight disorientation and delayed thought formation) and instability of character.

Headache allied with mental confusion and vomiting may give shape to a pseudotumoral clinical picture attributable to endocranial venous hypertension.

In an unusual case reported by *Leonardi et al.,* a female patient who was only 18 years old presented oculomotor paralysis. Two years after diagnosis, the polycythemia picture was further complicated by recurrent headache and vomiting together with diplopia. Venesection and X-ray therapy did not relieve the clinical picture. However, spinal puncture led to the disappearance of headache and diplopia, and treatment with busulfan resulted in considerable improvement of the blood picture (still apparent after three months).

Pseudotumoral symptoms are occasionally so impressive that the patient is subjected to ventriculography (*Drew and Grant*). In cases of this type examination of the fundus oculi is of special importance, since changes induced by polycythemia are usually observed at an early stage, sometimes before the other clinical signs. The absence of edema of the optic disk should be noted, though it may be present in polycythemia as a result of liquoral hypertension caused by disturbed reabsorption, the result of venous stasis (*Gaisböck*).

Involvement of the spinal cord and the peripheral nervous system is exceptional.

A 53-year-old woman described by *Grunberg et al.* presented lower extremity sensory disturbances of one year's standing. Four days before admission, she had been struck by a sudden, violent chest pain irradiating to the abdomen and followed by the onset of tetraplegia within a few minutes. Regression of the upper limb paralysis occurred an hour later. The clinical picture on admission was that of transverse cord section (total, flaccid paraplegia with anesthesia as far as the xiphoid process, and sphincter disturbances). A diagnosis of polycythemia was given. The cerebrospinal fluid (CSF) was xanthochromic and contained $1.20^o/oo$ albumin. Death occurred on the 17th day. Necropsy showed multiple venous thrombosis of the viscera and limbs. The brain was congested; the spinal cord was a pasty mass at D6 and for a height of 3/4 cm. The spinal veins at this level projected like black cords, while those in the remaining segments had a normal appearance. Histological examination of the spinal lesion showed complete nervous tissue disorganization, with systematic degeneration of the funiculi posteriores in the overlying and underlying segments.

This case has been interpreted by *Labauge et al.* as a typical expression of secondary softening of the cord due to polycythemia-induced venous thrombosis.

Turning to the peripheral nerves, it may be remarked that mono- multi-, and even polyneuritis pictures have been reported (*Liessens; Lugaresi and Ghedini; etc.*) with sensibility damage only, or with a complete sensory and motor symptomatology.

Treatment sometimes leads to regression. *Sturgis* has reported the case of a patient who knew that he had to undergo bloodletting whenever he had impaired sensation in his hands or feet. The evolution of such forms may, however, be unfavorable. *Liessens* is of the opinion that they are the result of ischemia of the nerve trunks, caused by sclerosis of the respective vessels, while others (*Chalgren and Johnson*) feel that nerve fiber hypoxia caused by increased blood viscosity is the determining factor.

Polyneuritis was observed by *Resnick and Unterberger* in a 61-year-old woman who presented polycythemia followed by pernicious anemia.

With regard to diagnosis, it should be borne in mind that neurological complications of polycythemia are extremely complex and variable, with hemorrhage or serious softening of the brain as possible terminal events. When confronted with symptoms of the kind described, particularly where there is further clinical evidence of polycythemia—special mention may be made of redness of the face and mucosae, with infection of the conjunctiva, and splenomegaly—the physician must obtain a hemogram and the hematocrit plasma/corpuscle ratio to determine the presence of the disease.

Differential diagnosis must constantly be directed to the possibility of so-called central polyglobulia. As its name suggests, this form is characterized by increased red cell counts, at times considerable, usually in the company of normal white cell and platelet levels; spleen enlargement is uncommon. This variety of polycythemia is held to be distinct from polycythemia vera, being no more than a simple increase in the globular elements of the blood secondary to lesion, normally cerebellar hemangioblastoma (*Freymann et al.*), in the central nervous system (CNS). Forty cases of association of this tumor and polycythemia appear in the world literature from 1934 to 1961 (*Waldmann et al.*). Comparison of the pre- and post-resection hematological pictures in 21 of these cases showed normalization of the number of circulating red cells, while in six cases polyglobulia accompanied recurrence of the neoplasm.

An interesting case was reported by *Bousser et al.* Redness of the face of one year's standing followed by endocranial hypertension with headache and vomiting, though without splenomegaly, was at first diagnosed as polycythemia vera with neurological complications in a 31-year-old male. The red cell count was 8,290,000 cells/mm^3 and the hematocrit was 76%. Following the failure of repeated administrations of ^{32}P and the appearance of bilateral optic disk edema, ataxia, and oculomotor paralysis, surgical management was adopted and a large, solid cerebellar hemangioblastoma resected.

A 38-year-old-male observed by *Brody and Rodriguez* complained of serious intermittent headache in the left temporal region, usually occurring as twice-daily episodes of about 15 minutes each, and ingravescent asthenia of the thigh muscles leading to seriously disturbed gait. Later, dysphagia appeared. Objective examination revealed slight depression of the deep reflexes, disturbed muscle coordination, and decelerated gait. Liquor hypertension was also noted. Three months later loss of weight, intention tremor of the left hand, and hyperemia and incipient edema of the optic disk appeared. The gait was markedly ataxic. The blood picture was one of frank polyglobulia, without pathological signs in the case of the white cells and platelets. Six months later the symptoms included considerable papillary edema, nystagmus, asthenia of all four limbs, and a tendency to fall to the left when standing. A ventriculogram showed frank dilatation suggestive of internal hydro-cephalus. Suspicion of cerebellar neoplasia (with secondary polyglobulia) led to craniotomy and the discovery of a hemangioblastoma. Surgical management was restricted to improvement of the cerebral circulation. Radiotherapy of the tumor coupled with bloodletting for two months was followed by evident normalization of the blood picture.

Cerebellar hemangioma may be associated with retinal hemangioma-tosis (Hippel-Lindau's syndrome) (*Bousser et al.*).

Histological examination, however, may show the tumor to be a hypernephroma metastasis (*Bousser et al.*). The 80 cases of tumor accompanied by polyglobulia culled from the 1934–61 literature by *Waldmann et al.* were equally divided between hemangioblastoma and hypernephroma, with both tumors present in 19 cases.

Solid hemangioblastomas consisting of extremely well vascularized masses of glial and foam cells are usually involved (*Cramer and Kimsey; Freymann et al.*), and the cells of this tumor are morphologically similar to those of hypernephroma (*Waldmann et al.*). This is important to the understanding of the pathogenic mechanism thought to give rise to polyglobulia, in the sense that the latter is held to be genuine, i.e. the result of increased marrow red cell production, and not relative, i.e. due to decreased plasma volume (*Freymann et al.*). It is, in fact, supposed that the rich endothelial tissue of cerebellar hemangioblastoma is the source of a presumably humoral agent that stimulates marrow erythropoiesis. Both *Jacobson et al.* and *Erslew* have clearly shown that such a stimulating principle ("erythropoietin") may be produced by a hypernephroma, while *Waldmann et al.* found a substance of this kind in the cystic liquid of a cerebellar tumor observed in a case of polyglobulia of central origin.

Other suggestions made concerning the pathogenesis of polyglobulia in cases of cerebellar tumor include damage to the hypothalamus caused by tumor pressure (*Haynal and Graf*) or by secondary hydrocephalus (*Primrose*) and depression of the respiratory center (*Holmes et al.*). The functional complexity of the hypothalamus is notorious and the associa-tion of lesions involving this organ and polyglobulia is known to be possible. Such lesions are attributable to various etiologies (cranial trauma, encephalitis, neoplasia, etc.). Gaisböck's syndrome, which ap-pears as polyglobulia, arterial hypertension, and cardiac hypertrophy (splenomegaly is initially absent but may sometimes appear later) has also been held to be the expression of diencephalic disturbance responsible for both the hypertension and the polyglobulia. Some workers regard the syndrome as a variety of polycythemia vera.

Pituitary tumors, particularly basophilic adenomas (Cushing's disease), are among the intracranial causes of polyglobulia.

Accurate diagnosis of polyglobulia of central origin must include consideration of the fact that the disease itself may, where red cell increases are particularly high, infrequently be the cause of neurological changes due to circulatory insufficiency or thrombosis (*Kaung and Peterson*).

The evolution of nerve involvement in polycythemia vera is a function of early diagnosis and timely treatment. Modern management is primarily based on oral or intravenous administration of a single 0.1 mc/kg of ^{32}P. Bloodletting may be useful in severe cases. Since the mean red cell life cycle is about 120 days, the action of the radioisotope, which is taken up by the bone marrow, will not be apparent for two to three months and the patient's blood picture will remain unchanged in the interim period. Once the benefit of the treatment has become apparent, periodic checkups, monthly at first, then every three to six months, must be made to give timely warning of relapse.

Beneficial treatment of neurological signs has been reported by *Paliard et al.; Calabresi and Meyer; Labauge et al.;* and others. *Labauge et al.* are of the opinion that a good response to treatment is a true diagnostic test for such signs. The effectiveness of ^{32}P administration is also demonstrated by the almost twofold increase in mean survival times (six to seven years before the introduction of ^{32}P (*Videbaek*), compared to 13 years and sometimes more today). The increased tendency of the disease to progress to leukemia is thought by some workers to be a result of increased survival times.

Some writers attribute this tendency to ^{32}P therapy, and cite the presence of various clinical factors, such as high initial white blood cell values and splenomegaly (*Tubiana et al.*). Thus venesection is urged as the sole form of treatment, with the administration of a low-iron diet or the periodic and suitably spaced administration of busulfan as optional supplementary measures (*Dameshek*).

Good results were obtained with glutamic acid in the management of chorea in the case reported by *Bogolepov*. Blood viscosity may usefully be decreased with Rheomacrodex according to *Holte*.

REFERENCES

ALAJOUANINE, T.; BOUDIN, G.; ANDRÉ, and GOUDAL, H.: Les manifestations nerveuses de la maladie de Vaquez. Bull. Soc. méd. Hôp., Paris 68:538–549 (1952).

ANDREWS, G.A.: Thrombocytopenic purpura complicating radioactive phosphorus treatment in patient with polycythemia vera. Amer. J. Med. 7:564–568 (1949).

BEAL, R.W.: Polycythaemia vera. Med. J. Austr. 46:841–845 (1959).

BIELING, K.: Menièrescher Schwindel bei Polyzythämie. Med. Klin. 29:1410–1411 (1940).

BOGOLEPOV, N.K.: Chorea in combination with gangrene of the fingers in polycythemia. Zhurn. Nevropat., Moscow 62:45–50 (1962).

BORISOVA: in Bogolepov.

BOUCHER, M.; PIALOUX, P. and TRÉLAT: Syndrome vestibulaire central au cours de la maladie de Vaquez. Ann. Oto-Laryng., Paris 70:469–472 (1953).

BOUSSER, J.; TCHERDAKOFF, P. and BOIVIN, P.: Hémangioblastome du cervelet et polyglobulie. Nouv. Rev. franc. Hémat. 1:493–502 (1961).

BREDEMANN, W.: Neuropsychiatrische Befunde bei Polycythemia rubra vera. Ärztl. Wschr. 14:285–288 (1959).

BROCKBANK, T. W.: Neurologic aspects of polycythemia vera. Amer. J. med. Sci. 178:209–215 (1929).

BRODY, J. I. and RODRIGUEZ, F.: Cerebellar hemangioblastoma and polycythemia (erythrocythemia). Amer. J. med. Sci. 242:579–584 (1961).

BURRIS, M. B. and ARROWSMITH, W. R.: Vascular complications of polycythemia vera; study of 68 cases. Surg. Clin. N. Amer. 33:1023–1028 (1953).

CALABRESI, P. and MEYER, O. O.: Polycythemia vera. I: clinical and laboratory manifestations. Ann. intern. Med. 50:1182–1202 (1959).

CHALGREN, W. and JOHNSON, D. R.: Peripheral neuritis due to polycythemia vera. Minnesota Med. 34:145–147 (1951).

CHRISTIAN, H. A.: The nervous symptoms of polycythemia vera. Amer. J. med. Sci. 154:547–554 (1916).

COCCONI, G.; DALL'AGLIO, P. and ANDREUCCI, V. E. : Patogenesi dell'insufficienza emostatica nella policitemia vera e nella trombocitopenia emorragica. Studio di un caso. Haematologica 50:1389–1420 (1965).

COURVILLE, C. B.: Changes in the vasculature of the encephalic gray matter in marked congestion (polycythemia vera). Bull. Los Angeles neurol. Soc. 23:134–141 (1958).

CRAMER, F. and KIMSEY, W.: Cerebellar hemangioblastomas; review of 53 cases, with special reference to cerebellar cysts and association of polycythemia. Arch. Neurol., Chicago 67:237–252 (1952).

CROIZAT, P.; REVOL, L. and VIBOUD, G. P.: La maladie de Vaquez (à propos de 62 observations). J. Méd., Lyon 41:1279–1345 (1960).

DAMESHEK, W.: Commenti alla terapia della policitemia vera. Aggiornamenti Emat., Rome 3:341–343 (1966).

DAMMERT, K. and KAIPANEN, W. J.: Acute erythremic myelosis as a terminal stage of polycythemia vera. Acta path. microbiol. scand. 50:156–162 (1960).

DREW, J. H. and GRANT, F. C.: Polycythemia as neurosurgical problem; review, with reports of 2 cases. Arch. Neurol., Chicago 54:25–36 (1945).

DUVOIR, M.; BERTRAND, I. and BERNARD, J.: Lésions encéphaliques dans un cas de maladie de Vaquez. Sang 9:103–105 (1935).

ERBSLÖH, F.: Veränderungen bei der Polycythämie. In Lubarsch and Henke, Handbuch der speziellen pathologischen Anatomie und Histologie, vol. XIII/2, pp. 1481–1492 (Springer, Berlin-Göttingen-Heidelberg 1958).

ERSLEV, A. J.: Erythropoietic function in uremic rabbits. Arch. intern. Med. 101:407–417 (1958).

FIEHRER, A.: Sang incoagulable et maladie de Vaquez. Sang 21:655–658 (1950).
FORSBERG, S. A.: Polycythaemia vera and essential thrombocythaemia. Two variants of the myelo-proliferative syndrome. Acta med. scand. 171:209–221 (1962).
FREYMANN, J. G.; ZACHS, S. I.; MARLER, E. A. and BURRELL, S. B.: Erythrocythemia associated with cerebellar hemangioblastoma. A study of blood volumes, ferrokinetics, pulmonary function, and pathology. Proc. 7th Congr. Int. Soc. of Hematology, Rome 1958, vol. II, pp. 231–233 (Il Pensiero Scientifico and Grune & Stratton, Rome-New York 1960).
FRIEDBERG, H. D.: The treatment of polycythemia vera by irradiation. J. Fac. Radiol. 10:77–79 (1959).
GAISBÖCK, F.: Die Polycythämie. Ergebn. inn. Med. Kinderheilk. 21:204 (1922).
GARRETT, M.: Polycythaemia vera. Irish J. med. Sci. 431:224–236 (1960).
GAUTIER-SMITH, P. C. and PRANKERD, T. A. J.: Polycythemia vera and chorea. Acta neurol. scand. 43:357–364 (1967).
GOLDSTEIN, K.: Polyzythaemia und Hirnerweichung. Med. Klin. 6:1492–1495 (1910).
GRUNBERG, A.; BLAIR, J. L. and RAWCLIFFE, R. M.: Unusual neurological symptoms in polycythemia rubra vera. Edinburgh med. J. 57:305–308 (1950).
HABER, J.: Psychosis in polycythemia vera. J. nerv. ment. Dis. 115:537–540 (1952).
HARVIER, P.; LAFITTE, A. and LAVARÈNE, G.: Maladie de Vaquez et chorée. Paris méd. 40:277–282 (1950).
HAYNAL, E. and GRAF, F.: The rôle of the hypophyseal-hypothalamic system in the pathogenesis of erythraemia and symptomatic polycythaemias. Acta med. scand. 139:61–77 (1950).
HILLER: in Bumke and Förster, Handbuch der Neurologie, vol. XI (Springer, Berlin 1936).
HOLMES, C. R.; KREDEL, F. E. and HANNA, C. B.: Polycythemia secondary to brain tumor; report of two cases. Sth. med. J. 45:967–972 (1952).
HOLTE, W.: Blodviskositet hos polycytaemipatienter med neurologiske symptomer. Ugeskr. Laeg. 130:1259–1263 (1968).
HUTCHISON, R. and MILLER, C. H.: A case of splenomegalic polycythemia with report of postmortem examination. Lancet, i: 744–746 (1906).
JACOBSON, L. O.; GOLDWASSER, E.; FRIED, W. and PLZAK, L.: Role of the kidney in erythropoiesis. Nature, Lond. 179:633–634 (1957).
JOHNSON, D. R. and CHALGREN, W. S.: Polycythemia vera and nervous system. Neurology, Minneap. 1:53–67 (1951).
KAUNG, D. T. and PETERSON, R. E.: 'Relative polycythemia' or 'pseudopolycythemia.' Arch. intern. Med. 110:456–460 (1962).
KOTNER, L. M. and TRITT, J. H.: Chorea complicating polycythemia vera; report of case. Ann. intern. Med. 17:544–548 (1942).
KRAMER, W.: Neurologic disorders in polycythemia vera. Ned. T. Geneesk. 105:1277–1281 (1961).
LABAUGE, R.; IZARN, P. and CASTAN, P.: Les manifestations nerveuses des hémopathies. Rapport LXI Congr. Franç. de Psychiatrie et de Neurologie, Nancy 1963 (Masson, Paris 1963).
LAFON, R.; TEMPLE, J. P. and MINVIELLE, J.: Hémiplégie régressive au cours d'une polyglobulie. Persistance d'une thrombose de la cérébrale antérieure. Rev. neurol. 92:376–383 (1955).
LAWRENCE, J. H.: Polycythemia. Physiology, diagnosis and treatment (Grune & Stratton, New York 1955).
LENGSFELD, W.: Zerebrale Erscheinungen bei myeloischer Leukämie, bedingt durch Viskositätssteigerung (Gleichzeitig ein Beitrag zur Nirvanolwirkung). Jahrb. Kinderheilk., vol. 126, pp. 289–306 (Karger, Berlin 1930).
LEONARDI, F.: STIRPE, M. and ZENNARO, P.: Sindrome pseudotumorale in un caso di policitemia vera rubra (morbo di Vaquez). Boll. Ocul. 40:3–10 (1961).
LEVI, F.: Policitemia rubra. Riv. crit. Clin. med., Florence 6:784–789 (1905).
LEVIN, M.: Erythremia (polycythemia) with psychosis. Amer. J. Psychiat. 10:407–410 (1930).

LHERMITTE, J.: Les manifestations nerveuses de la polyglobulie. Erythrémie cryptogéné-tique. Maladie de Vaquez. Gaz. Hôp., Paris 103:661–667 (1930).

LHERMITTE, J. and PEYRE, E.: La narcolepsie-cataplexie, symptôme révélateur et unique de l'erythrémie occulte. Maladie de Vaquez. Rev. neurol. 1:286–290. (1930).

LIESSENS, P.: Manifestations neurologiques au cours de la maladie de Vaquez. Acta neurol. belg. 51:300–308 (1951).

LUGARESI, E. and GHEDINI, G.: Le complicanze neurologiche del morbo di Vaquez. A proposito di un caso personale. G. Psichiat. Neuropat. 89:1345–1351 (1961).

MAGNI, G. P.: La funzione cocleo-vestibolare nel morbo di Vaquez. Arch. ital. Otol. 72:171–183 (1961).

MILLIKAN, C. H.; SIEKERT, R. G. and WHISNANT, J. D.: Intermittent carotid and vertebral-basilar insufficiency associated with polycythemia. Neurology, Minneap. 10:188–196 (1960).

MÜLLER, E.: Ueber psychische Störungen bei Polyzythämia. Folia haemat., N.F. 9:233–241 (1910).

NELSON, D. and FAZEKAS, J. F.: Cerebral blood flow in polycythemia vera. Arch. intern. Med. 98:328–331 (1956).

NORMAN, I. L. and ALLEN, E. V.: Vascular complications of polycythemia. Amer. Heart J. 13:257–274 (1937).

OSLER, W.: Chronic cyanosis with polycythemia and enlarged spleen: a new clinical entity. Amer. J. med. Sci. 126:187–201 (1903).

PALIARD, F.; CROIZAT, P. and SCHOTT, B.: Choréo-athétose récidivante, révélatrice de maladie de Vaquez. Lyon méd. 90:353–354 (1958).

PARKES WEBER, F.: Erythremia with migraine, gout and intracardiac thrombosis. Lancet ii: 808–831 (1934).

PATRASSI, G. and JONA, E.: Policitemia con gangrena spontanea degli arti; rapporti fra policitemia e morbo di Bürger. Riv. Clin. med. 37:166–191 (1936).

PRIMROSE, D.A.: Polycythemia in association with hydrocephalus. Lancet ii: 1111–1112 (1952).

RESNICK, M. E. and UNTERBERGER, H.: Pernicious anemia, polycythemia vera and polyneuritis. Delaware med. J. 37:238–239 (1965).

ROSENTHAL, R. L.: Blood coagulation in leukemia and polycythemia; value of heparin clotting time and clot retraction rate. J. Lab. clin. Med. 34:1321–1335 (1949).

SCHOEN, R. and DOERING, P.: Die Polycythaemia rubra vera; in Heilmeyer and Hittmair, Handbuch der gesamten Hämatologie, vol. III, pp. 226–268 (Urban & Schwarzenberg, Munich-Berlin 1960).

SECONDI, R. DE: Sopra un caso di policitemia con gravi complicazioni cerebrali. Rif. med. 56:441–447 (1940).

SHIELD, L. K. and PEARN, J. H.: Platelet adhesiveness in polycythaemia rubra vera. Med. J. Austr. 56:711–715 (1969).

SLOAN, L.H.: Polycythemia rubra vera; neurologic complications; report of four cases. Arch. Neurol., Chicago 30:154–165 (1933).

STEFANINI, M. and DAMESHEK, W.: Le malattie emorragiche (Italian translation by Dr. C. Buoni) (Arti e Scienze, Rome 1965).

STIRPE, M.: Il fondo oculare nelle anemie ed emoblastosi. Osservazioni sulla casistica esaminata nel Policlinico di Roma durante il decennio 1955–1964. Boll. Ocul. 44:577–591 (1965).

STURGIS: in Johnson and Chalgren.

TINNEY, W.S.; HALL, B.E. and GIFFIN, H.Z.: Central nervous system manifestations of polycythemia vera. Proc. Staff Meet. Mayo Clin. 18:300–303 (1943).

TIZIANELLO, G.: Emorragia spontanea della leptomeninge e poliglobulia. Giorn. Med. Alto Adige 2:855–868 (1940).

TUBIANA, M.; FLAMANT, R.; ATTIE, E. and HAYAT, M.: A study of hematological complications occurring in patients with polycythemia vera and treated with P32 (based on a series of 296 patients). Blood 32:536–548 (1968).

VAQUEZ, M.H.: Sur une forme speciale de cyanose s'accompagnant d'hyperglobulie excessive et persistante. C. R. Soc. Biol. 4:384 (1892).

VIDEBAEK, A.: Polycythaemia vera; course and prognosis. Ugeskr. Laeg. 112:795–799 (1950).

WALDMANN, TH.A.; LEVIN, E.H. and BALWIN, M.: Association of polycythemia with a cerebellar hemangioblastoma: production of an erythropoieses-stimulating factor by the tumor. Amer. J. Med. 31:318–324 (1961).

WICK, H.: Polycythaemia vera mit neurologischen Komplikationen bei einem 12 jährigen Kind. Schweiz. med. Wschr. 99:186–189 (1969).

WINKELMANN AND BURNS: in Haber.

WINTHER, K.: Polyglobulie avec stase papillaire. Arq. Neuro-Psiquiat. 10:374–378 (1952).

WINTROBE, M.M.: Clinical hematology (Lea & Febiger, Philadelphia 1961).

Chapter III

NEUROLOGICAL SYMPTOMS
IN ERYTHREMIC MYELOSIS

The appearance of neurological signs in the acute form of erythremic myelosis (Di Guglielmo's disease) is primarily dependent on the degree of anemia and fever. When the disease first becomes evident, the anemia runs a rapidly ingravescent course with red cell values that may fall below 1,000,000 rbc/mm^3. Very high fever is observed immediately in some cases, clearly caused by infection resulting from low neutrophil granulocyte levels.

The possibility of hemorrhage should be borne in mind also. Basically this is attributable to thrombocytopenia and its picture is usually similar to that of leukemia. The data in the literature suggest that involvement of the nervous system is infrequent, since only a few cases of meningeal and retinal hemorrhage have been reported (*Lazzaro*). Subarachnoid bleeding in the occipital lobe was observed by *Di Guglielmo*.

Anatomical and histological evidence of erythremic and reticulo-endothelial cell infiltration in the encephalon and dura mater is also known.

Actual plugging of the cerebral capillaries with nucleated red cells was noted in a patient with generalized systemic erythremic myelosis described by *Paradiso and Reitano*. Outstanding involvement of the tectorial and basal dura mater was observed also. Infiltration of the dura mater in a case presenting neoplastic features was reported by *Lanza and Pafumi*. The subsequent course was marked by cranial and ophthalmic chloroma, while the histological findings showed simple histo-erythroblastic tissue in the bone marrow, lymph glands, spleen, dura mater, cranial and ophthalmic masses, ovaries, and in a retroperitoneal mass.

A complicated pseudotumoral brain symptomatology was noted in a case of acute anerythremic erythremia reported by *Loscialpo Ramundo*.

Anemia and hemorrhage may be responsible for nerve damage in chronic erythremic myelosis.

63

Di Guglielmo and Ferrara have reported stupor, signs of cerebral damage, and blindness due to retinal extravasation in a case of acute erythroleukemia that progressed to terminal intestinal hemorrhage. Anatomical and histological examination showed myeloid cell (primarily erythroblastic) infiltration of the brain and other organs.

REFERENCES

GUGLIELMO, G. DI and FERRARA, A.: Eritroleucemia acuta. C. R. III Congr. Soc. Int. Euro-
péenne Hémat., Rome 1951, pp. 471–473 (E.M.E.S., Rome 1952).
GUGLIELMO, G. DI: Le malattie eritremiche ed eritroleucemiche (Il Pen siero Scientifico,
Rome 1962).
LANZA, G. and PAFUMI, A.: La verietà neoplastiforme della malattia di Di Guglielmo. (Eri-
tremia acuta neoplastiforme col quadro clinico di cloroma). Haematologica 22:835–890
(1940).
LAZZARO: in Baserga and De Nicola, Le malattie emorragiche, p. 786 (Soc. Ed. Libraria,
Milan 1950).
LOSCIALPO RAMUNDO, D.: Considerazioni su un caso di eritremia acuta aneritremica and
evoluzione pseudotumorale cerebrale. Rass. Clin. Terap. 65:301–308 (1966).
PARADISO, F. and REITANO, R.: Malattia di Di Guglielmo con quadro anatomo-patologico di
mielosi sistematica diffusa. Boll. Soc. Med. Chir., Catania 7:99 (1939).

Chapter IV

NEUROLOGICAL SYMPTOMS
IN PORPHYRIA

Porphyria is usually the expression of a constitutional defect in porphyrin metabolism (*Di Pasquale and d'Eramo*). The porphyrins themselves are involved in hemoglobin exchange, since this compound is a chromoprotein formed of a colorless protein, globin, and a chromophoric prosthetic group, heme, which in turn is composed of protoporphyrin and bivalent iron.

Porphyrins are cyclic compounds with a basic structural nucleus of porphin. This parent substance is not found in nature and is formed by four pyrrole nuclei joined into a ring structure by means of $-CH=$ bridges (fig. 5). Substitution of the eight β-position H atoms with methyl, ethyl, acetyl, vinyl, or propione radicals leads to the formation of various products (etioporphyrin, uroporphyrin, coproporphyrin, and protoporphyrin), the isomers of which are determined by the position occupied by the radicals.

Porphyrin synthesis begins with the association of an ammonia base (glycine) with substances from the glucose metabolism cycle ("acetate,"

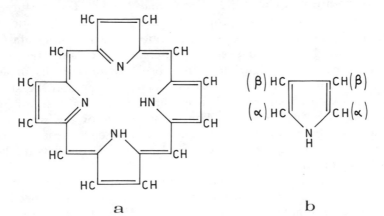

a   b

Fig. 5. (*a*) Porphyrin; (*b*) pyrrole ring.

pyruvic acid, α-ketoglutaric acid, and succinic acid), leading to the formation of δ-aminolevulinic acid (ALA). Two molecules of ALA condense to form porphobilinogen (PGB) or "common pyrrole precursor" (*Falk et al.*). Four PBG molecules combine with the $-CH=$ bridges to form uroporphyrinogen III. A decarboxylase converts this substance to coproporphyrinogen III and this is converted to protoporphyrin IX. Uro- and coproporphyrins are secondary products of the spontaneous oxidation of uro- and coproporphyrinogen. The above process leads to series III porphyrins only. However, both series I uro- and coproporphyrins are normally found in the body.

Under normal conditions, not less than 25 g of porphyrins are present in bone marrow, bone, and the white matter, together with smaller quantities dispersed throughout the body as a whole. About 300 mg are synthesized every day (*Rubino*), primarily in the bone marrow (i.e. in the main hemopoiesis center), though other data presented by the same writer suggest that maximum porphyrin levels are to be found in the liver. The normal adult excretes 300–600 μg/day (about two-thirds series I and one-third series III), very little of which is of alimentary or bacterial origin.

Increased porphyrin may be of marrow or hepatic origin. In the first case, the resulting disease is known as porphyria erythropoietica (or cutaneous or congenital porphyria or Gunther's disease). In the second case (porphyria hepatica), there are several forms: intermittent acute porphyria (a neurovisceral form), porphyria cutanea tarda, acquired or symptomatic porphyria cutanea tarda, porphyria mista, and latent porphyria.

Thirty-nine certain cases of porphyria erythropoietica were reported in the literature up to 1959 (*Caruso and Previti*). Tissue storage of porphyrins reaches massive proportions and gives a characteristic brown color to the bones and teeth (erythrodontia); marrow punctate values may be many hundred times normal. Increased circulating red cell and plasma levels are also high. The urine is brownish or reddish-purple and contains from a few to 100 or more mg porphyrins per day. Fecal values are high. *Garrod* suggests that erythrodontia is a sign of excess production during fetal life. The pathogenesis of the disease is at present attributed to erythron metabolic deficiency, resulting in the formation of large quantities of series I porphyrins (useless for hemoglobin synthesis) in many erythroblasts.

The natural history commences with onset before five years of age in most cases and pursues a chronic course with acute phases, electively in the spring or summer. The main feature of the clinical picture is the appearance of serious bullous dermatitis on parts exposed to the light, attributable to uroporphyrin light sensitivity. Hemolytic anemia with splenomegaly is observed in many cases also.

Porphyria hepatica is much more common. It is usually hereditary and transmitted as a dominant, non-sex-linked characteristic (*Waldenström*[c,d]*; Curnow et al.; Mouren et al.; etc.*). Three main features distinguish the porphyrin picture: absence of marrow lesions, massive porphyrian invasion of the liver, and the excretion of porphyrin precursors (ALA and PBG). Very high PBG and low uroporphyrin values are observed in the liver in the acute intermittent form. This picture is reversed in porphyria cutanea tarda and intermediate levels are observed in porphyria mista. Considerable urinary excretion of porphyrin precursors with small quantities of uroporphyrin is observed in the acute intermittent form, in association with increased stool proto-, copro-, and uroporphyrin values. Uro- and coproporphyrin excretion is also noted in both urine and feces in porphyria cutanea tarda, together with small quantities of ALA and PBG in some cases.

Porphyria hepatica is biochemically explained as the result of an enzyme defect involving either of two systems associated with porphyrin synthesis (*Rubino*). In the acute intermittent form, PBG is blocked, resulting in the storage and abnormal excretion of PBG and ALA. In porphyria cutanea, the block involves coproporphyrinogen-decarboxylase (transition to protoporphyrin), accompanied by the accumulation and excretion of type III copro- and uroporphyrins. Porphyria acuta and congenital porphyria cutanea tarda are marked by the genetic enzyme defect, coupled with certain precipitating factors. In acquired porphyria cutanea, on the other hand, with the exception of recently identified toxic forms, the importance of the liver as the pathogenic factor is beyond discussion, though the presence of some as yet undetermined factor must be postulated in the place of a genetic factor (*Rubino*). Hyperferremia, first noted by *Bolgert et al.*, may also be pathogenic in porphyria cutanea tarda. The clinical, anatomical, pathological, and biochemical analogies of this condition with hemochromatosis are known (*Langhof and Mildschlag; Lamont and Hathorn; Tuffanelli; Petrozzi and Nixon; etc.*) and some workers consider that porphyria may be a result of liver damage following excess iron deposit. Porphyrin synthesis block followed by overproduction of copro- and uroporphyrins, poor iron utilization for heme synthesis, and consequent iron storage has also been suggested (*Burnham and Fosnaugh*). The most recent proposal is that of *Scerrato and Calandra*, who postulated blockage of the mitochondrial enzyme system controlling the bonding of iron with the protoporphyrin molecule.

The uroporphyrin picture in porphyria cutanea tarda is similar to that observed in porphyria erythropoietica and explains the sensitivity to light inherent in the disease picture. In addition to signs of liver damage and occasional diabetes, the symptoms include skin changes, though the deformities and mutilations typical of porphyria erythropoietica are never reached.

PBG is accumulated in acute intermittent forms and may be logically held responsible for the typical acute neurovisceral crises. It is now considered (*Goldberg et al.; Goldberg*) that, in addition to porphyrins, PBG gives rise to a factor, as yet unidentified, which is involved in the myelinization of nerve fiber. Accumulation of porphobilinogen leads to a deficiency of this factor and this would explain the nervous and psychological symptoms, which are here almost as common as the abdominal visceral symptoms. If, however, in line with recent views, we exclude the formerly held suggestion that porphyrins and PBG have a spastic effect on the intestinal muscles and vessels, central nervous system (CNS) and peripheral changes (seen in terms of the hypothesis mentioned above and not as the result of toxic mechanism) may in themselves serve to explain the neuropsychological and the abdominal symptoms of acute porphyria, as well as the cardiovascular syndrome observed in about 40% of cases.

Nervous disturbances in acute porphryia have been attributed to diminished acetylcholine synthesis (*Rimington*). Benefit is, in fact, derived from the cholinesterase-inhibiting effects of neostigmine. Results observed in chick embryos treated with Sedormid led *Aldrich et al.* to suggest that purine production block may occur in acute porphyria. This would make more ALA available for porphyrin synthesis, but would also interfere with nucleic acids and result in nerve damage. *Gray* has recently put forward a similar view, namely that the acute porphyrin picture may be attributable to a fundamental metabolic disturbance responsible for both abnormal porphyrin excretion and neurovisceral signs. The latter are not directly referable to abnormal porphyrin exchange and may be only the expression of changes in nerve metabolism (*Ackner et al.*). As *Gray* points out, the fact that neurovisceral signs display a dramatic onset, reaching maximum intensity within a few hours, in the acute crises of intermittent porphyria may be relevant in this respect. The similarity between porphyrin pigments and vitamin B_{12} (*Bonnet et al.*) and between the neuropsychological picture of pernicious anemia and acute porphyria have suggested disturbed metabolism of vitamin B_{12} as a cause (*Jori*), since it is theoretically possible that the vitamin is routed by the liver (via the purine nuclei?) into the metabolic path that leads from the porphyrin precursors to the nerve fiber myelinization principle mentioned earlier. It may be recalled that, as in porphyria, pernicious anemia patients also present abdominal episodes marked by pseudo-occlusion.

Anatomical and histological examination will show central and peripheral nerve demyelinization in intermittent acute porphyria, and interruption of the axons has been observed (*Drury; Gibson and Goldberg; etc.*). Nerve cell changes (chromatolysis, vacuolization, and protoplasm pigmentation), particularly of the anterior gray columns and the spinal ganglia, have been reported by *Courcoux et al., Boulin et al.[a]*, *Hierons, Giannini, and Ten Eyck et al.* and are considered to be retrograde (i.e. secondary to involvement of the peripheral nerves) by several workers (*Lapresle[b]*). Ischemic damage to both the cerebral white matter and the peripheral nerves has been described (*Denny-Brown and Sciarra*). Abdominal and cardiovascular involvement is seen as a result of damage to the fibers and nuclei of the vagus, and the fibers and ganglia of the autonomic nervous system and the reticular substance.

Intermittent acute porphyria is the commonest form of the disease. Onset is usually in the third to fourth decade of life and females appear to be most often affected. The course is marked by acute episodes separated by clinically silent intervals of varying length. Biologically and clinically indistinguishable spontaneous and induced crises are observed and may alternate in the same patient. Inducement may be attributable to physical effort, cold, psychological trauma, menstruation, infection, surgery, alcoholism, liver disease, though exogenous toxic substances are most commonly responsible: barbiturates, hypnotic drugs containing sulfur (sulfonal, trional), Sedormid (isopropylallylacetylurea), analgesics (especially those with a pyrazolone base and some synthetic hypnoanalgesic drugs of the meperidine group (e.g., Dolantin), sulfa drugs, griseofulvin, anesthetics, narcotics, mercurial diuretics, progestins, estrogens, nitrobenzols, lead, and arsenic. Pregnancy may prove an aggravating factor (*Jamain and Guyot*).

The abdominal syndrome consists of the classic triad described by Gunther: abdominal pain, constipation, and vomiting, with colic as the most frequent sign (present in 85% of acute cases: *Waldenström[a,d]*; *Goldberg*). Pain is usually violent and may last for hours or even days. The whole of the abdomen is usually affected, though local pain simulating a wide range of abdominal diseases may be observed. During these episodes, the abdomen is tractable, While palpation is well tolerated and may even bring relief. Slight tension of the abdominal wall or signs of meteorism are occasionally reported (*Watson*). Intractable constipation is an inconstant companion of colic (*Waldenström[a,d]*; *Goldberg*) and may last for several days, followed by the excretion of dark-red stools (rich in porphyrins) that turn black on exposure to the air. Diarrhea is not unknown (*Waldenström*[d]; *Viglioglia et al.; Goldberg*). Vomiting is more common than constipation, but is by no means always present.

Laparotomy, following a mistaken diagnosis of acute abdomen (*Vannotti*), and radiography (*Beclin and Cotton; Calvy and Dundon*) have demonstrated intestinal spasms alternating with dilated, atonic areas.

As has been stated, the neuropsychological syndrome is almost as common as the abdominal syndrome (*Waldenström*[a,d]; *Goldberg*): 80% of intermittent acute porphyria patients present nervous system involvement, associated or alternating with abdominal crises. Barbiturates appear to render neuropsychological disturbances more severe and more frequent (*Goldberg*).

The neuropsychological syndrome includes signs of peripheral nerve damage (the picture is one of polyneuritis), involvement of the CNS, and psychological disturbances in the true sense.

Polyneuritis (both the peripheral nerves and the anterior gray columns are damaged) is the most common nerve sign in porphyria and is virtually confined to the motor system: flaccid-type paralysis or paresis is observed (limited to simple muscular asthenia in some cases), associated with loss or reduction of osteo-tendinous reflexes, muscular hypotonia, and hypotrophy, frequently of a serious nature, and degenerative electrical reaction in many cases. Paralysis may be either widespread or extremely local. Any group of muscles may be involved, though some writers have observed that the upper limbs are the site of choice (*Magun and Tölken; Steinbrecher; Greve*). Neither symmetry nor ascendency is normally present (*Waldenström*[c]), though cases with tetraplegia and respiratory paralysis have been noted (*Schmid et al.; Castaing et al.*), or an evident Landry-type ascending paralysis (*Courcoux et al.; Hart and Collard; Lapresle*[b]; *Cerrito et al.*). Descending types have also been reported (*Boulin et al.*[a]). A case reported by *Spota and Alvarez Morales de Roballos* included flaccid tetraplegia (with muscular atrophy and equine attitude of the feet), associated with bilateral involvement of the scapulo-humeral musculature and limitation of the hip joints. Superficial sensory disturbances and frank signs of bulbar damage were also observed. A Guillain-Barré syndrome is occasionally reported, with albumino-cytological dissociation of the cerebrospinal fluid (CSF) (*Pino*). In many cases the motor defect involves individual peripheral nerves (radial, external popliteal sciatic nerves) (*Boulin et al.*[b]).

Lapresle[a] reports a case in which a picture of polyneuritis involving especially the upper extremities included radial nerve damage which gave the fingers the "horn-like" attitude typically observed in lead poisoning. This attitude was provoked by extending the arms. This was followed by a fall of the hands to flexion, primarily to the left rather than to the right side, with the middle and fourth finger set on a lower plane than that of the other fingers.

Cranial nerve damage is less common. The literature suggests a frequency of a little less than 30%, while involvement of the limbs appears in about 50% of cases of acute porphyria. Ocular paralysis, optic atrophy, paralysis of the facial nerve, dysphagia, and paralysis of the vocal cords have been observed.

Apart from exceptional cases (*Discombe and D'Silva*), sensibility is unaffected. However, all writers emphasize the frequent and sometimes striking muscular pain that precedes and accompanies motor deficits, together with intense, widespread paresthesia in some instances (*Capone et al.*). 10% of the series of *Aronsen*, cited by *Waldenström*[d], presented neuralgic signs.

CNS involvement is much less common. Generalized, jacksonian-type epileptic crises have been observed in 10% of patients with acute porphyria (*Goldberg; De Grailly et al.; Dhirawani*) and may constitute the first sign of the underlying disease (*Gajdos and Gajdos-Török*). Fatal grand mal was observed in a case reported by *Perrault et al.* Monolateral or bilateral Babinski's reflex has been noted (*Courcoux et al.; Hoesch; etc.*), and in some cases accentuated Achilles reflexes (*Watson; etc.*) or indeed their preservation, together with the loss of all other reflexes (*Roth; De Gennes et al.*), have been reported. Initial coma is occasionally observed (*Hoagland*) and cerebromeningeal hemorrhage may complicate the course of the crisis (*Hoesch; Roult*).

Whittaker has described a woman in whom an acute attack was accompanied by the sudden onset of considerable extrapyramidal rigidity in all limbs and uncoordinated movements; afterward, a two-day period of coma was observed and death occurred five months later. Necropsy demonstrated extensive demyelinization of the cerebral cortex and the basal ganglia.

In regard to the psychological signs, it has been remarked on many occasions that the porphyric patient usually exhibits an uncommon form of behavior, typified by insomnia, headache, irritability, and eccentricity with a tendency to depression. In some cases, attempted suicide by acute poisoning, followed by the sudden appearance of acute porphyria, has clarified both prior abdominal episodes and the abnormal psychological conduct of the patient (*De Gennes et al.*). Psychological disturbances associated with the visceral and neurological signs of intermittent acute porphyria may range from a simple and extremely frequent state of disquiet and insomnia to delirium (present 36% to 38% of patients, according to *Waldenström*[a,d] and *Goldberg*), hysteria, maniacal behavior, and hallucinations. Hallucinatory psychosis is a serious prognostic sign and often the prelude to coma and death. Schizophrenia and Korsakoff-type syndromes have also been observed (*Roth; Vannotti*). On some occasions, the psychological signs appear in isolation and bear no relationship to the abdominal and neurological symptoms; they may even dominate the clinical picture. Confusion with purely psychotic forms is, therefore, by no means impossible.

The CSF is unremarkable in acute porphyria, but encephalographic changes (*Kiloh and Nevin; O'Leary*) may be in direct proportion to the seriousness of the attacks (*Sikes; Dow; Rey-Bellet; Greve; Papy et al.*). These changes include: high voltage, slow activity, bilateral synchronous and generalized paroxystic activity, and sudden and brief appearance of slow waves in different and various loci.

Trophic disturbances are observed on rare occasions (*De Gennes et al.*).

Baker and Messert have observed respiratory dysrhythmia of central origin consisting of involuntary hyperventilation. This was particularly severe during sleep and during periods of mental depression. The subsequent history included marked alkalosis and coma.

Acute porphyria with marked neurological signs was observed in three generations by *Mouren et al.* The observation recalls the dominant hereditary familial cases reported by *Waldenström*[c,d] since 1937. The first patient, a 30-year-old man, presented a clinical picture consisting of colic pain of one year's standing, with constipation (and sometimes vomiting), consisting of two- to three-day episodes; appendectomy had failed to produce marked regression of pain. The recent history included progressive loss of weight, psychological disturbances, and motor-type polyneuritis. The suspicion of acute porphyria was confirmed in the laboratory. Investigation of the patient's family revealed that the daughter was afflicted with ill-defined abdominal disturbances and presented urinary PBG, while the mother, aged 63, had presented an acute digestive episode with diarrhea and vomiting; she had also been paralyzed in the right lower extremity one morning on rising (this condition had since incompletely regressed). Lastly, a maternal aunt of the patient had died at 32 years from a mysterious and rapid disease. This appeared to have been acute porphyria with a neurological syndrome of the Landry ascendent paralysis type: the death certificate, in fact, read: "colitis, intestinal infection, polyneuritis, death due to ascending paralysis."

Familial neurological involvement (a sister with an encephalomeningeal picture, psychological disturbances, and abdominal pain; fatal polyneuritis in a cousin) accompanied a case of intermittent acute porphyria (with complete tetraplegia, areflexia, and diaphragm paralysis) in a 46-year-old woman observed by *Bertoye et al.*

Arterial hypertension (up to 200 mm Hg) is the most common sign in the cardiovascular syndrome and is usually accompanied by sinus tachycardia (up to or over 160 beats per minute). Coronary electrocardiographic (ECG) changes are sometimes matched by an angina symptom pattern, associated with Raynaud-type peripheral circulation disturbances (*Deparis et al.; Lapresle*[a]). Retinal spasm and transient amaurosis may occur *Waldenström*[a,b]; *Gajdos and Gajdos Török.*).

Lipparini et al. have reported a case of amaurosis with recurring episodes of polyneuritis and generalized alopecia (probably attributable to toxic effects on the diencephalon).

Other clinical signs in intermittent acute porphyria include: fever (in 20–30% of cases, particularly during abdominal crisis); leucocytosis (present in 10% of cases, particularly in relationship to abdominal disturbances); blood chemistry changes. Hyponatremia, hypocalcemia, and alkalosis are observed in cases of repeated vomiting. *Hellman et al.*, cited by *Leavell and Thorup*, suggest that hyponatremia and the occasionally observed hypochloremia are caused by imbalanced secretion of antidiuretic hormone. Also included are signs of renal damage and insufficiency (oliguria, anuria, hyperazotemia, etc.), which should be properly included in the circulatory syndrome, since they are due to decreased plasma flow and renal filtrate caused by afferent artery spasm (*Crepet and Gobbato*). However, the part played by the abnormal quantity of porphyrins excreted through the renal filter cannot be overlooked; Occasionally there are observed signs of liver damage.

Acute crises, with abdominal and nervous disturbances, are sometimes observed in porphyria cutanea tarda, though they are constantly absent in the acquired or symptomatic form. In mixed porphyria, liver signs proper to porphyria cutanea tarda and dermatological changes (which may be exceptionally observed also in the intermittent acute form) are associated or variously alternated with the acute abdominal or the neuropsychological syndrome.

Diagnosis of hepatic porphyria from the complete symptom picture is relatively easy. Some, by no means rare, cases of acute porphyria present a unilateral or predominant (abdominal, neurological, psychological, circulatory) symptom pattern. In these cases differential diagnosis must range over a large variety of abdominal, neurological, psychological, and other diseases, with the result that the same case may be variously diagnosed from time to time. We cite the case of a patient observed by *Watson*, whose first acute abdomen episode was ineffectually treated by appendectomy. Thyroidectomy was carried out many years later on account of asthenia, tachycardia, and neuropsychological erethism. Next, slight skin pigmentation and debility was erroneously diagnosed as Addison's disease and treated accordingly. Lastly, a typical neurological and abdominal symptom picture appeared, followed by complete regression.

Judging from the small number of references in the literature, the strictly neurological signs would seem less susceptible to mistakes in diagnosis; though pictures simulating acute toxic polyneuritis, a Guillain-Barré syndrome, acute anterior poliomyelitis (particularly in the presence of fever in a young subject), myopathy, serum paralysis, or encephalitis (particularly in cases with sleep disturbances) may occasionally be observed. The association of a neurological syndrome, abdominal pain, and neurotic or schizophrenic disturbances render the diagnosis of porphyria more probable (*Cross*).

The psychological signs in acute porphyria are much more likely to result in serious diagnostic error, and porphyria patients are commonly discovered as inmates of psychiatric hospitals (*Roth; De Gennes et al.; Dean and Barnes*). Systematic research carried out by *Dean and Barnes* resulted in the discovery of several cases of porphyria in a hospital for mental diseases. As already pointed out, the psychological signs may dominate the whole picture during an acute crisis, resulting in the diagnosis of a wide range of purely psychotic diseases: maniacal psychosis, delirium tremens, Korsakoff syndrome, and schizophrenia (*Vannotti*). Hysteria is the most common of these mistaken diagnoses (*Garcin and Lapresle*) and may well be induced by the habitual temperamental instability common to the porphyria patient and by the very nature of the colic pains. These, though violent, are not accompanied by abdominal defense, whereas initial paralysis of the limbs may be accompanied by apparently normal reflexes.

Chronic lead poisoning must always be kept in mind in the differential diagnosis of the abdominal and neurological forms of acute porphyria, since, during its acute phases, it repeats in a minor form the typical features of an acute porphyria crisis: pain, constipation, vomiting, and paralysis. The differential signs include hemolytic anemia, very frequent oliguria caused by reduction of renal flow, and basophilic red cells, as well as the occupational nature of the disease, which affects printers, foundry-men, painters, or those working with accumulators or engaged in new forms of plastic manufacture. Other signs include the "lead line" on the gingival margin and pathological blood and urine lead values (over 100 μg per 100 cm^3 and per liter, respectively).

Neurological signs have been personally observed in one case of mixed porphyria and in one case of acute porphyria.

The first patient (*d'Eramo and Di Pasquale*), a 39-year-old male, presented epileptic signs of eight years' standing, together with episodic left supraorbital neuralgia as a common concomitant of abdominal pain crises. The psychological picture included signs of depression and anxiety, while the clinical picture was that of the visceral signs of porphyria cutanea tarda and acute intermittent porphyria. The first was responsible for bullous skin changes in areas exposed to light—the outcome of these changes was observed—and liver damage. The second was responsible for recurrent abdominal colic (the first attack, marked by episodic epigastric and right lumbar pain, with vomiting, constipation, and reddish urine, suggested renal colic and the patient had been admitted for surgery), sinus tachycardia, coronary electrocardiographic changes (fig. 6), fever (with occasional peaks up to 40°C paralleling the episodes of abdominal pain), and leukocytosis. Splenomegaly, a very

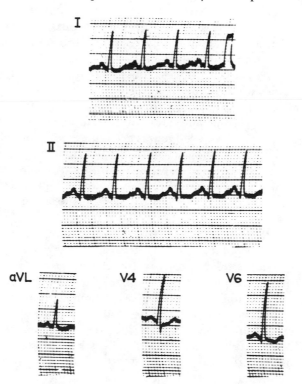

Fig. 6. Mixed porphyria: ECG changes (personal observation).

unusual finding, was also observed. Followup was not long protracted but seemed to indicate that splenectomy had brought both clinical and biochemical improvement in a porphyria picture possibly induced by splenic damage to the liver parenchyma. The spleen enlargement in this case was not secondary to portal hypertension and was histologically classified as of the fibrous-congestive type, with outspoken centrofollicular hyperplasia.

The second patient, a 33-year-old man, presented depression with occasional bouts of euphoria (these signs were usually out of proportion to the underlying disease). The patient himself requested laparotomy for a supposed disease of the appendix and, in spite of its negative result, resorted only to surgeons whenever his abdominal disturbances appeared, in the hope of achieving surgical relief. After contriving to get himself readmitted to the Surgical Department, he avoided all contact with us, even to the point of running away, because of a mixture of fear and disagreement with the diagnosis of porphyria which we had given.

This patient's clinical picture consisted of recurrent abdominal colic with constipation and fever with occasional peaks over 38°C. His temperature commonly remained high between the abdominal episodes and this fact, together with a distinct, positive tuberculin skin reaction, had led other physicians to suggest tubercular mesenteric lymphadenitis. The first episode of abdominal colic had reasonably suggested the consideration of intestinal subocclusion, and the patient had been admitted to a surgical clinic and later referred to us. The last abdominal attack of which we have knowledge was accompanied by bloody diarrhea with notable secondary anemia. A distinctive feature of the clinical picture was the appearance of brownish skin pigmentation under both eyes during the acute stages. Because it was coupled with arterial hypotension, the sign had first led to the consideration of Addison's disease.

Leaving aside the further course of the liver damage, the prognosis is good for porphyria cutanea. The acute form, however, is fatal in about 50% of cases (*Waldenström*[a,d]), as a result of respiratory infection and, more particularly, respiratory or bulbar paralysis. (*Thiodet*). Acute cardiocirculatory insufficiency is only occasionally responsible, and then only in cases where myocardial disease is already present (*De Grailly et al.*). On the other hand, many severe cases (e.g. that reported by *Spota and Alvarez Morales de Roballos*) may follow a benign course. It would seem true, however, that cases whose symptomatology is solely abdominal stand the best chance of running a fully satisfactory course (*Ventura*).

No patient with porphyria congenita has ever been observed to survive middle age. The disease has a slowly progressive course with infection and ingravescence of anemia as the most serious complications. Splenectomy may be a successful management for anemia. Postoperative decreases in light sensitivity and porphyrin excretion are sometimes observed. These are presumably attributable to decreased marrow activity following the cessation of splenic hemocatheresis.

There is no specific therapy for acute porphyria and measures designed to prevent the onset of acute episodes are thus of special importance. The discovery of a case in the active stage must be followed by examination of urinary PBG and stool proto- and coproporphyrin values in the patient's relatives, since above-normal levels will be found in healthy carriers (*Prato et al.*). Both patient and carriers must be forbidden the use of substances capable of causing acute episodes. Any infection must be made the subject of early, meticulous, and sufficient treatment. Alcoholic drink should be avoided. The risks attendant on pregnancy should be explained.

Oral chlorpromazine in fractioned doses totalling 100–150 mg per 24 hours (*Goldberg; Melby; Filippini*) would seem to be the drug of choice during acute attacks. Convulsions can be successfully managed with chloral hydrate and paraldehyde. Pain may be sometimes allayed by opiates, by Demerol (50–100 mg intramuscular) or by ganglion blocking agents (200–250 mg intravenous or 500–1000 mg intramuscular tetra-ethylammonium chloride). The fluid-salt balance must be restored in cases of severe vomiting. Respiratory paralysis must be handled with an iron lung. Symptoms referable to sympathetic hypertonia (arterial hyper-tension, tachycardia, constipation) are treated with sympatholytic drugs. The successful use of chelating agents (BAL, EDTA) has been reported (*Peters et al.; etc.*), though other workers have reported failures with these drugs. *Rasetti and Pettinati* note that the effect of chelating agents on porphyrin metabolism will be partly conditioned by the body metal-ion balance and the action of the agent on such ions. Cortisone therapy may be attempted when other treatments have failed (*Jori*), but must be interrupted if the clinical picture fails to improve or if there is deterioration with respect to neuropsychological disturbances. Good results have also been reported by ovulation inhibitors (*Haeger-Aronsen; Perlroth et al.; Hopmann; Rubino and Rasetti; etc.*). However, cases have been reported where these same drugs brought about attacks of acute porphyria (*Contro et al., etc.*).

An abundant intake of liquids (about three liters per day) either by mouth or by phleboclysis is advisable in acute crises. Hemodialysis, exchange blood transfusion, or venesection should be adopted in particularly severe cases to ensure rapid removal of toxic metabolic products.

Calcium gluconate should be administered, since its formation of complex bonds will encourage porphyrin metabolite deposit in bone, with a consequent fall of blood levels. Defective adenosine triphosphoric acid synthesis may be presumed and should be treated by the administration of adenosine monophosphate. Vitamins (B_1, B_2, nicotinic acid, and B_{12}), enzymes (intravenous cytochrome), and drugs to protect the liver should also be given. On the rare occasions in which skin manifestations are observed, patients must be kept away from sources of light. Anabolic drugs may usefully be given after an acute attack.

REFERENCES

ACKNER, B. G. C.; COOPER, J. E.; GRAY, C. H.; KELLY, M. and NICHOLSON, D. C.: Excretion of porphobilinogen and 5-aminolaevulinic acid in acute porphyria. Lancet i:1256–1260 (1961).

ALDRICH, R. A.; HAWKINSON, V.; GRINSTEIN, M. and WATSON, C. J.: Photosensitive or congenital porphyria with hemolytic anemia; clinical and fundamental studies before and after splenectomy. Blood 6:685–698 (1951).

ARONSEN: in Waldenström[d].

BAKER, N. H. and MESSERT, B.: Acute intermittent porphyria with central neurogenic hyperventilation. Neurology, Minneap. 17:559–566 (1967).

BECLIN and COTTON: in Jori.

BERTOYE, M. A.; VINCENT, P.; BALOT, J. F.; MONIER, P. and WOERLHE, R.: La porphyrie aiguë intermittente de l'adulte (à propos de 14 observations). J. Méd., Lyon 50:1413–1418 (1969).

BOLGERT M.; CANIVET, J. and SOURD, M. LE: La porphyrie cutanée de l'adulte; étude de neuf cas et description. Sem. Hôp., Paris 29:1587–1608 (1953).

BONNET, R.; CANNON, J. R.; JOHNSON, A. W.; SUTHERLAND, I.; TODD, A. R. and SMITH, C. L.: The structure of vitamin B_{12} and its hexacarboxilic acid degradation product. Nature, Lond. 176:328–330 (1955).

BOULIN, R.; GARCIN, R.; NEPUEX and ORTOLAN: a) Porphyrinurie primitive à forme paralytique. Presse méd. 45:1755–1757 (1937). b) Sur un cas de porphyrinurie primitive à forme paralytique. Bull. Soc. méd. Hôp., Paris 53:1079–1084 (1937).

BURNHAM, T. K. and FOSNAUGH, R. P.: Porphyria, diabetes and their relationship. A case report. Arch. Derm., Chicago 83:717–722 (1961).

CALVY AND DUNDON: in Jori.

CAPONE, C.; CENCI, G. P. and POLITANÒ, E.: La sindrome neurologica della porfiria acuta. Policlinico, Sez. prat. 64:505–511 (1957).

CARUSO, P. and PREVITI, A.: Contributo allo studio della porfiria eritropoietica: due casi con anemia emolitica, splenomegalia, ipofunzio nalità surrenalica. Min. pediat. 12:250–265 (1960).

CASTAING, R.; BOURGEOIS, M.; VITAL, CL.; CHEVAIS, R.; GILLARDEAU, G.; GARRIGUE, J. C. and CARDINAUD, J. P.: Porphyries aiguës: étude de 4 observations nécessitant une réanimation respiratoire. Soc. de Neuro-Psychiatrie de Bordeaux, meeting 14 November 1965. J. Méd., Bordeaux 143:114 (1966).

CONTRO, L.; DELLI SANTI, N.; MORBELLI, E. and PETRINI, C.: Crisi di porfiria acuta intermittente scatenata dall'uso di contracetivi orali (segnalazione di un caso clinico). Minerva med. 62:2238–2240 (1971).

CERRITO, B.; BIONDI, L. and BARBA, G.: Su un caso di polineuropatia da porfiria epatica. Rif. med. 82:13–17 (1968).

COURCOUX, A.; LHERMITTE, J. and BOULANGER-PILLET: La paralysie extenso-progressive hématoporphyrique; étude anatamo-clinique. Presse méd. 37:1609–1613 (1929).

CREPET, M. and GOBBATO, F.: Atti XXI Congr. Med. Lavoro, Merano.

CROSS, T. N.: Porphyria-deceptive syndrome. Amer. J. Psychiat. 112:1010–1014 (1956).

CURNOW, D. H.; MORGAN, E. H. and SARFATY, G. A.: Acute intermittent porphyria. A family study. Austr. Ann. Med. 8:267–271 (1959).

DEAN, G. and BARNES, H. D.: Porphyria: a South African screening experiment. Brit. med. J. i:298–301 (1958).

DENNY-BROWN, D. and SCIARRA, D.: Changes in nervous system in acute porphyria. Brain 68:1–16 (1945).

DEPARIS, M.; CANIVET, J.; BONNIOT, R. and ROSSIGNOL, P.: Sur un cas de porphyrie aiguë. Étude clinique et biochimique d'une attaque. Bull. Soc. méd. Hôp., Paris 66:705–715 (1950).

DHIRAWANI, M. K.: Porphyria: report of two cases of acute hepatic porphyria with review of literature. Indian J. med. Sci. 14:359–369 (1960). ˙

DISCOMBE, G. and SILVA, J. L. D': Acute idiopathic porphyria. Brit. med. J. ii:491–493 (1945).

Dow, R. S.: The electroencephalographic findings in acute intermittent porphyria. Electroenceph. clin. Neurophysiol. 13:425–437 (1961).

DRURY, R. A. B.: Nerve biopsy in acute intermittent porphyria. J. Path. Bact. 71:511 (1956).

ERAMO, N. D' and PASQUALE, L. DI: Su un caso di porfiria mista. Atti XIX Congr. Naz. Soc. Ital. Emat., Pavia 1963, pp. 637–638 (Tip. Viscontea, Pavia). Osservazioni in un caso di porfiria mista. Splenomegalia fibroso-congestizia con iperplasia centrofollicolare: splenectomia. Epatologia 9:133–154 (1963).

FALK, J. E.; DRESEL, E. J. B. and RIMINGTON, C.: Porphobilinogen as porphyrin precursor, and inconversion of porphyrins, in tissue system. Nature, Lond. 172:292–294 (1953).

FILIPPINI, L.: La terapia della porfiria intermittente acuta. Med. tedesc. 3:39–40 (1967).

GAJDOS, A. and GAJDOS-TÖRÖK, M. A.: Porphyrines et porphyries—Biochimie et clinique (Masson, Paris 1969).

GARCIN, R. and LAPRESLE, J.: Manifestations nerveuses des porphyries. Sem. Hôp., Paris 26:3404–3422 (1950).

GARROD, A. E.: Inborn errors of metabolism (H. Frowde, London 1923).

GENNES, L. DE; BRICAIRE, H. and TUBIANA, M.: La porphyrie aiguë intermittente. Ann. Med. 50:56–71 (1949).

GIANNINI, A.: Su un caso di porfiria acuta (rilievi clinici e terapeutici). Riv. Neurobiol. 4:1–32 (1958).

GIBSON, J. B. and GOLDBERG, A.: Neuropathology of acute porphyria. J. Path. Bact. 71:495–509 (1956).

GOLDBERG, A.; PATON, W. D. M. and THOMPSON, J. W.: Pharmacology of porphyrins and porphobilinogen. Brit. J. Pharmacol. 9:91–94 (1954).

GOLDBERG, A.: Acute intermittent porphyria. A study of 750 cases. Quart. J. Med. 28:183–209 (1959).

GRAILLY, R. DE; LÉGER, H.; LEURET, J. PH. and AUBERTIN, J.: Porphyrie aiguë et troubles cardio-vasculaires. Sem. Hôp., Paris 36:1471–1479 (1960).

GRAY, C. H.: The relationship between the neurological and biochemical lesions in acute intermittent porphyria. Acta med. scand. 179 (supplm. 45): 41–47 (1966).

GREVE, W.: Beitrag zu den neuropsychiatrischen Verlaufsformen der akuten hepatischen Porphyria. Nervenarzt 37:545–552 (1966).

HAEGER-ARONSEN, B.: Various types of porphyria in Sweden. S. afr. J. lab. clin. Med. 9:288–295 (1963).

HART, F. D. and COLLARD, D.: Acute idiopathic porphyria presenting as progressive paresis of Landry type. Brit. med. J. i:278–279 (1950).

HELLMAN, E. S.; TSCHUDY, D. P. and BARTTER, F. C.: Abnormal electrolyte and water metabolism in acute intermittent porphyria. The transient inappropriate secretion of antidiuretic hormone. Amer. J. Med. 32:734–746 (1962).

HIERONS, R.: Changes in the nervous system in acute porphyria. Brain 80:176–192 (1957).

HOAGLAND, P.: Acute porphyria; report of 2 cases with neurologic manifestations. Proc. Staff Meet. Mayo Clin. 17:273–280 (1942).

HOESCH, K.: Über akute Porphyrie. Z. ges. inn. Med. 63:321 (1942).

HOPMANN, R.: Akute intermittierende ovulozyklische Porphyrie und ihre Behandlung. Dtsch. med. Wschr. 93:76–81 (1968).

JAMAIN, B. and GUYOT, P.: Porphyrie aiguë intermittente et grossesse. Rev. franç. Gynéc. 60:595–601 (1965).

JORI, G. P.: Disordini del metabolismo porfirinico. Recenti Progr. Med. 36:288–334 (1964).

KILOH, L. G. and NEVIN, S.: Acute porphyria with severe neurological changes. Proc. roy. Soc. Med. 43:948–949 (1950).

LAMONT, N. McE. and HATHORN, M.: Increased plasma iron and liver pathology in Africans with porphyria. S. afr. med. J. 34:279–281 (1960).

LANGHOF, H. and MILDSCHLAG, G.: Aktinisch-traumatisch-bullöse Porphyrin dermatose kombiniert mit beginnender Hämochromatose. Arch. Derm. Syph., Berl. 199:21–32 (1954).

LAPRESLE, J.: a) La porphyrie aiguë intermittente (Arnette, Paris 1950). b) Neuropathologie de la porphyrie aiguë intermittente. Bull. Soc. méd. Hôp., Paris 115:1125–1134 (1964).

LEAVELL, B. S. and THORUP, O. A. JR.: Fundamentals of clinical hematology (Saunders, Philadelphia-London 1966).

LIPPARINI, L. et al.: Un caso di porfiria acuta intermittente a manifestazioni addominali e nervose e con alopecia generalizzata reversibile. Arch. Pat. Clin. med. 42:45–52 (1965).

MAGUN, R. and TÖLKEN, O.: Beitrag zum neurologischen Bild der akuten Porphyrie. Medizinische 18:754–757 (1958).

MELBY et al.: in Dimier, H. G.; Lavarello, A. O.; Moron, M. A. and Huberman, E. D.: Porfiria. Prensa med. argent. 47:38–42 (1960).

MOUREN, P.; PASTOR, J. and GUILLEMIN, R.: Porphyrie aiguë avec manifestations neurologiques au cours de trois générations. Marseille méd. 99:116–119 (1962).

O'LEARY, J. L.: Changing status of electroencephalography in neurologic practice. Neurology, Minneap. 5:827–846 (1955).

PAPY, J. J.; ROGER, J.; DANIEL, F.; PONCET, M. and GASTAUT, H.: Aspects électroencéphalographigues et corrélations électrocliniques dans la porphyrie aiguë intermittente. L'Encéphale 57:383–406 (1968).

PASQUALE, L. DI and ERAMO, N. D': Le porfirie. Patologia e clinica. Recenti Progr. Med. 33:66–101 (1962). La terapia delle porfirie. Clin. ter. 22:979–997 (1962).

PERLROTH, M. D.; MARVER, H. and TSCHUDY, D. P.: Oral contraceptive agents and the management of acute intermittent porphyria. J. amer. med. Ass. 194:1037–1042 (1965).

PERRAULT, M.; KLOTZ, B.; CANIVET, J. and CAROIT, M.: Porphyrie aiguë; particularités anatomo-bio-cliniques concernant le porphobilinogène et les porphyrines urinaires. Bull. Soc. méd. Hôp., Paris 69:1048–1059 (1953).

PETERS, H. A.; WOODS, S.; EICHMAN, P. L. and REESE, H. H.: The treatment of acute porphyria with chelating agents; a report of 21 cases. Ann. intern. Med. 47:889–899 (1957).

PETROZZI, C. and NIXON, R. K.: Hemochromatosis and porphyria cutanea tarda. Henry Ford Hosp. med. Bull. 13:285–288 (1965).

PINO, R. F.: Guillain-Barré syndrome associated with porphyrinuria. Ann. intern. Med. 53:600–607 (1960).

PRATO, V.; ALLARA, C.; MAZZA, U. and MASSARO, A. L.: Studi sulla ereditarietà della porfiria acuta. Minerva med. 56:3236–3240 (1965).

Rasetti, L. and Pettinati, L.: Chelanti e metabolismo porfirinico. Minerva med. 57:219–223 (1966).

Rey-Bellet, J.: L'E.E.G. dans la porphyrie aiguë intermittente. Schweiz. med. Wschr. 33:1134–1143 (1964).

Rimington, C.: Neurological disorders in porphyria. Atti VII Congr. Int. Neurologia, Rome 1961, vol. I:21–28 (Soc. Graf. Romana, 1961).

Roth: Neuropsychiatric aspects of porphyria. Psychosom. Med. 7:291–301 (1945).

Roult, A.: Thèse Paris (1942).

Rubino, G. F.: Le porfirie (Ediz. Minerva Medica, Torino 1961).

Rubino, G. F. and Rasetti, L.: Azione dei contracettivi sulla porfiria epatica e sul metabolismo porfirinico. Minerva med. 59:1491–1498 (1968).

Scerrato, R. and Calandra, P.: Sul significato dell'ipersideremia nella patogenesi della porfiria cutanea tarda. Rass. clin.-scient., Milan 44:323 (1968).

Schmid, R.; Schwartz, S. and Watson, C. J.: Neuere Ergebnisse auf dem Gebiete der Porphyrien. Acta haemat., Basel 10:150–164 (1953).

Sikes, Z. S.: Electroencephalographic abnormalities and psychiatric manifestations in intermittent porphyria. Dis. nerv. Syst. 21:226–229 (1960).

Spota, B. B. and Alvarez Morales Roballos, B. A. de: Determinaciones neurologicas de la porfiria, polineuropatia extenso-progresiva. Incidencia genetica. Sem. méd., B.Aires 116:795–801 (1960).

Steinbrecher, W.: Chronische Polyneuritis bei toxischer Porphyrie. Fortschr. Neurol. Psychiat., vol. 27:601–604 (Thieme, Stuttgart 1959).

Ten Eyck, F. W.; Martin, W. J. and Kernohan, J. W.: Acute porphyria: necropsy studies in nine cases. Proc. Staff Meet. Mayo Clin. 36:409–422 (1961).

Thiodet: in Lapresle[b].

Tuffanelli, D. L.: Porphyria cutanea tarda associated with hemochromatosis. U. S. armed Forces med. J. 11:1210–1216 (1960).

Vannotti, A.: Porphyrins. Their biological and chemical importance (Hilger & Watts, London 1954).

Ventura, S.: Porfirinopatie; in Introzzi Trattato italiano di medicina interna, part III, vol. II, pp. 1469–1487 (Abruzzini, Rome 1961).

Viglioglia, P. A.; Linares, R. O.; Viglioglia, J. and Vidiella, J.: Porfiria mutilante. Prensa méd. argent. 45:3671–3677 (1958).

Waldenström, J.: a) Studien uber Porphyrie. Acta med. scand. 82 (supplm.): 1–254 (1937). b) Neurological symptoms caused by so-called acute porphyria. Acta psychiat. neurol. 14:375–379 (1939). c) Studies on the incidences and heredity of acute porphyria in Sweden. Acta genet., Basel 6:122–131 (1956). d) The porphyrias as inborn errors of metabolism. Amer. J. Med. 22:758–773 (1957).

Watson, C. J.: Porfiria. In Cecil and Loeb, Trattato di medicina interna, vol. I, pp. 703–707 (S.E.U., Rome 1954).

Whittaker: in Jori.

Chapter V

NEUROLOGICAL SYMPTOMS
IN COAGULATION
AND PLATELET DISEASES

Neurological symptoms are comparatively uncommon hemorrhagic diseases. With the exception of some cases of Henoch-Schönlein disease (Henoch's purpura) and the rupture of nervous microhemangiomas in Osler's hemorrhagic hereditary telangiectasia (*Borchers and Mittelbach*), hemorrhagic complications involving the nervous system have not been reported for vascular purpura, scurvy, or congenital or familial vascular fragility.

The literature contains only a few references to neurological involvement in Henoch-Schönlein disease. *Erbslöh* cites the case reported by *Wiskot,* in which a 7-year-old girl presented episodic cerebropathic signs against a background of serious neurological and psychological changes. *Erbslöh* notes two stages in the course of such nervous alterations. In the first, there is nervous tissue diapedesis; in the second, there is inflammation and necrosis of the vessel walls, followed by thrombus formation. It should be mentioned that *Erbslöh,* like *Heilmeyer and Begemann* and *Levinson,* treats Henoch-Schönlein disease as an allergy, basically localized in the capillaries, arterioles, and small arteries, and recognized by vasal dilatation and hyperemia stasis. This picture, in fact, corresponds to the first stage described by *Erbslöh. Alajouanine et al.[b]* have reported a case of peripheral nerve lesions caused by intraneural extravasations. Flaccid paraparesis, with degenerative electrical reaction and sensory loss, together with slight paresis of the upper extremities, was observed by *Busch and Jankoff* in a 58-year-old woman. Histological examination of the encephalon showed fibrous atheromatous vascular changes (flaking of the elastica, hyperplasia of the intima, and atheromas), together with perivasal space edema and small deposits of lipofuscin in the nerve cells. Grossly distended vessels well packed with blood and surrounded by a small sleeve of red cells were observed in the left locus niger and the foot of the pedunculus cerebri on the same side.

Frank vasal congestion was noted histologically at the anterior roots of the spinal cord (in the lower thoracic and the lumbar sacral segment), while a fragment of the proximal segment of the sciatic nerve appeared unimpaired. Bearing in mind the fundamentally polyneuritic nature of the neurological picture, however, *Busch and Jankoff* suggest that the lesions are too peripheral to cause serious damage to the proximal segments and the nerve cells.

Neurological complications are also rare in coagulation diseases. In hemophilia, however, nerve involvement is not uncommon and neurological complications were present in 12 patients (11.4%) of the 105 cases on the records of the Montpellier Institute of Hematology (*Labauge et al.*). Both the peripheral nerves and the central nervous system, CNS, (encephalon and the spinal cord) may be involved in this disease.

Neurological complications are not uncommon in the different forms of thrombocytopenia. These usually involve the encephalon and the meninges, whereas the spinal cord and the peripheral nerves are affected only in exceptional cases.

In cases of hemorrhagic diathesis, neurological involvement is usually attributable to pressure exercised by collections of blood on nerve structures or to the direct action of hemorrhages.

Ischemic contracture of muscles involved in a hemorrhage site is a possible cause of muscle damage in pictures of widespread hemorrhage of the soft parts. With regard to the peripheral nerves, a disturbance of their blood supply may be secondary to hemorrhage within various surrounding tissues.

Peripheral nerve damage in hemophilia is observed (in order of decreasing frequency) in the femoral, sciatic, external popliteal sciatic, median, cubital, radial, and facial nerves. Paralysis of the femoral nerve forms part of the picture of hematoma of the psoas muscle, which may be difficult to distinguish from that of an acute peritoneal syndrome.

Peripheral paralysis in hemophilia responds well to treatment, with disappearance of motor and sensibility changes paralleling the regression of hemorrhage. Such treatment consists of the administration of antihemophilic plasma fractions, followed by motor reeducation of the muscles involved.

Where hemostatic treatment is not given or is delayed, serious sequelae may be observed (*Labauge et al.*).

In a case of hemophilia reported by *Borchers and Mittelbach* massive hemorrhage of the right forearm muscles (the limb was bluish and hot and movements were extraordinarily painful) was followed by paresis of the ulnar and median nerves, coupled with "glove-like" sensibility changes and muscular ischemic contracture. This led to the formation of the claw hand seen in Volkmann's syndrome.

With regard to the spinal cord, cases of hematomyelia or compression of nerve tissue due to sub- or epidural hematoma have been observed. Their prognosis is not necessarily poor, since early and intense anti-hemorrhagic treatment may produce improvement, including the disappearance of all signs of neurological involvement (*Imhoff*). Surgical management may also be kept under consideration, since sufficient intra- and immediate postoperative hemostasis may now be obtained with the therapeutic means already mentioned, as well as with local medication. Laminectomy and removal of sub- or epidural clots pressing the cord have been reported by *Schiller et al., Jones and Knighton, Mac Farlane et al.,* and *Sumner.* In the case described by *Mac Farlane et al.* laminectomy involved 12 vertebrae, from D5 to L4. Postoperative hematoma, however, is still the major risk attached to such operations.

Terminal intracranial hemorrhage has been observed in as many as 70% of some series (*Labauge et al.*). Such hemorrhage is more common in childhood, due, undoubtedly, to the greater frequency of accidents at that age (*Silverstein*[a]). Obstetric trauma also may be responsible. *Labauge et al.* observed two hemophilic neonates in whom intracranial hemorrhage occurred at birth, one following the use of forceps. In contrast, the prognosis is more favorable in infancy than in adulthood (*Guillain and Rouguès; Labauge et al.*).

In the 31 cases reported by *Silverstein*[a], hemorrhage was sub- or epidural in 14, subarachnoid in 11, intracerebral in 11 and intracerebral with ventricular flooding in four.

The clinical picture is that classically observed in cerebromeningeal hemorrhage. Particular attention must be given to convulsions. These are caused by irritation of the cortex and may be responsible for limb hematoma. The risk of convulsion should generally be prevented in such patients by the administration of sedatives (*Silverstein*[a], *Labauge et al.*).

Intracranial hemorrhage is a common cause of death in hemophilia. Though early and suitable antihemophilic treatment may be followed by regression, recurrence, at times with a fatal outcome, is not uncommon (*Aita*). A typical case of recurrent meningeal hemorrhage has been reported by *Baer et al.* Patients who survive intracranial episodes are commonly afflicted with sequelae.

Labauge et al. found cortical atrophy by means of pneumoencephalography in a 4-year-old boy with serious hemophilia A. Following dystocic labor and the use of forceps, this patient presented signs of meningeal hemorrhage, together with umbilical hemorrhage, in the immediate postpartum period. At the age of three months, left hemiplegia was still present, and was accompanied by facial paralysis and left external squint. These workers have also observed transient unconsciousness, typical epilepsy episodes, spastic hemiplegia, and frankly retarded weight, statural, and mental development. The last three sequelae were associated in a 3-year-old boy. This patient had presented meningeal hemorrhage four days after birth, detected by the appearance of convulsions (the cerebrospinal fluid (CSF) was hemorrhagic and a large cephalohematoma was also present). One month later, right hemiparesis appeared.

Diagnostic lumbar puncture is not considered dangerous in the hemophilic patient, provided antihemophilic treatment is given first (*Silverstein*[a], *Labauge et al.*).

Intracerebral hemorrhage may be rapidly fatal and can only be handled medically. The prompt and beneficial effect of fresh plasma is emphasized by *Fessey and Meynell.* Arteriographically diagnosed sub- or epidural blood masses which do not respond to medical treatment may be surgically removed after craniotomy. Naturally, antihemophilic cover must be provided during the operation and continued without pause during the postoperative period. Successful surgical management was reported by *Singer and Schneider* in a 3-month-old boy with a subdural hematoma in the temporal region. *Ferguson et al.* also reported a successfully treated case.

Neurological complications may be observed in the hemorrhagic disease of the newborn also.

The main feature of this disease is a serious deficiency in certain coagulation factors (proconvertin, prothrombin, and possibly factors IX and X) caused by vitamin K deficiency. However, it should be noted that all neonates present a physiological tendency to hemorrhage because of their low intestinal formation of vitamin K and, particularly in the case of the premature, because of the state of relative hepatic insufficiency.

Hemorrhage usually appears on the second or third day of life during the peak of coagulation disorders. In the absence of fatal anemia, regression is spontaneous at the end of the first week.

In many cases intracranial hemorrhage is the most serious and the most frequent expression of visceral involvement. Following obstetric trauma, particularly podalic delivery (*Panella et al.*), hemorrhage results from capillary lesions which would be completely innocent in themselves. Except in the case of the premature child, the white substance is rarely involved. Subdural and subarachnoid hemorrhages are most common, the site of choice being the convex surface and the tentorium of the cerebellum, around the cerebellum and the bulb. Ventricular and choroid plexus hemorrhages have been observed, particularly in the premature child.

The neurological picture in this disease is primarily marked by motor disturbances: clonic contractures; relative absence of movement; laziness in feeding and feeble crying; muscular hypertonia, with trismus and opisthotonos crises, though hypotonia is occasionally noted; paralysis of the cranial nerves and, more commonly, nystagmus; yawning and hiccups; repeated vomiting, mimicking pyloric stenosis and responding to spinal puncture; later, convulsions, often with hyperthermia, consisting of usually generalized alternating tonic (longer) and clonic forms—varying degrees of contracture and internal squint are observed between crises, while the sensorium is constantly clouded (*Fanconi; Baserga and De Nicola*). Temperature disturbances (hyper- or hypothermia, or both), respiratory disturbances (alternating apnea and cyanosis caused by abnormal stimulation of the respiratory and vasomotor centers), and liquor changes (xanthochromia or frankly hematic appearance) are also observed. Tension of the fontanel accompanied by conjugated deviation of the head and eyes may suggest ventricular flooding.

Both retinal edema and hemorrhage and pupillary changes (mydriasis or myosis) may be observed. Stiffness of the nucha has also been recorded.

The neurological aftermath of hemorrhagic disease of the newborn may include Little's disease, cerebral hemiplegia and diplegia, imbecility, idiocy, and deafmutism.

In addition to other hemorrhagic signs (cutaneous, umbilical, melena, etc.), a considerably increased prothrombin time value is essential in diagnosing the nature of the neurological signs. In asymptomatic cases, evidence of the potential presence of the disease must be found in the laboratory (*Ferlazzo*). Clotting time is generally normal or only slightly increased. Bleeding time, clot retraction, and platelet counts are within the limits of normal. Differential diagnosis must not overlook sepsis and serious jaundice as possible causes of symptomatic hypoprothrombinemia.

Vitamin K usually normalizes prothrombin time after about 12 hours and is followed by the disappearance of hemorrhage. Quicker results may be obtained in particularly serious cases by blood transfusions or the injection of plasma. Even a small quantity of blood (15–20 cc) will be sufficient to normalize coagulation for a short time (*Fanconi*). It would seem that blood transfusions have a hemostatic effect even in vitamin-K resistant cases.

Cortisone may be usefully employed in the presence of increased hematic fibrinolysis. This drug and antifibrinolytic drugs (Trasylol) are indispensable where particularly high values are observed (precocious hemorrhage in the neonate).

The most important prophylactic measure is early and well-conducted breast feeding. Vitamin K may usefully be given to the neonate in cases of dystocic labor and delayed milk secretion, as well as to all premature children. It should be noted, however, that too high and too frequently repeated doses of vitamin K may lead to enclosed-body anemia or nuclear jaundice, particularly in the premature child.

Therapeutically induced K-hypovitaminosis due to the administration of dicumarol or its derivatives should be remembered. Here, intracranial hemorrhage, often preceded by hematuria, may form one of the major complications (*Gehrmann; Rotman and Zander; etc.*) and is observed when total prothrombin activity (Quick test) falls below 20%. The spinal cord may also be involved (*Cloward and Yuhl; Alderman; Winer et al.; etc.*).

The hematorrhachis observed by *Alderman* may be mentioned because of its exceptional nature. Changes in the vessel walls encourage the onset of hemorrhage, which means that atherosclerosis, diabetes, and hypertension are predisposing factors. The same may be said for protracted anticoagulant treatment (*Pollard et al.*), particularly in the case of Osler's disease (*Duff and Shull*). Treatment consists of the administration of vitamin K and continuous plasma perfusion. The latter must be begun early to create an immediate supply of prothrombin.

Neurological damage may also result from heparin therapy in myocardial infarct. Evidence of multiple hemorrhage in the gray and white spinal cord substance was observed by *Borchers and Mittelbach* in one case after four days of such treatment.

With the exception of hemophilia and fibrin stabilizing factor deficiency, nervous system hemorrhage is very rare in congenital coagulation factor deficiencies. *Rhoads and Fitz-Hugh* observed fatal subdural hematoma in one case.

Congenital afibrinogenemia is a relatively rare cause of intracranial hemorrhage. Fatal subdural hemorrhage was reported by *Schönholzer* in a boy of 15 years. The collection of blood covered the surface of the frontal lobe and infiltration of the right hemisphere was also noted.

Von Willebrand's disease (angiohemophilia) may show cerebral hemorrhage (*Quick and Hussey; Soulier and Larrieu; Marx and Fruhmann; Cornu; Ottaviani et al.*[b]).

Neurological complications may also occur in consumption coagulopathies (*Weber*). These—also known as defibrination syndromes—are marked by disordered coagulation resulting from excessive intravascular clotting and the consumption of circulating coagulating factors, often associated with a hemorrhagic diathesis.

As stated, intracranial hemorrhage may be responsible for neurological signs in thrombocytopenia, whereas involvement of the spinal cord and peripheral nerves is unusual. This incidence picture is repeated in other hemorrhagic diseases, with the exception of hemophilia where the position is reversed.

This difference may be explained by the fact that hemophilia is characterized by a deficiency of plasma antihemophilic factors concerned in intrinsic thromboplastinogenesis. In the case of rupture of a vessel (e.g. following trauma), this deficiency may be remedied by tissue factors endowed with thromboplastic activity, resulting in an adequate extrinsic thromboplastinogenesis. This would explain the low frequency of cerebral accidents in hemophilia, since the nerve tissue's high thromboplastin content cancels the effect of the plasma deficiency proper to the disease. Thromboplastin activity is virtually nil in joint tissue and synovial fluid, however, so that hemarthrosis is a likely finding in hemophilia.

Cerebral involvement may occur in all types of thrombocytopenia. The outstanding picture associated with acute leukosis and marrow aplasia may lead to serious cerebral hemorrhage with flooding of the ventricles, appearing clinically as collapse, coma, and rapid death. Particular reference may be made to the more commonly observed idiopathic forms (Werlhof's disease). Here cerebral hemorrhage was more frequent when splenectomy and cortisone treatment were not practiced. Today, however, other sites are more in evidence: in a series of 66 cases reported by *Ballerini et al.* skin and mucosal hemorrhage was observed in 65%, but in only 5% of the series (three cases) was involvement of the nervous system noted.

It should not be forgotten that such hemorrhages may escape clinical examination. Necropsy, indeed, may often reveal hemorrhage of the nervous system rendered clinically silent by its site or by limited extravasation. Such cases often concern small or very small disseminated purpuric suffusions in the cerebrospinal area, forming part of the widespread visceral hemorrhagic damage caused by frank hemostatic involvement in the acute phase of Werlhof's disease. *Sturgis*, indeed, has found nerve center or meningeal hemorrhage in all cases subjected to necropsy.

The anatomic picture in such hemorrhages is by no means uniform and may include cerebral purpura (not always fatal and sometimes accompanied by meningeal purpura), cerebral hemorrhage, subarachnoid hemorrhage, and subdural hematoma. It has been suggested that in thrombocytopenia the site frequency pattern is not that of typical cerebral hemorrhage: the personal and literature data presented by

Serafini et al. indicate a 27% frequency of basal hemorrhages as opposed to 72% in other brain sites.

Hemorrhage is Werlhof's disease may be considered attributable to platelet deficiency (usually when values fall below 20,000/mm³) and to hemostatic vasal factor deficiency caused either by known causes (such as serotin or platelet vasoconstrictive factor) or by other biochemical functions and properties as yet incompletely understood. The hemostatic defect is of the vasal type (widespread skin hemorrhages, increased bleeding time, and decreased capillary resistance), but clotting times are normal. Petechiae, that is, hematic extravasation following vasal rupture, may be considered the typical hemorrhagic sign in Werlhof's disease. The meta-arterioles and the precapillary and capillary sphincters are the sites of choice. These petechiae are the basis of the brain and spinal cord purpuric lesions observed in the acute terminal phase. Their limited extent may be the result of the procoagulant action of nerve tissue lipids, since these are partly capable of correcting the thromboplastin deficiency of the plateletless clot.

Intracranial hemorrhage is rarely an isolated event in Werlhof's disease, nor is it often the dominant feature in any part of its course. It more commonly accompanies the serious visceral hemorrhages (hemoptysis, hematuria, metrorrhagia, etc.) observed in the terminal period, and appears as the cause or as one of the causes of death in 60% of cases (*Chalgren; Walton; Millikan et al.; Simpton and Robson; Aballi; Meyers; Silverstein*[5]). Meningeal hemorrhage is, in any event, more serious, since it is almost always followed by dramatic involvement of the nervous system, coma, and death.

Recent reports (*Astrup and Sjölin; Moltke*) suggest that this is the result of a high meningeal fibrinolytic factor content. The platelet deficiency is thus associated with premature breakup of the fibrinic clot caused by enhanced fibrinolysis (*Ballerini et al.*).

The symptom picture of both cerebral and meningeal hemorrhage is far from constant. Initial permanent headache, low visual acuity, and photophobia may either regress spontaneously or proceed to a more complete symptom picture with clear signs of brain involvement (jacksonian epilepsy, hemiparesis or hemiplegia, hemianopsia, and aphasia). Convulsions are not uncommon and anisocoria and paralysis of the cranial nerves have also been observed.

Ala and Shearman observed both a Guillain-Barré syndrome and autoimmune hemolytic anemia in one case and they suggest that different autoimmune diseases may coexist in the same patient.

The neurological diagnosis will be based on the clinical examination (signs of hemorrhage in other sites) and lumbar puncture, mandatory in meningeal syndromes since it excludes inflammation and indicates the age of the hemorrhage, depending on whether the liquid is frankly hemorrhagic or xanthochromic. Suspected subdural or intracranial hematoma can be investigated with carotid angiography. Both examinations must, of course, be done under hemostatic cover to prevent hemorrhage at the puncture site; carotid angiography, indeed, may lead to cervical hematoma as a result of puncture. Laboratory assessment of the coagulation processes and the platelet picture will be useful also.

Diagnosis is particularly difficult when intracranial hemorrhage is the first sign of thrombocytopenia and here the laboratory evidence will be of particular importance. In a case reported by *Franklin et al.* intracranial hemorrhage was traced to intracerebral arterial aneurysm.

The prognosis for intracranial hemorrhage is poor, particularly in aged subjects with vascular system changes. However, slight and circumscribed nervous system hemorrhages may regress completely without sequelae. Since, as stated, some forms of nerve involvement are clinically silent, this regression may occur more frequently than can be shown. Yet sequelae are not uncommon. Typical multiple sclerosis (checked by stable recovery of the underlying disease) followed splenectomy in a young woman who had presented numerous hemorrhagic episodes with signs of cerebral and spinal involvement (*Ballerini et al.*).

Hemorrhagic internal pachymeningitis was observed intraoperatively and at postmortem respectively in two cases reported by *Ciani and Fabri.* This alteration was compressing the cerebral substance and appeared to be the result of subdural hemorrhagic extravasation organization.

Improvements in treatment (splenectomy and cortisones) have had a fundamental influence on prognosis. Untreated neurological hemorrhage is almost invariably fatal.

Medical treatment, however, is not entirely satisfactory. Concentrated platelet suspensions must be prepared from fresh blood and therefore require a great deal of difficult work. Blood transfusions supply only a small number of platelets and must be carried out with siliconate materials or "nonabsorbent" plastic to avoid platelet adhesion. Cortisones effectively diminish hemorrhage time but do not result in an increase in platelet levels: the adult dose is 50–80 mg oral deltacortisone (prednisone) or 300–400 mg intravenous hydrocortisone hemisuccinate (*Labauge et al.*).

In cases of idiopathic thrombocytopenia, or when signs of hypersplenism are present, the failure of cortisones to reduce intracranial hypertension may indicate emergency splenectomy. In spite of the very unfavorable conditions in which it must be carried out, this may be life-saving (*Laubage et al.; etc.*). Intracranial hemorrhage pools may be evacuated by means of craniotomy. As in cases of hemophilia, intra- and postoperative hemostatic cover is essential. Improved local hemostasis may usefully be obtained with controlled hypotension during the operation.

Terminal cerebral hemorrhage was the most striking event in a personal case of Werlhof's disease in an 18-year-old girl. The disease was of about one year's standing. It first appeared as skin ecchymosis following minimal trauma and nose-bleeding (the latest episode requiring anterior nasal plugging) and resulted in the patient's hospitalization. Signs of serious cerebral hemorrhage with ventricular flooding appeared suddenly on the fifth night. Extremely violent headache, dysarthria, right lower facial paresis, flaccid right limb paralysis, coma, and, lastly, generalized muscular contracture with occasional left extremity clonus appeared within the space of about two hours. Frank pupillary anisocoria with marked left mydriasis and right myosis were also observed.

Subarachnoid hemorrhage was revealed by intense headache and vomiting in a second personal case, that of a 39-year-old woman. The CSF was hypertensive and hemorrhagic. Slight anemia and a few signs of skin hemorrhage, together with retinal hemorrhage unaccompanied by visual disturbances, were also noted. Splenectomy produced rapid resolution of the clinical picture.

Subarachnoid hemorrhage was the terminal event in a third personal patient, a 24-year-old woman with marrow aplasia and thrombocytopenia. The following symptoms were noted: headache, stupor, nuchal rigidity, Kernig's sign and gun-hammer posture of the lower limbs. The CSF was hypertensive and diffusely hemorrhagic. Retinal hemorrhage was accompanied by almost no visual acuity.

Neurological symptoms may also be observed in primary or idiopathic hemorrhagic thrombocythemia, a rare disease of recent classification.

This is a chronic and usually fatal disease, observed most often in subjects in their fifties. The basic symptom picture includes hemorrhage (particularly of the nasal, oral, and gastrointestinal mucosae), thrombosis, splenomegaly, and thrombocytosis. Platelet levels are never less than 1,000,000/mm³ and in many cases exceed 2,000,000; values as high as 12,000,000 have been reported. Lower values sometimes reported may be attributed to increased circulating platelet destruction probably secondary to thrombi formation (*Levine and Swanson*). Giant platelets may be observed.

Hypochromic anemia with anisopoikilocytosis is observed in most cases. Alternatively, slight erythrocytosis is accompanied by a generally moderate increase in white cell levels. It is thought that hemorrhage in this disease is secondary to thrombosis formation, with blood stasis and vasal wall distention upstream from the clots leading to vasal rupture (*Revol*). Other possibilities include local fibrinogenopenia caused by thrombosis (*Arlotti and La Paglia*) or fibrinolysis caused by platelet synthesis of a fibrinolytic substance, the concentration thus increasing as platelet levels increase (*Bile et al.*).

Hemorrhagic thrombocythemia must be distinguished from the more common secondary thrombocythemia usually associated with polycythemia vera and the early stages of myeloid leukemia, as well as with infection, neoplasia, endocrine disease, and sometimes with sarcoidosis. Here platelet levels are usually below 600,000/mm³ and the typical thromboelastograph signs of the hemorrhagic form are absent. The formation of venular and arteriocapillary thromboses is a typical feature of these forms too.

Brain and peripheral nerve changes and meningeal hemorrhages are included in the hemorrhagic thrombocythemia picture.

Brain involvement is relatively frequent and has a protean and generally transient paroxystic symptomatology: violent headache accompanied by dizziness, transient hemianesthesia, lateral hemianopsia, fleeting aphasia. Other reports include hemiplegia or monoplegia (*Kissel et al.[a]; Korenman*), sometimes followed by postumi. Cerebellar symptoms (*Kissel et al.[a]*) and Wallenberg's syndrome (*Kissel et al.[b]*) were noted. Convulsions have been reported by *Shaw and Oliver; Ozer et al., and Korenman. Labauge et al.* reported two cases of almost narcoleptic and even cataplectic manifestations. In one, the picture included oneirism, voluminous splenomegaly, and a maximum platelet level of 975,000/mm³. The administration of 6 mc of ^{32}P normalized platelet levels and led to the disappearance of the subjective signs. ECG changes representing a disturbance of the wakefulness system also regressed following ^{32}P in the other case.

Protean and fleeting, though recurrent, brain symptoms, and frequent neurologic symptom diversity in the same case, similar to that described for the cerebral ischemic changes observed in polycythemia vera, are typical of hemorrhagic thrombocythemia and indicate the ischemic nature of the nerve disturbances, though brain hemorrhage may be observed occasionally. Regression after ^{32}P treatment is another typical feature. The symptomatological inconstancy of the neurological picture is evidenced by the first case reported by *Thieffry*. This was a 12-year-old boy with 4,000,000 platelets/mm³, who presented fleeting and more and more frequently repeated neurological disturbances. The initial picture was of painful micturition with recurrent lateral hemi-anopsia, together with local paresthesia on the face and an arm, with similar episodes less than one year and four years later. The two cases of successful treatment with ^{32}P reported by *Labauge et al.* may be compared with that reported by *Kissel et al.*ᵃ Here, complete neurologi-cal regression was obtained in a 43-year-old woman with a platelet level of 1,200,000–2,500,000/mm³, who had presented two episodes of anar-thria, central type right facial paralysis, and right brachial monoplegia, and one, the last, of right brachial paresis with paresthesia.

Cases have been reported in which the neurological disturbances, as already mentioned, have been followed by sequelae, or in which there has been no regression of the nervous symptoms (*Lorrain*). Thrombosis of the large cervical or encephalic vessels must be presumed in such cases. This is in accord with the affinity between nerve involvement in hemorrhagic thrombocythemia and with some aspects of similar involve-ment in polycythemia vera. It may be noted that both diseases are expressions of a myeloproliferative process.

The peripheral nervous system is very rarely affected. Single cases of facial paralysis have been reported (*Thieffry*)—in this case the symptom was repeated three times in nine months and was constantly preceded by skin hemorrhage—paresis of the femoral nerve (*Kǎse et al.*), polyneuritis (*Alajouanine et al.*ᵃ), and radicular damage (*Korenman*). Although ana-tomical details are lacking, it would seem that involvement of the nerve trunks must be connected with thrombosis of the vasa nervorum or hemorrhage of the nerve sheaths.

Meningeal hemorrhage must be considered as exceptional.

Neurological improvement due to ^{32}P treatment will be apparent only when the platelet level has fallen as a result of the action of the isotope in the marrow. Until this occurs, no changes in the nerve picture will be observed. The treatment is no defense against recurrent attacks, and timely warning of incipient increases in platelet levels must be gained by periodic checkups.

A case of persistent postsplenectomy hyperthrombocythemia reported by *Dazzi and mercuriali* included a neurological picture of focal symp-toms (recurrent distal paresthesia, transient dysarthria, and fleeting right hemiparesis) and intracranial hypertension with bilateral papillary stasis, severe headaches, and cerebral type vomiting. Coupled with normal ventriculographic data and the benign course, this last complication had led to the interpretation of the picture as one of cerebral pseudotumor.

Appendix. Moschcowitz's disease

Thrombotic thrombocytopenic purpura or hemolytic thrombocytopenic microangiothrombosis was first described by *Moschcowitz* in 1924. Its clinical and anatomic pictures were subsequently mapped out by *Symmers*. While most workers align this rare form with the collagen diseases (*Symmers and Gillet; Lucherini; etc.*), the clinical picture has some special features, and morphological differences between its signs and those of the collagen diseases undoubtedly exist (*Breton et al.; etc.*). Clearly Moschcowitz's disease must be considered an independent form and its inclusion of hemolytic anemia, thrombocytopenia, and hemorrhage as symptoms classify it as a blood disease in the broad sense. A clear understanding of its neural complications is undoubtedly useful in the differential diagnosis of those complications observed in hemorrhage of a strictly hemopathic nature.

The etiology of the disease is still unclear, though most workers suppose its basis to be a Schwartzmann-Sanarelli type acquired change in reagent capacity due to stimuli other than those of the antigen-antibody reaction (*Keller; Roessle*). The normally acute course and the anatomic data (serious and widespread capillary arteriole hyaline thrombosis and occasional symmetric necrosis of the renal cortex) appear to support this view.

The symptoms mentioned above, together with fever, early renal damage, and possible liver involvement (*Patrassi and Menozzi*), are commonly accompanied by neurological signs (53% of the 63 cases of *Antes*). The protean symptomatology includes: general signs (nausea, vomiting, violent headaches, indistinct vision, profound asthenia, etc.), hemi- or monoplegia, aphasia, cranial nerve paralysis, sensibility defects (sometimes hemianesthesia), paresthesia, convulsions (usually general), and psychological disturbances. Changes in the visual field (*O'Brien and Sibley*), pupil abnormalities, and early papillary edema may also be observed. The general signs are commonly present in the initial period. The clinical overture sometimes consists of nerve site and psychological signs (*Breton et al.; etc.*), though these symptoms usually appear at a later stage.

The neurological symptomatology is both protean and fleeting (*Patrassi; Bertoni et al.; Bied and Ehrhart*). The 24-year-old man described by *Bertoni et al.* presented right hemiparesis and speech disturbance as the neurological onset. The former disappeared rapidly but reappeared after about one hour on the opposite side. Periods of perfect psychological lucidity alternated with frank mental confusion. Other neurological symptoms followed: hypoacusis, central type left facial deficiency, slow corneal reflexes, rhinolalia, paresis of the vocal cords, etc. A general epileptic crisis also occurred; after two days it reoccurred and was followed, on the same day, by two jacksonian-type episodes involving the left hand. In the case recently reported by *Bied and Ehrhart,* an onset picture of intermittent left upper limb motor disturbance was followed by confusion and an inconstant pattern of right facial paralysis. The subsequent course included epilepsy with intercrisis hypertonia, hyperreflexia, and bilateral Babinski's sign. Though these disturbances later regressed, variably severe epilepsy crises increased in frequency. One such crisis was accompanied by left facial paresis with rightward conjugate deviation of the eyes and hand. Other crises were preceded by apnea and palpebral clonus. This stage marked the onset of terminal delirium.

Necropsy reveals typical Moschcowitz neurovascular changes accompanied by signs of hemorrhage and soft necrotic sites. Subarachnoid hemorrhage was observed in a case described by *Adams et al.* Usually vasal changes are found in the gray substance of the hemispheres and in the cerebral trunk (*Adams et al.; O'Brien and Sibley*), though in three cases *Adams et al.* observed predominant involvement of the subcortical white substance. Necrosis limited to the district of the left middle cerebral artery was observed by *Breton et al.*

In the case reported by *Bertoni et al.* gross examination of the brain showed slight semioval central white substance congestion in the area of the pial vessels, with slight edema and very slight congestion in various cerebral and cerebellar districts. The histological picture included numerous gray substance thromboses, and the widely edematous nerve structure spread in the form of vacuoles around the thrombosed vessels, accompanied by slight signs of inflammatory infiltration.

Treatment—cortisones and, occasionally, splenectomy—is usually ineffective, though high doses of cortisones sometimes yield good results (*Planques et al.*). Long survival after splenectomy is occasionally reported (*Meacham et al.; etc.*), and *Bernard et al.* have shown that early splenectomy may lead to encouraging results. Satisfactory results after exchange blood transfusions (*Planques et al.*) and heparin (*Bernstock and Hirson*) have been observed *Allanby et al.* state that *Bernstock and Hirson*'s patient later died in spite of repeated heparin treatment. They also report successful results in a case treated with an association of heparin and magnesium. Resort to heparin may be justified by the observation of consumption coagulopathy, as in the case reported by *Muller et al.*

REFERENCES

ABALLI, A. J.: Bleeding disorders of the newborn infant. Gener. Prac. 24:90–104 (1961). (1961).

AITA, J. A.: Neurologic manifestations of general diseases (C. Thomas, Springfield, Ill. 1964).

ALA, F. A. and SHEARMAN, D. J. C.: A case of autoimmune haemolytic anaemia, thrombocytopenia and Landry-Guillain-Barré syndrome. Acta haemat., Basel 34:361–369 (1965).

ALAJOUANINE, T.; CASTAIGNE, P.; FOURNIÈRE; CAMBIER, J. and AUZÉPY: a) Multinévrite avec gangrène ischémique des doigts chez une femme présentant une thrombocytémie; guérison après application de P 32. Rev. neurol. 98:772–777 (1958).

ALAJOUANINE, THUREL and MAURICE: b) in Busch and Jankoft.

ALDERMAN, D. B.: Extradural spinal-cord hematoma; report of case due to dicumarol and review of literature. New Engl. J. Med. 255:839–842 (1956).

ARLOTTI, O. and LAPAGLIA, S.: Le trombocitemie. In Baserga, A.: Attualità in Ematologia, vol. II, pp. 397–427 (Abruzzini, Rome 1958).

ASTRUP, T. and SJÖLIN, K. E.: Thromboplastic and fibrinolytic activity of human synovial membrane and fibrous capsular tissue. Proc. Soc. exp. Biol., N.Y. 97:852–853 (1958).

BAER, S.; GOLDBURGH, H. and PEARLSTINE, B.: Recurrent intracranial hemorrhages in patient with hemophilia. J. amer. med. Ass. 121:933–935 (1943).

BALLERINI, G.; CANTELLI, T. and TENZE, L.: Le manifestazioni emorragiche delle piastrinopenie a livello del sistema nervoso centrale. Minerva med. giuliana 3:56–57 (1963).

BASERGA, A. and NICOLA, P. DE: Le malattie emorragiche (Soc. Ed. Libraria, Milan 1950).

BILE, G.; BIASI, R. DE and RUBERTELLI, M.: Le trombocitemie (Ediz. Haematologica, Pavia 1965).

BORCHERS, H. G. and MITTELBACH, F.: Neurologische Störungen bei Blutkrankheiten. Internist, Berl. 2:105–117 (1961).

BUSCH, K. T. and JANKOFF, J.: Neurologische und neuropathologische Beiträge zur Schönlein-Henochschen Krankheit. Psychiat. Neurol. med. Psychol., Lpz. 13:321–324 (1961).

CHALGREN, W. S.: Neurologic complications of hemorrhagic diseases. Neurology, Minneap. 3:126–136 (1953).

CIANI, N. and FABRI, S.: Sulle localizzazioni emorragiche encefalo-meningee nelle porpore piastrinopeniche. Contributo anatomo-clinico. Note Psichiat. 58:671–704 (1965).

CLOWARD, R. B. and YUHL, E. T.: Spontaneous intraspinal hemorrhage and paraplegia complicating dicumarol therapy. Neurology, Minneap. 5:600–602 (1955).

CORNU, P.: Thèse Paris (1959).

DAZZI, P. and MERCURIALI, A.: Pseudotumor cerebri in corso di trombocitemia postsplenectomia. G. Psichiat. Neuropat. 96:179–196 (1968).

DUFF, I. F. and SHULL, W. H.: Fatal hemorrhage in dicumarol poisoning, with report of necropsy. J. amer. med. Ass. 139:762–776 (1949).

ERBSLÖH: in Busch and Jankoff.

FANCONI, G.: Die Störungen der Blutgerinnung beim Kinde (Thieme, Stuttgart 1941).

FERGUSON, G. G.; BARTON, W. B. and DRAKE, C. G.: Subdural hematoma in hemophilia: successful treatment with cryoprecipitate. Case report. J. Neurosurg. 29:524–528 (1968).

FERLAZZO, A.: Lineamenti clinici e terapeutici della malattia emorragica del neonato. Gaz. san., Milan 37:410–421 (1966).

FESSEY, B. M. and MEYNELL, M. J.: Haemorrhage involving the central nervous system in haemophilia: account of the management of five cases. Brit. med. J. ii:211–212 (1966).

FRANKLIN, E. C.; POWELL, M. J. and KRUEGER, E. G.: Subarachnoid hemorrhage from an aneurysm in a patient with thrombocytopenic purpura. Neurology, Minneap. 7:293–295 (1957).

GEHRMANN, G.: Neurologische Komplikationen bei Antikoagulantienbehandlung. Med. Welt, Stg. 22:327–329 (1971).

GRASSO, E. and CONCA, G.: Le malattie emorragiche nell'infanzia (Ediz. Minerva Medica, Turin 1958).

GUILLAIN, G. and ROUQUÈS, L.: Les manifestations nerveuses de l'hémophilie. Bull. méd., Paris 58:161–166 (1944).

HEILMEYER and BEGEMANN: in Busch and Jankoff.

IMHOFF, H. H.: Über das Vorkommen von hämophilen Blutungen am und im Zentralnervensystem. Z. menschl. Vererb. Konstitlehre 30:466–484 (1951).

JONES, R. K. and KNIGHTON, R. S.: Surgery in hemophilia with special references to the central nervous system. Amer. J. Surg. 144:1029 (1956).

KÄSF, F.; BEJŠOVEC, M. and MATOUŠEK, J.: Neurologische Komplikation bei einer primären hämorrhagischen Thrombozytamie. Z. ges. inn. Med. 21/23:761 763 (1966).

KISSEL, P.; DUREUX, S. B.; SCHMITT, J. and TRIDON, P.: a) Les complications nerveuses des thrombocytémies. Rev. neurol. 98:766–772 (1958).

KISSEL, P.; SCHMITT, J.; BARRUCAND, D. and MARCHAL, C. C.: b) Syndrome de Wallenberg au cours d'une thrombocytémie chronique chez une splénectomisée. Ann. méd., Nancy 3:1004–1012 (1964).

KORENMAN, G.: Neurologic syndromes associated with primary thrombocythemia. J. Mt. Sinai Hosp. 36:317–325 (1969).

LABAUGE, R.; IZARN, P. and CASTAN, P.: Les manifestations nerveuses des hémopathies. Rapport LXI Congr. Franç. de Psychiatrie et de Neurologie, Nancy 1963 (Masson, Paris 1963).

LEVINE, J. and SWANSON, P. D.: Idiopathic thrombocytosis. A treatable cause of transient ischemic attacks. Neurology, Minneap. 18:711–713 (1968).

LEVINSON: in Busch and Jankoff.

LORRAIN, P.: Complications nerveuses des thrombocytémies. Thèse Nancy (1957).

MAC FARLANE, R. G.; MALLAM, P. C.; WITTS, L. J.; BIDWELL, E.; BIGGS, R.; FRAENKEL, G. J.; HONEY, G. E. and TAYLOR, K. B.: Surgery in hemophilia; the use of animal antihemophilic globulin and human plasma in thirteen cases. Lancet ii:251–259 (1957).

MARX, R. and FRUHMANN, G.: Dominante, milde Hämophilie AB mit verlängerter Blutungszeit-eine Untergruppe der Pseudohämophilien. Klin. Wschr. 23:1109–1118 (1958).

MEYERS, M. C.: Results of treatment in 71 patients with idiopathic thrombocytopenic purpura. Amer. J. med. Sci. 242:295–302 (1961).

MILLIKAN, C. H. *et al.*: A classification and outline of cerebral vascular diseases. Neurology, Minneap. 8:397–434 (1958).

MOLTKE, P.: Plasminogen activator in animal meninges. Proc. Soc. exp. Biol., N.Y. 98:377–379 (1958).

OTTAVIANI, P.; DETTORI, A. G. and MANAI, G.: a) La malattia trombocitopenica (Ediz. Minerva Medica, Turin 1956).

OTTAVIANI, P.; MANAI, G. and MANDELLI, F.: b) L'angioemofilia (Leonardo Ediz. Scientifiche, Rome 1961).

OZER, F. L.; TRUAX, W. E.; MIESCH, D. C. and LEVIN, W. C.: Primary hemorrhagic thrombocythemia. Amer. J. Med. 28:807–823 (1960).

PANELLA, I.; CIANCI, S. and MAROTTA, N.: La malattia emorragica del neonato: considerazioni anatomo-cliniche e statistiche sul materiale della Clinica Ostetrico-Ginecologica di Catania. Gaz. san., Milan 37:265–267 (1966).

POLLARD, J. W. *et al.*: Problems associated with long-term anticoagulant therapy. Observations in 139 cases. Circulation 25:311–317 (1962).

QUICK, A. J. and HUSSEY, C. V.: Hemophilic condition in girl. Amer. J. Dis. Child. 85:698–705 (1953).

REVOL, L.: La myélose hyperthrombocytaire (thrombocytémie hémorragique). Sang 21:409–423 (1950).

RHOADS, J. E. and FITZ-HUGH, T.: Idiopathic hypoprothrombinemia: an apparently unrecorded condition. Amer. J. med. Sci. 202:662–670 (1941).

ROTMAN, M. and ZANDER, E.: Hémorragies intracrâniennes complications du traitement anticoagulant. Praxis 60:459–464 (1971).

SCHILLER, F.; NELIGAN, G. and BUDTZ-OLSEN, O.: Surgery in haemophilia; case of spinal subdural haematoma producing paraplegia. Lancet ii:842–845 (1948).

SCHÖNHOLZER, G.: Die hereditäre Fibrinogenopenie. Dtsch. Arch. klin. Med. 184:496-510 (1939).

SERAFINI, U.; NOFERI, G.; BARTOLI, V. and BENCINI, A.: Il problema diagnostico dell'apoplessia cerebrale. Riv. crit. Clin. med. 59:381 (1959).

SHAW, S. and OLIVER, R. A. M.: Primary haemorrhagic thrombocythaemia. Proc. roy. Soc. Med. 51:768–772 (1958).

SILVERSTEIN, A.: a) Intracranial bleeding in hemophilia. Arch. Neurol., Chicago 3:141–157 (1960). b) Intracranial hemorrhage in patients with bleeding tendencies. Neurology, Minneap. 11:310–317 (1961).

SIMPSON, D. A. and ROBSON, H. N.: Intracranial haemorrhage in disorders of blood coagulation. Austr. N.Z. J. Surg. 29:287–303 (1960).

SINGER, R. P. and SCHNEIDER, R. C.: The successful management of intracerebral and subarachnoid hemorrhage in a hemophilic infant. A case report. Neurology, Minneap. 12:293–294 (1962).

SOULIER, J. P. and LARRIEU, M. J.: Déficit en facteur antihémophylique B avec allongement du temps de saignement. Sang 28:138–141 (1957).

STURGIS, C. C.: Hematology (C. Thomas, Springfield, Ill. 1955).

SUMNER, D. W.: Spontaneous spinal extradural hemorrhage due to hemophilia. Report of a case. Neurology, Minneap. 12:501–502. (1962).

THIEFFRY: in Labauge *et al.*

WALTON, J. N.: Subarachnoid hemorrhage of unusual etiology. Neurology, Minneap. 3:517–543 (1953).

WEBER, M. B.: Neurologic complications of consumption coagulopathies. Neurology, Minneap. 18:185–188 (1968).

WINER, B. M.; HORONSTEIN, S. and STARR, A. M.: Spinal epidural hematoma during anticoagulant therapy. Circulation 19:735–740 (1959).

WISKOT: in Busch and Jankoff.

Appendix. Moschcowitz's disease

ADAMS, R. D.; CAMMERMEYER, J. and FITZGERALD, P. J.: Neuropathological aspects of thrombocytic acroangiothrombosis; clinico-anatomical study of generalized platelet thrombosis. J. Neurol. Neurosurg. Psychiat. 11:27–43 (1948).

ALLANBY, K. D.; HUNSTMAN, R. G. and SACKER, L. S.: Thrombotic microangiopathy. Recovery of a case after heparin and magnesium therapy. Lancet i:237–239 (1966).

ANTES, E. H.: Thrombotic thrombocytopenic purpura; a review of the literature with report of a case. Ann. intern. Med. 48:512–536 (1958).

BERNARD, R. P.; BAUMAN, A. W. and SCHWARTZ, S. I.: Splenectomy for thrombotic thrombocytopenic purpura. Ann. Surg. 169:616–624 (1969).

BERNSTOCK, L. and HIRSON, C.: Thrombotic thrombocytopenic purpura. Remission on treatment with heparin. Lancet i:28–29 (1960).

BERTONI, L.; BASEVI, D. and GHIDINI, O.: La microangiotrombosi emolitica piastrinopenica. Malattia di Moschcowitz (contributo clinico). Haematologica 49:926–944 (1964).

BIED, B. and EHRHART, C.: A propos d'un cas de maladie de Moschcowitz. Sem. Hôp., Paris 8:520–528 (1968).

BRETON, J.; GUAZZI, G. C.; MACKEN, J. and TVERDY, G.: Les manifestations cérébrales de la maladie de Moschcowitz (microangiopathie thrombotique). Rev. neurol. 107:432–452 (1962).

KELLER: in Bertoni *et al.*

LUCHERINI, T.: In tema di ordinamento clinico-nosologico delle collagenopatie. Rass. clin.-scient. 40:161–172 (1964).

MEACHEM, G. C.; ORBISON, J. L.; HEINLE, R. W.; STEELE, H. J. and SCHAEFER, J. A.: Thrombotic thrombocytopenic purpura: a disseminated disease of arterioles. Blood 6:706–719 (1951).

MOSCHCOWITZ, E.: An acute febrile pleiochromic anemia with hyaline thrombosis of the terminal arterioles and capillaries. An undescribed disease. Arch. intern. Med. 36:89–93 (1925).

MULLER, J. M.; COUDERC, P.; KOLODIE, L.; CORDONNIER, D.; MASSOT, C.; SCHAERER, R. and MARTIN, H.: La maladie de Moschcowitz: coagulopathie de consommation? Presse Med. 77:1885–1899 (1969).

O'BRIEN, J. L. and SIBLEY, W. A.: Neurologic manifestations of thrombotic thrombocytopenic purpura. Neurology, Minneap. 9:55–64 (1958).

PATRASSI, C.: Su di un caso di porpora trombotica trombocitopenica. Abstracts of reports 7th Congr. Int. Soc. of Haematology, Rome 1958, p. 263 (Tip. S. Giuseppe, Rome 1958).

PATRASSI, G. and MENOZZI, L.: Su di un caso di'porpora trombotica trombocitopenica. Acta med. patavina 18:147–167 (1958).

PLANQUES, J.; ARLET, J.; BIERME, R.; BOUISSOU, H.; FABRE, J. and FABRE-ACKERMANN, C.: Maladie de Moschcowitz. Étude clinique et anatomopathologique d'un cas. Sem. Hôp., Paris 41:1424–1429 (1965).

ROESSLE: in Bertoni *et al.*

SYMMERS, W. S. C. and GILLET, R.: Polyarteritis nodosa, associated with malignant hypertension, disseminated platelet thrombosis, 'wire loop' glomeruli, pulmonary silicotuberculosis, and sarcoidosis-like lymphadenopathy. Arch. Path. 52:489–504 (1951).

SYMMERS, W. S. C.: Thrombotic microangiopathy; histological diagnosis during life. Lancet i:592–596 (1956).

Chapter VI

NEUROLOGICAL SYMPTOMS
IN LEUKEMIA

Nerve signs in leukemia have been under study for many years. As early as 1823, *Burns* noted a strange enlargement of the brain in a subject whose death was attributed to chloroma. A succession of later reports by *Liebreich* (1861), *Eisenlohr* (1878), *Fraenkel* (1895), *Benda* (1898), *Dock and Warthin* (1904), *Baudouin and Parturier* (1910), *Casolino* (1913) led gradually to the diverse and well-documented case series available today. Careful examination of the anatomical, pathological, and clinical aspects of nerve system involvement in leukemia has led to the isolation of several variously serious pictures, known collectively as neuroleukemic affections.

The postmortem data are far from being in harmony with the clinical data with respect to the *frequency* of such involvement. Nerve damage is, in fact, frequently observed at necropsy. *Trömner and Wohlwill*, for example, observed leukemic infiltrations in 12 out of 13 cases, and an examination of the statistical data by *Diamond* suggested that histological evidence of hemoblastic cell infiltration or hemorrhage resulting in nerve damage will be found in 90% of leukemic patients. However, the clinical silence of nerve lesions is well known. When they do appear, they may give rise to confusing pictures for which no exact diagnosis can be found.

Frequency assessments will also vary widely in value if consideration is given to all nerve syndromes irrespective of their pathogenesis, or only to those due to leukemic infiltration of the cerebrospinal axis, that is, excluding all aspecific changes due to hemorrhage, thrombosis, or degeneration secondary to anemia. Some workers, indeed, stress the fact that inflammation may be the cause of neurological involvement in leukemia.

Revol et al. omit meningeal and predominantly meningeal signs from their large series (594 cases), since cerebrospinal fluid (CSF) examination had not always been carried out and since leukemic meningeal damage can be proved only by the finding of immature blood cells in the liquor

100

sediment. These workers also omit cases with mild neurological signs, cases of herpes zoster, episodes characterized by respiratory disturbances or neurovegetative signs, and massive terminal neurological episodes.

Recent evidence suggests that nerve system involvement is more common in acute than in chronic leukemia. Damage due to infiltration was observed in 9.9%, 16%, and about 25% of the acute infantile leukemia series reported by *D'Angio et al., Chaptal et al.*[a], and *Sullivan*[a], respectively. *Shaw et al.* found 16.6% involvement in a series composed of both children and adults, and 15.7% of the 261 acute leukemic children and adults studied by *Bernard et al.*[a] presented neuromeningeal involvement undoubtedly attributable to the underlying disease. Furthermore, these workers consider this value too low, since part of their series was studied only in the initial stage. As many as 32.3% of the acute leukemia series reported by *Polli* displayed neurological signs. Evidence of nervous infiltration was observed in 30% of 201 acute leukemic children by *Corrie et al.*, and 55% of cases of acute lymphocytic leukemia studies by *Evans et al.*[b] showed signs of neurological involvement.

Necropsy evidence of meningeal involvement was noted by *Thomas* in 38–44% of acute lymphatic leukemia and 16–17% of acute myeloid leukemia cases.

Neurological symptoms are considered infrequent in chronic myeloid leukemia (*Labauge et al.*). According to *Schwab and Weiss*, clinical evidence of central nervous system (CNS) and peripheral nerve lesions may be expected in 20% of cases. However, this is considered too high a percentage by *Rouquès, Storti*, and others. Even lower frequency values are claimed for chronic lymphatic leukemia.

Infants, notoriously the prime candidates for acute leukemia, are more frequently afflicted by neurological complications than children or adults, and males are more commonly affected than females.

Differences in frequency percentages are thus readily explained, since reported values are conditioned by the nature (postmortem or clinical) of the data collected, by the type of leukemia studied (acute or chronic, myeloid or lymphatic), by age and sex distribution in the series under examination, and by the criteria adopted by individual writers. *Revol et al.* reported nerve involvement in only 4.2% of their series (5.5% in the acute cases considered separately), because they considered well-identified motor deficiencies as the only acceptable evidence of neurological damage.

The difference in acute and chronic nerve sign frequency values must be related to the particular expression and course of these two forms. Apart from the particular aggressiveness of the hemopathic process, modern treatment is incriminated in the striking incidence of nerve signs in acute leukemia by most writers. Nevertheless, such treatment has prolonged the mean life expectancy of acute leukemia patients (*Pierce*[b]; etc.). The existence of the so-called hematoencephalic barrier leads to lower antileukemic drug concentrations in the cerebrospinal fluid than in the blood. The central nervous system lesions have more time to develop and to become apparent. Nor is such a development sufficiently hindered by the drugs themselves, since these, in contrast to their complete therapeutic effect in other tissues, are unable to impede the survival of leukemic cell sites within the nerve structures (*Dameshek and Gunz*).

This may explain the striking frequency of neurologic (particularly meningeal) signs so commonly reported in acute leukemia. Also supporting this view is the fact that nerve symptoms more commonly appear in treatment-induced clinical and hematological remission periods.

Other workers (*Nies et al.*) have suggested that the apparent increase in the frequency of meningeal changes in leukemia may be explained by the fact that now CSF is more frequently checked.

Necropsy shows three fundamental types of nerve system change: leukemic infiltration, hemorrhage, and malacic and degenerative lesions. Infiltration is the most common and most typical finding. Mixed infiltration and hemorrhage pictures are often observed, particularly in acute leukemia.

Such infiltrations may be diffused (simple infiltrations) or neoplastiform (tumoral infiltrations) (*Rouquès*), though the two forms are not clearly distinct. The tumoral form may be the last stage of a simple infiltration.

Simple infiltrations may be observed in the meninges, the cerebrospinal axis, the spinal ganglia, and in both the cranial and spinal peripheral nerves. In some cases infiltrations in the dura mater can be detected histologically only. In other cases gross examination shows them as a slight thickening or yellowish coloration of the membrane or, more rarely, as large nodules with a diameter varying from 0.5 cm to 2 cm. In a case reported by *Fialho and Gollo*, the dura mater was almost completely occupied by nodules. Hemorrhage and infiltration may exist concurrently. The internal and the external surfaces of the dura are most commonly involved at the level of the cranium and the spinal cord, respectively.

Infiltration of the arachnoid is usually widespread and involves both the encephalic and spinal districts. The areas of the membrane corresponding to the convexity of the encephalon, the cranial base, and the cerebral trunk are particularly affected. Arachnoid infiltrations often extend to the pia mater, though the encephalic cortex is almost always unimpaired (*Laszlo et al.*) or at least only exceptionally involved (*Labauge et al.*).

Infiltration of the dura mater is frequently observed. It was present in 65% of the acute leukemia series reported by *Moore et al.*, while infiltration of the leptomeninx was noted in only 30% of the cases.

Either nodular or simple infiltration may be observed in the cerebro-spinal axis. *Moore et al.* and *Thomas* noted leukemic nodules in 19% and 10–12% of their respective acute leukemic series. The signs include sleeves around the vessels packing the perivasal spaces, or clearly defined, often multiple and sometimes confluent parenchymal nodular masses visible on gross examination, with diameters from 5 mm to 2 cm (*De Ajuriaguerra et al.*; *Dameshek and Gunz*). There have been few reports of simple infiltration. In an exceptional case reported by *De Ajuriaguerra et al.*, a true "leukosic encephalopathy" was expressed as widespread leukemic infiltration of the brain, the cerebral trunk, and the cerebel-lum. Uniform infiltration of the internal capsule was observed in one case of chronic leukemia by *Tapie and Cassar*.

Simple infiltration involves the brain more frequently than the cerebral trunk, cerebellum, or spinal cord. The white substance is the site of choice; involvement of the gray substance is comparatively rare. It is not known whether infiltration is of local origin or due to diapedetic invasion of nerve tissue: the frequent appearance of mitotic figures in the infiltrate and the centrifugal spread of infiltration sites (*Leidler and Russell*) are evidence in favor of the former view. Infiltration of nerve tissue, however, is commonly associated with leukostasis and perivasal infiltration. Leukostasis is related to the pleocytosis proper to the underlying disease and may take on the appearance of true leukemic thrombosis. In this connection *Giraud et al.*[b] note the essentially cellular structure of the fibrin-poor clot and the absence of vasal wall reaction.

Yet leukostasis is also observed in the CNS gray substance and this, as we have seen, is only exceptionally infiltrated. It may be asked, therefore, why leukostasis in this site is not followed by diapedesis and hence by infiltration of nerve tissue. Some workers, *Bernard et al.*[b], consider that such infiltration proceeds from the arachnoid spaces via the perivasal sheaths, and not through the walls of vessels within the parenchyma.

This brief note on the origin of leukemic infiltration of nerve tissue leads to the wider question of the histogenesis of human leukemia. Some workers consider this a disease of the reticular histiocyte system, with generalized proliferation of undifferentiated mesenchymal cells fol-lowed by either myeloid or lymphatic hematopoiesis and relative course.

Bufano and his school place leukemia in the so-called "systemic-tending histiocyte sarcomatosis" group with other systemic blood diseases, on the grounds of a common pathogenesis. Other workers, however, regard leukemia as anatomically limited to the hemolymphopoietic organs and capable of systemic expansion within these limits. A metastatic origin (through diapedesis, as stated above) has been suggested for leukemic infiltration, though some writers (*Lanza*) consider that colonization would be the more appropriate term, since it would more exactly express the tendency of leukemic cells "to vegetate both inside and outside the capillaries without adopting a clear-cut neoplastic attitude." (According to *Dameshek*, chronic lymphatic leukemia is an accumulation disease resulting from an abnormal, disordered, generalized, and self-maintaining proliferation of small lymphocytes, infiltration being but a part of this process.)

With respect to the cranial nerves, the 7th and 8th pairs are most commonly infiltrated, though they may also be involved as a result of leukemic damage to the middle ear. Cranial nerve involvement is very common, particularly in acute leukemia. Damage to the spinal nerves, however, is less frequent: the roots of the sciatic nerve and the cauda equina appear to be the sites of choice. Infiltration of the peripheral nerve trunks is less common.

Infiltration of both the cranial and spinal nerve roots is localized in the perineurium and the perineural sheath, with occasional propagation along the septa. This may explain the frequent involvement of the external surface of the spinal dura mater at the nerve-exit points (*Rouquès*). Infiltration of the trigeminal (*Trömner and Wohlwill; Tarro*) and the spinal ganglia (*Dickenman and Chason*) has also been observed.

The somewhat rare tumoral infiltrations in leukemia have an epidural or an osteoperiosteal origin. Their development in the form of a tumoral mass leads to compression of the underlying nerve centers. The spine is the site of choice, though cerebral localizations are occasionally reported (*Bass; Winkler; Rouquès; Moore et al.*). The 15 or so cases in the literature present a picture of neoplastiform infiltration in the spinal epidural space, on and usually inseparable from the external surface of the dura mater. The internal surface of the dura, the soft meninges and the spinal cord are generally unimpaired, though this was not so in the case reported by *Bernard et al.*[b] Infiltrating tissue may attain a thickness of 1 cm and completely surround the meninges and spinal cord in the form of a sleeve. This, in turn, surrounds the nerve and vessel formations of the epidural space and may exit from the vertebral foramina (*Labauge et al.*). The dorsolateral tract is the site of choice and several vertebrae are usually involved (nine in a case reported by *Kissel et al.*). *Hatta* reports an exceptional case in which infiltration extended from the cervical to the lumbar tracts.

Histological examination most commonly shows myeloblasts to be the only component of the tissue and it may be noted that neoplastiform infiltration is primarily observed in myeloid leukemia. This finding assimilates tumoral infiltration to chloroma, itself a particular expression of myeloid leukemia.

Leukemic infiltration has a frankly tumorous appearance in chloroma. The typical greenish color of the neoplastic masses is due to abnormal cell metabolic synthesis of a substance—choleglobin—formerly classified as a type of protoporphyrin. In addition to the spine, the sternum, ribs, anterior skullcap, and base of the skull may be the sites of osteoperiosteal infiltration. Infiltration of the temporal and retro-orbital areas, with possible exophthalmos, is a distinctive feature of chloroma and is responsible for the typical "chloroma face." The greenish color of the tumors can also be seen through the skin.

Chloroma is observed most often in infancy, though adults may be affected. Cranial infiltration would seem more common in infants, though its incidence is by no means insignificant in some adult series (*Confino*). *Confino's* results show that in the adult the site of choice is within the dorsal portion of the vertebral canal.

CNS disturbances in chloroma are considered to be primarily compressive, since the neoplastiform infiltration, having reached the dura mater, does no more than peel it from the skeleton, without infiltration or perforation (*Kolomoitseva and Machonkova*). The only result, therefore, is compression of the underlying nerve structures. In some cases, however, the dura may be perforated, though it is not considered that this change necessarily leads to nerve tissue infiltration, which is rare in any event. One case of infiltration of the infundibulum and five of infiltration of the spinal cord have been reported by *Critchley and Greenfield*.

Compression is also held responsible for the more frequent and typical involvement of the cranial nerves in chloroma (particularly the oculomotor nerves and the 7th and 8th pairs). Infiltration of the roots and peripheral trunk is considered exceptional.

Chloromatous tissue very occasionally forms between the paravertebral muscles and then extends toward the vertebral canal or outward, sometimes compressing the peripheral nerves (*Klein and Steinhaus; Rouquès*).

Revol et al. described a case of myeloid leukemia with a massive presacral tumoral infiltrate (it was not specified whether the infiltrate had chloromatous characteristics), which had induced a cauda equina syndrome.

Nervous system hemorrhage in leukemia is most common in acute cases and its normally sudden onset may precipitate the terminal stage. Infants or young subjects are the most common victims: two-thirds of the cases collected by *Rouquès* were under 25 years of age. A relationship between the severity of hemorrhage and the terminal leukocyte count has been observed (*Phair et al., etc.*).

In contrast to the position in hypertension and atherosclerosis, leukemic hemorrhage may be observed in every part of the cerebral parenchyma, though the white substance (more particularly that of the temporal globes) is the site of choice. The most common picture is of hemorrhage sites of medium diameter, surrounded by smaller purpuric hemorrhages, while massive hemorrhage is rare. Isolated purpura is uncommon. A finding peculiar to leukemia is that of the nodule surrounded by a hemorrhagic ring. The effect is that of a cockade with a central, grayish nodule surrounded by a dark red hemorrhagic area (*Bertrand*).

Subarachnoid and subdural hemorrhages are commonly reported. These may be associated with cerebral hemorrhage, which sometimes results in ventricular flooding.

Hemorrhage of the spinal cord is rare. *Giraud et al.*[a] observed one case with purpuric involvement of the medullary cone and the roots of the cauda equina. Hemorrhage of the peripheral nerve trunks has also been reported.

Leukemic infiltration of the brain and meninges may also lead to cerebral edema. This was present in four out of 82 cases examined postmortem by *Leach.* Widespread edema may often be one of the anatomical causes of the endrocranial hypertension observed in leukemia.

It is uncertain whether cerebral edema should be considered a consequence of leukemic infiltration of nerve tissue (*Labauge et al.*). It seems likely that infiltration is also pathogenic for cerebral hemorrhage during terminal leukemic proliferation crises. In 45% of such cases, the typical histological picture of the cerebral tissue includes intravascular leukostasis, nodular infiltrates complicated by recent hemorrhage, necrosis or rupture of vascular walls, and aneurysmatic type dilatation. According to *Moore et al.* the pathogenetic mechanism consists of intravascular leukostasis followed by diapedesis and the formation of a leukemic infiltrate. This in turn leads to hemorrhage caused by dissociation of the vessel wall.

In a case of acute basophilic leukemia in a 49-year-old woman reported by *Quattrin et al.*, the necropsy picture was one of frank subarachnoid hemorrhage and hemorrhagic changes of the cerebral substance. Histological examination of the nerves showed extensive perivasal infiltration originating in the adventitia and composed of histoid cells. These workers posit a connection between hemorrhagic episodes and perivasal infiltration. They suggest that wear on the small vessels in various sites, particularly in the brain and the digestive tract mucosa, is the fundamental cause of the serious hemorrhagic diathesis which often complicates this type of leukemia.

A careful study of vasal changes caused by leukemic infiltration was made by *Frugoni* in 1908 in a case of myeloid leukemia accompanied by a large muscular hematoma. Histological examination showed a thick muscular myeloid infiltration and serious changes in the vessel walls within the infiltrated areas. "Staining of the elastic fibers showed that the myeloma was eroding and infiltrating the vessel wall in several places, that the wall itself was being partially interrupted and replaced by invading tissue resulting in partial discontinuity of the endothelium and direct communication between the lumen and the surrounding tissue, and, lastly, that the elastic framework of the vessel wall was so altered and broken down in some places as to be more or less completely destroyed."

However, the main cause of cerebral hemorrhage in leukemia must be sought in thrombocytopenia. This is particularly true of massive and fatal hemorrhages. Platelet levels below $60,000/mm^3$ were observed in 31 out of 41 cases of intracranial hemorrhage during leukemia collected by *Groch et al.* In nine cases of meningeal hemorrhage observed by *Shaw et al.* platelet levels were less than $10,000/mm^3$; in four patients values were even below $1,000/mm^3$. Of course, hemorrhage is promoted by the coagulation abnormalities observed in leukemia too (hypoprothrombinemia, afibrinogenemia, or fibrinogenopenia).

Certain brain vessel changes occasionally observed in the leukemic patient—hyperplasia of the endothelium and hyalinosis of the media—may also play a part in the onset of cerebral hemorrhage (*Diamond; Ninni and Rovello*). Note also the view held by *Feissinger and Marie*, that leukemic cells may produce a proteolytic enzyme which damages the vessel wall.

Aspecific malacic and degenerative lesions may be observed in both the brain and the spinal cord. These include chromatolysis, nuclear eccentricity, fatty degeneration, and necrosis. Leukemic infiltration is certainly involved in the onset of such changes, though they are thought to be the consequence of leukemic thrombosis. This conclusion may be drawn from the great extent of axon and myelinic changes around the vessels, as well as their segmentary nature (*Dereymaeker*).

Some responsibility for these changes must be assigned to toxic causes also, sometimes in association with infection, and to serious anemia. Several workers (*Minnick; Muller; Nonne; etc.*) have reported findings of a combined sclerosis of the spinal cord identical to that observed in pernicious anemia. These data, however, are denied by *Rouquès*.

Nerve tissue thrombosis, attributable to hyperleukocytosis and increased blood viscosity, is common in chronic myeloid leukemia. Here the typical picture is one of an association of cell infiltrates and thrombosis, whereas in lymphatic leukemia cell infiltration predominates. Microscopic examination shows the ivory-yellow thrombus to be formed of closely packed myeloid cells, separated by a thin fibrin network. Nerve tissue thrombosis in chronic myeloid leukemia is particularly intense and widespread and explains the existence of sometimes disseminated and very extensive necrosis sites in the thickness of such tissue, as well as hemorrhagic infarcts (*Giraud et al.*[b]).

Extensive softening of the dorsal and lumbar tracts of the spinal cord was observed by *Büsing* in a case of acute myeloid leukemia in an 18-year-old boy.

Disseminated cortical and subcortical necrotic sites in the cerebral and the cerebellar hemispheres was reported by *Petronio et al.* in a case of eosinophilic leukemia. Microscopic examination showed thrombosis and blockage of the small brain vessels as a result of the presence of leukemic cells.

Finally, it should be noted that tetraventricular hydrocephalus associated with meningeal infiltration, particularly of the basal arachnoid, is sometimes reported (*Sullivan*[a]; *Hunt et al.; Moore et al.*).

The extremely protean symptomatology of nerve system involvement in leukemia has complicated the identification of separate clinical pictures, since simultaneous or successive involvement of several areas of the nervous system is a typical feature of the disease. It is useful, topographically, to classify signs into syndromes of cerebral, spinal cord, and peripheral nerve damage.

In acute leukemia, neuroleukemic signs are sometimes observed at an early stage, whereas in chronic forms they often appear later and may be the terminal event. However, nerve symptoms, particularly those caused by infiltration, may appear in periods of therapeutic remission, especially in acute leukemia. Less common, though of undoubted clinical interest because of the resultant problems of diagnosis, are those cases in which neurological symptoms are the first sign of the underlying disease.

Both *Weil* and *Storti* have reported cases in which paraplegia was the first sign of acute leukemia. Facial nerve paralysis was the first manifestation in single cases observed by *Andreani et al., Poppi and Morgante,* and *Radicchi,* in two cases observed by *Dameshek and Gunz,* and in several reported by *Revol et al.* Convulsions and coma were the initial signs in the case of acute leukemia reported by *Bass.* In a case of acute leukemia observed by *Castan and Dehing,* the clinical overture consisted of coma, widespread hemorrhage, and adenopathy 15 days after antipoliomyelitis vaccination. Neurological manifestations formed the initial clinical picture in six out of seven cases of leukemia reported by *Giroire et al.*, and serious paraparesis was the initial sign in a case recently noted by *Cavazzuti et al.* Out of 103 acute leukemia patients observed by *Geronimi et al.,* ten were admitted with neurologic syndromes (intracranial hypertension in seven cases, paraplegia in two and subarachnoid hemorrhage in one).

Leukemia-induced cerebral damage may give rise to various clinical signs: meningeal symptoms, true encephalic signs (hemiplegia and convulsions are the most common), intracranial hypertension, and psychological signs.

Meningeal symptoms caused by cellular infiltration (usually infiltration of the arachnoid) or by hemorrhage are relatively common in leukemia, particularly in the acute form (17.8% *Schwab and Weiss;* 20% *Rodriguez;* 30% *Hardisty and Norman*). Infants (*Anderson and Taft*)— particularly males (*Boggs et al.*)—are most commonly affected.

Infiltration generally establishes itself gradually and the symptom picture varies from case to case. Simple headache may be observed (as in a case of lymphatic leukemia studied by *Horton*) or there may be true states of meningeal irritation, with headache, vomiting, nuchal rigidity, and the corresponding semeiologic signs (*Kernig; Brudzinski; etc.; Baudouin and Parturier; Barker; etc.*). In general, however, the clinical picture is incomplete and limited to some of the classic symptoms. Headache and vomiting are virtually constant, while nuchal rigidity and signs connected with radicular damage appear in only a few cases. Often meningeal symptoms are not accompanied by fever. In spite of its incompleteness, however, the meningeal symptomatology is usually outstanding in the overall clinical picture and the widespread use of such terms as "leukemic meningitis" or "meningosis leucaemica" (*Gasser*), or, more correctly, "meningeal leukemia," is fully justified.

Occasionally meningeal involvement is the first sign of the underlying disease (*Vlach et al.; Girard et al.*). More commonly it appears when leukemia is well established or even during a therapeutic remission of an acute form. Its frequency seems independent of both the prior duration of the disease (*Shaw et al.*) and of the medicaments employed in obtaining remission (*Pierce*[b]). In a case of chronic granulocytic leukemia observed by *Kwaan et al.*, meningeal involvement was the first manifestation of an acute myeloblastic transformation.

Though few in number, cases have been reported in which a typical acute meningitic clinical picture followed leukemic infiltration of the arachnoid (*Croizat et al.; Gélin and Rosan; Litteral and Malamud; Léchelle; etc.*). A suppurative acute meningitis picture, however, is quite exceptional (case no. 2 reported by *Gilbert and Rice* and case no. 1 by *Vlach et al.* and by *Chaptal et al.*[b]). In the case reported by *Chaptal et al.*[b], the CSF was frankly purulent. The liquor cell population, which consisted of immature white cells, was 4,000/mm³. Negative results were obtained from a culture of the liquor. Intrathecal amethopterin produced clinical and biological improvement of the meningeal symptom picture.

In cases of this kind, a precise diagnosis of the meningeal change can be obtained only by examination of the CSF. This serves to exclude inflammation and to indicate leukemia. Finding immature white cells in the liquor sediment, sometimes in mitosis (*Spriggs and Boddington*), is fundamental and will be of particular importance in cases where the meningeal symptoms are the first clinical sign of a hitherto unrecognized leukemia.

Liquor cell values are inconstant in leukemic infiltration of the meninges; as many as 11,000 cells/mm³ have been observed (*Shaw et al.*). These cells have the same features, including chromosomal constitution (*Mastrangelo et al.*), as those of the white series found in the patient's peripheral blood or bone marrow. In a case of eosinophilic leukemia reported by *Forkner*, the liquor contained only eosinophilic cells. Great care must be exercised in cytologic interpretation of the liquor cells, however, since morphological similarities exist between immature cells of the white series and those of medullomeningeal proliferation processes (medulloblastomas and reticuloendotheliopathies of meningeal origin). Accidental puncture of the vertebral bodies may also lead to the passage of bone marrow blast cells into the liquor space (*Spriggs*). *Lereboullet* has also stressed the fact that unusual cell features may be observed in the liquor as a result of atypical macrophagic reactions in an albuminous environment loaded with disintegration products or red cells. Philadelphia (Ph¹) chromosomes were observed in the liquor leukemic cells in the case of *Kwaan et al.*

Furthermore, increased pressure and albumin values (3.72 g ⁰/₀₀ (*Shaw et al.*) and even 11.50 g ⁰/₀₀ (*Bernard et al.*) are usually observed. Increased protein levels are not constantly parallel to increased liquor cell values, and the two signs are often dissociated. Hypoglycorrhachia is sometimes observed (*Schwab and Weiss; Williams et al.*). Its pathogenesis is obscure, though most writers postulate cells with high glycolytic activity in the liquor.

Electrophoretic study of the CSF in meningeal leukemias by *Rothman et al.* showed decreased prealbumin values along with increased proteinorrhachia. The latter finding was attributed by these writers to enhanced movement of albumins from the plasma on the basis of an increased liquor–serum albumin ratio.

Examination of the CSF must be routine practice in leukemia since it may demonstrate the presence of clinically silent meningeal changes (*Spriggs*). A negative finding, however, does not absolutely exclude meningeal involvement even when coupled with an absence of clinical signs. The examination should therefore be repeated periodically. Obviously, such an examination must be made in all cases in which meningeal involvement is suspected, so that a timely warning of leukemia with an initially meningeal clinical picture may be obtained.

No special features distinguish the liquor symptomatology of meningeal hemorrhage in leukosis. Again, meningeal syndromes, including those of a hemorrhagic nature, like any other form of intracranial hemorrhage, sometimes form the first clinical sign of leukemia. Intracranial hemorrhage, particularly when otherwise inexplicable in a young subject, will always lead to a suspicion of leukemia (*Duvoir and Philippe; Hutinel and Martin; Revol et al.; Labauge et al.*).

As stated, there is a rapidly ingravescent effect of intracranial hemorrhage in leukemia. Virtually intractable and typically apoplectic pictures with a fulminating course are commonly observed.

Often intracranial hemorrhage is part of a widespread hemorrhagic picture involving several districts (skin, mucosae, digestive tract, urinary apparatus, etc.). This condition is frequently severe and difficult to control.

Hemiplegia is observed in 32% of cases (*Schwab and Weiss*), particularly in acute leukemia. This is usually the result of infiltration of the brain or cerebral hemorrhage, though these conditions may coexist. Normally the onset of infiltration is gradual, whereas that of hemorrhage is sudden. Cerebral hemorrhage, with its resultant hemiplegia and coma, is an extremely serious event in leukemia (*Tapie and Cassar; Bass; Farrel; Monges et al.; Ninni and Rovello; Cafaro; etc.*). Its course and prognosis are similar to those of intracranial hemorrhage, which have already been described.

In a personal case of acute myeloid leukemia in a 14-year-old girl, a symptom-free cerebral hemorrhage in the cortical-subcortical area of the right frontal lobe was discovered at necropsy. This formed part of a widespread hemorrhagic picture consisting of numerous diffused skin ecchymoses and purpura of the gastroduodenal mucosa.

Convulsions are more frequent in acute leukemia and in children than in older subjects. Generalized tonic or clonic convulsions, with loss of consciousness and coma, are the rule (*Bass; Lucherini; Viets and Hunter; Bernard and Talamon; etc.*). Tongue biting and urine and stool incontinence are also observed (*Goudemand et al.*). Jacksonian type epilepsy was the first clinical sign of acute leukosis in a case observed by *Fabian and Naegli*. Convulsions were the first sign of acute leukemia in the case reported by *Bass* and in another noted by *Rossi*. Persistent coma with muscular hypertonia, possibly the result of a convulsion crisis, heralded acute leukosis in a 5-year-old boy with signs of meningeal involvement observed by *Christiaens and Nuyts*. Convulsion is attributed to cerebral infiltration, though slight widespread meningeal hemorrhage is also noted.

Left upper extremity clonus appeared suddenly a few hours before death in a personal case of acute leukemia in a 63-year-old woman. The clinical picture included ulceronecrotic changes in the mouth and abdominal ecchymoses. Necropsy was not performed.

Less frequent encephalic manifestations include: sensibility disturbances (hemianesthesia (*Brandt*)), sensory disturbances (lateral hemianopsia (*Talamon*)), monoparesis (caused by pressure on the upper pyramidal pathways at the anterior central gyrus or the semioval center (*Maggia and Grandesso*), extrapyramidal signs (*Wells and Silver*), cerebral trunk syndromes (fig. 7) (*Picard; Ravetta and Rezzonico*), decerebration syndrome (*Bernard and Talamon*), chorea (*Bernard et al.* [b]) and choreoathetosis (*Revol et al.*).

A picture of chorea with a markedly rheumatic pattern, later diagnosed as a result of leukemia, was observed by *Bernard et al.* [b] The CSF contained a large number of immature white cells, and intrathecal amethopterin produced a dramatic improvement, including the complete disappearance of the choreal symptom.

Acute leukemia, hematologically demonstrated, in a 4-year-old girl observed by *Revol et al.* presented a picture of choreoathetosis, particularly of the head and right upper extremity. Intractable to X-ray therapy and ordinary sedatives, this condition remained stationary for several months and was still present at the patient's death, which occurred about one year after the onset of leukemia.

Ravetta and Rezzonico noted gradual involvement of the cerebral trunk in a 33-year-old woman with chronic myeloid leukemia. On admission, the patient had a stunned appearance, had difficulty in expressing herself, and complained of diplopia. The neurological examination showed: uncertain and fleeting maintenance of the erect position even with the eyes open (worsened in Romberg's test), hesitant gait (without support, though only for a limited distance) with swaying of the body and reeling, particularly to the right, blindfold gait possible for only a few steps, inability to turn the eyeballs to the right, static and dynamic left facial deficiency, left hypoacusis, uncertain hypoesthesia in the left trigeminal district, deterioration of speech with a tendency to palinphrasia, difficulty in swallowing liquids (sometimes with loss of liquid through the left nostril), inability to put out the tongue, sluggishness of the soft palate, poor left limb active motility (during examination these limbs commonly fell heavily on the bed), weak grip, weak dorsal flexion of the foot, slight atrophy of the left trapezial muscle, depressed left osteotendinous reflexes, slight weakening of lower abdominal reflexes, left Babinski and Oppenheim reflexes, slight dysmetria (more apparent on the left), and variable left hypopallesthesia. Necropsy was not done. The clinical data, however, were interpreted as evidence of a nerve lesion at the level of the bulbus and the pons, primarily on the left side, with involvement of the rhombencephalic nerve nuclei, the superior cerebellar peduncles (at the decussation) and the pyramidal pathways (below the decussation). Thrombosis or hemorrhage was considered an unlikely cause (no disturbance of blood clotting was noted). Thus the nerve signs were attributed to leukemic infiltration, particularly because of their gradual onset and their appearance during a hematologically demonstrated acute period of the underlying disease.

Cerebellar syndromes are reported occasionally. Intracranial hypertension and immature white cells in the liquor were noted in a single-hemisphere syndrome observed by *Bernard et al.*[b] Cerebellar symptoms appeared one month before death in the case of acute lymphatic leukemia reported by *Chaptal et al.*[a] Necropsy showed infiltration of the pia mater of the brain and spinal cord, primarily perivasal infiltration of the cerebellum, and large hemorrhagic sites in the vermis.

Pictures testifying to involvement of the infundibulum, the ashen tuber, and hypophysis have been reported by *Joseph and Levin, Allies, Zuelzer and Flatz, Borchers and Mittelbach, Steffey, Dameshek and Gunz, Rosenzweig and Kendall, etc.* The signs have included polyphagia, with a tendency toward increased weight and sometimes obesity, diabetes insipidus, and hypersomnia (sometimes to the point of narcolepsy, as in a case reported by *Grifoni*). Diabetes insipidus as the clinical overture to leukemia was noted by *Dameshek and Gunz.* Edematous exophthalmos appeared to be the result of massive infiltration of the pituitary capsule in a patient observed by *Giroire et al.*[b]

Although intracranial hypertension was rarely reported in the period

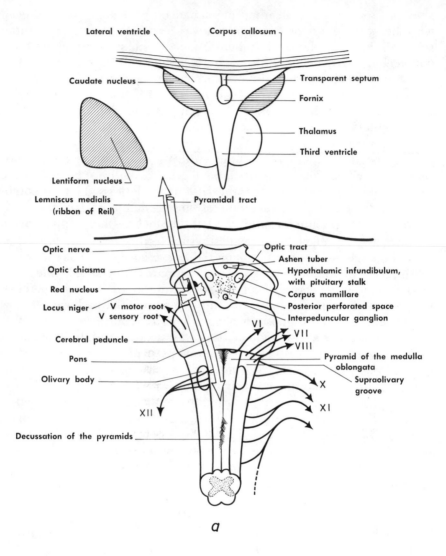

Fig. 7. Brain stem: (*a*) anterior area (showing cerebromedullary connections); (*b*) lateral area; (*c*) posterior region (floor of the 4th ventricle) (from Figs. 53, 54, 55, and 137 in *Masquin and Trelles*).

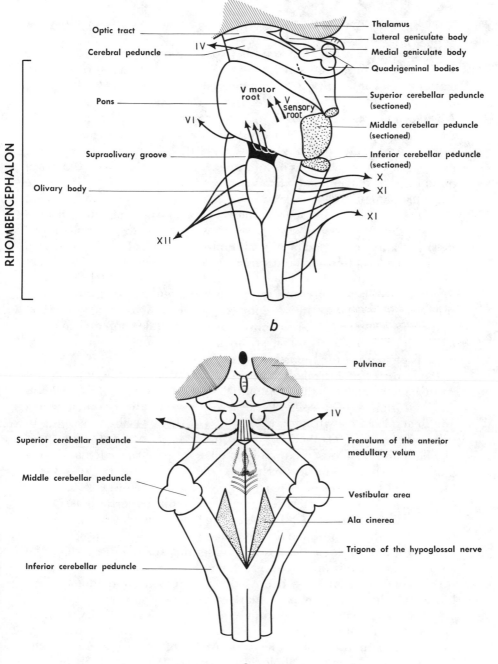

RHOMBENCEPHALON

Optic tract

Cerebral peduncle

Pons

Supraolivary groove

Olivary body

IV

Thalamus

Lateral geniculate body

Medial geniculate body

Quadrigeminal bodies

V motor root

V sensory root

Superior cerebellar peduncle (sectioned)

Middle cerebellar peduncle (sectioned)

VI

Inferior cerebellar peduncle (sectioned)

X

XI

XI

XII

b

Pulvinar

IV

Superior cerebellar peduncle

Frenulum of the anterior medullary velum

Middle cerebellar peduncle

Vestibular area

Ala cinerea

Trigone of the hypoglossal nerve

Inferior cerebellar peduncle

c

prior to modern antileukemic therapy, it is more frequently observed today.

De Ajuriaguerra et al., for example, could find only nine cases in the 1952–59 literature. A personal, though partial, examination revealed at least 14 cases in this period, namely: one reported by *Poncher et al.*, probably the first in the literature; one by *Bernard and Seligmann;* two by *Hamilton and Elion;* one by *Pierce*[a]*;* two by *Sansone;* and seven by *Sullivan*[a]*;* (Anderson Hospital, University of Texas). Even so, the number of cases is small and considerably less than that of recent years. These include: 12 out of 372 cases of infantile leukemia (*D'Angio et al.*); 10 out of 34 cases of leukemia (*Williams et al.*); 25 out of a series of 150 acute leukemia patients (*Shaw et al.*); 29 out of 261 cases of leukemia (*Bernard et al.*[b]). A diagnosis of "pseudo-tumoral leukemic meningoencephalitis" was given by *Goudemand et al.* to a series of ten acute leukemia cases, mostly infants in a period of clinical remission, seven of whom presented intracranial hypertension, and three presented convulsions. Also a case of intracranial hypertension was reported by *Cafaro* in 1964.

Intracranial hypertension is typical of acute leukemia, particularly in children. This increase in its reported frequency is related to the fact that modern treatments allow more time for it to develop and to make itself clinically apparent. The syndrome may often be noted during periods of therapeutic remission (*Pierce*[b]).

The most common manifestations of intracranial hypertension are irritability, headache, nausea, vomiting, signs of meningeal involvement, and confusion or even coma. Paralysis of the 6th pair of cranial nerves and generalized convulsion crises, or loss of the lower limb osteotendinous reflexes and peripheral paralysis of the facial nerve (*Goudemand et al.*) have also been observed. Uni- or bilateral papillary edema, accompanied by exudation or hemorrhage is common (16 out of 25 cases with intracranial hypertension reported by *Shaw et al.*). However, papillary edema in leukemia is not a sure sign of intracranial hypertension (*Leidler and Russell; Bernard et al.*[b]*; Labauge et al.*), since it may be caused by infiltration of the optic nerve (*Borgeson and Wagener; Frank, T. J. F.*), venous distension due to leukostasis, or serious anemia. It may even be an unusual expression of retinal hypertension caused by cortisone therapy. Likewise, the absence of papillary edema does not exclude intracranial hypertension, particularly in the young subject.

Rapid expansion of the cranial perimeter, radiologically demonstrated as separation of the sutures, is a typical sign of intracranial hypertension in the child. The seriousness of the condition can be judged directly from the radiological evidence. This may be obtained at a very early stage and may even precede the appearance of clinical signs.

Changes in the sella turcica have also been noted (*Sansone*). This is a rare finding, however, and would appear to be more common in older children whose sutures are less likely to separate (*Sullivan*).

Repeated examination of the sutures will provide useful evidence for prognosis. Treatment may lead to regression of the separation along with improvements in the clinical and biological signs.

Suture separation, however, is not an absolute sign of intracranial hypertension. *Hitzig and Siebenmann* report an unusual case in which the separation was due to infiltration of the periosteum of the suture edges.

The intracranial hypertension syndrome may also include: vision disturbances, paresthesia, loss of muscular strength, absence of deep tendon reflexes (*Sansone*), squint (*Poncher et al.*), and facial paralysis (*Hamilton and Elion*). Involvement of the infundibulum and tuber (hypertension, obesity) (*Sansone; Sullivan*) has also been reported.

A notable increase in pressure will be found on examination of the liquor: values over 15 cm (nine of 25 cm and two as high as 60 cm) were observed in the entire series of *Shaw et al.* Other liquor changes are the same as those discussed in connection with meningeal leukemias.

The EEG picture commonly includes widespread dysrhythmia, while local distress is unusual (*Shaw et al.; Bernard et al.*). *Krump* observed serious and outspoken EEG changes without neurological signs in a series of acute leukemia cases. Cerebral ventriculography is rarely done, but has been known to show slight dilatation of the lateral ventricles (*Williams et al.*).

The necropsy data indicate that intracranial hypertension is caused by infiltration of the meninges, resulting in CSF circulation block. Infiltration of the meninges, particularly of the basal arachnoid, may be followed by tetraventricular hydrocephalus, as noted above. This is caused by blockage of the cisternae of the basis cerebri, as was shown radiographically by *Sansone*.

If widespread, cerebral edema plays an important part in the onset of intracranial hypertension (*Labauge et al.*) and may be associated with infiltration of the encephalon and meninges.

The prognosis for intracranial hypertension in leukemia is poor. Although therapeutic remission may be obtained, signs of increasing severity (headaches, atrophy of the optic nerve and blindness, involvement of the deep cerebral structures) usually appear quickly.

A case of aleukemic lymphoblastomatosis in a 15-year-old boy observed by *Gadrat et al.* included a clinical picture of intracranial hypertension, expressed as bilateral paralysis of the abducent nerve and bilateral edema of the optic disk, together with at first left and later bilateral exophthalmos. Meningoencephalic involvement was demonstrated by the EEG data and the liquor findings (200 cells/mm³; 61% lymphoblasts). Other features of the case included an unusually rapid increase in height, attributed to a possible hemoblastic site in the diencephalon, and subcutaneous infiltration nodules on the chest and abdomen and in the inferior pole of the left testicle.

Psychological changes (apathy, ready loss of attention, melancholy, anxiety) are common in leukemia, though usually they are vague and of little importance. Occasionally, however, striking psychological signs such as agitation and mental confusion are observed (*Parkes Weber*).

In a personal case of acute myeloid leukemia in a 32-year-old man, the outspoken psychopathological picture was characterized by severe anxiety, with depression (weeping, mutism, suicidal desires) or acute psychomotor excitement (verbigeration and motor agitation; in one such crisis the patient broke a ward window with his fist).

The subsequent picture was of cerebral hemorrhage with terminal coma. The postmortem examination disclosed a large hemorrhagic site formed by the confluence of several small hemorrhages at the radiate crown of the two frontal poles. The hemorrhage also partially involved the white substance of the proximal subcortical portion of the parietal lobes. In addition, the patient presented frequent and violent headaches and retinal hemorrhage.

Increased blood ammonia levels have been reported in leukemia, particularly in the chronic forms (*Fuld; Halff; Larsen and Manning; Bockel et al.; Rezzonico and Repetto; etc.*). This is an exclusively leukocyte type, unaccompanied by diffusion into the plasma, so that the nervous system is not involved (*Bockel et al.*). Hyperuricemia, however, has been held responsible for nerve damage and the appearance of psychological disturbances (*Cambier et al.*).

Spinal cord syndromes in leukemia are much less frequent. The symptomatology may be that of subacute transverse myelitis, with either paraplegia or tetraplegia, depending on the site (*Schultze; Kast; Spitz; Baudouin and Parturier; Geitlin; etc.*).

Sometimes spinal cord involvement is the first clinical sign. Alternatively, it may be the last and most serious episode of complex CNS involvement in an already known leukemic picture. A case of this kind was reported by *Maggia and Grandesso.* A 26-year-old man with acute lymphoadenosis presented peripheral left facial paresis one month after the onset of the underlying disease. This was followed by paresis of the right facial and abducent nerves, and later by bilateral amaurosis (which regressed after X-ray therapy) and flaccid paraparesis of the lower limbs, accompanied by very high liquor leukemic cell values. Necropsy revealed hydrocephalus and cerebral edema, together with microscopic evidence of leukemic cell conglomerates in the lower dorsal tract of the spinal cord.

Spinal cord compression has been reported by a number of writers (*Bassol; Critchley and Greenfield; Reese and Middleton; Rouquès; Kolomoitseva and Machonkova; Bernard et al.*[b]*; Labauge et al.; Revol et al.; Cafaro; etc.*). This is caused by deep infiltration of the spinal cord or the meninges or, on rare occasions, by neoplastiform infiltration, whether chloromatous or not. Such infiltration, as stated above, is of epidural or osteoperiosteal origin and is commonly sited in the spine. In exceptional cases, compression may be caused by crushing or spontaneous fracture of vertebral bodies following infiltration by leukemic tissue.

Compression is exercised on both the nerve structures and the vessel formations, and circulation disturbances are of prime importance in producing spinal cord changes.

Usually the symptoms of spinal cord compression appear gradually. In the initial stage there is violent, lancinating radicular pain, radiating beltwise and to the lower limbs, and sometimes associated with paretic-spastic gait. Later there is frank paraparesis or paraplegia accompanied by segmentary sensibility disturbances, sphincter incompetency (usually appearing as urinary retention or fecal incontinence), leading to a complete spinal cord section syndrome with trophic disturbances. The latter often may be particularly serious, as in the case of vertebral chloroma reported by *Kolomoitseva and Machonkova,* in which numerous and extensive skin eschars in the kidney area rapidly spread and deepened, reaching the skeleton.

In vertebral chloroma—an unusual form more commonly seen in the adult—the radicular symptoms often may be associated with signs of cranial nerve damage (facial paralysis, buzzing in the ears, uni- or bilateral deafness). These signs are a typical expression of the multisited development of this form and indicate compression caused by chloroma, to the exclusion of nonhemopathic causes. It might be noted that the neurological symptoms often may precede the appearance of peripheral blood signs of leukemia. In a surgically diagnosed case observed by *Chaes and Kalemcik,* the peripheral blood picture remained normal until the death of the patient.

Differential diagnosis will be assisted by the fact that patients with nonchloromatous tumoral infiltration are usually young and that compression develops more rapidly (*Labauge et al.*). The preparalytic radicular pain symptom is always much shorter (maximum duration: four months) than in chloroma. In some cases this stage may last only a few days or a few hours, and in a case observed by *Bernard et al.*[b] the onset of paraplegia was of a frankly apoplectic type.

In cases of meningeal cavity block the picture will include albuminocytologic dissociation of the liquor (taken from under the block), negative Queckenstedt-Stookey test, and arrest of lipiodol or the gaseous medium above the compression on myelography. The presence of immature white cells in the CSF is associated with leukemic infiltration of the meninges. It will be rare for such cells to be found in the liquor sediment in cases of neoplastiform infiltrations (Garcin et al.; Bernard et al.[b]).

Compression was noted as the first clinical sign in a case of hemocytoblastic leukemia observed by *Balestra and Morandini,* in which there were also signs of cranial nerve, infundibulum, and tuber damage.

A clinical picture resembling that of combined degeneration of the spinal cord (Lichtheim's syndrome) is occasionally observed in leukemia and has been related (*Roger and Olmer*) to the already mentioned, though not universally accepted, anatomical pictures of combined sclerosis of the cord. Lastly, cases of ascending paralysis have been reported (*Cornil et al.*).

An uncommon example of spinal damage limited to the medullary cone was observed by *Chini* in a case of subacute paramyeloblastic leukemia in a 29-year-old woman. The sudden appearance of the neurological syndrome in this case was, in the absence of necropsy, attributed to hematomyelia. The CSF was normal. The initial nerve signs were hypoesthesia and paresthesia of the perineum, external genitalia, buttocks, and upper middle surface of the thighs. These were followed by urination disturbances, initially in the form of difficulty in commencing, while at a later stage there was both urinary and fecal incontinence. The partial positivity of all serum tests for syphilis was interpreted as aspecific (the Wassermann test was negative in the liquor). The patient also presented hemorrhagic exudative pleuritis and lung excavation, probably of leukemic origin.

Hematomyelia was suspected in a personal case of acute leukemia in a 26-year-old man who presented outstanding skin and mucosal hemorrhage, including rhinorrhagia related to vasal varices and leukemic infiltration of the nasal mucosa. About three months after onset, a picture of spinal cord section suddenly formed, with flaccid paraparesis, complete anesthesia as far as D8, and sphincter paralysis. The paraparesis was immediately preceded and accompanied in its initial stages by radicular pain, which spread to the lower limbs. The CSF was hemorrhagic. Death occurred nine days after the onset of paraparesis. Necropsy was not done.

Peripheral nerve damage is not commonly observed in leukemia, though cranial nerve involvement is fairly frequent, especially in acute forms (22 out of the 102 cases of neuroleukemia reported by *Brandt*).

Facial paralysis is the most common sign. This may be unilateral (*Tapie and Cassar; Bass; Critchley and Greenfield; Zunin; Revol et al.; Dameshek and Gunz; etc.*) or, more frequently, bilateral (*Eisenlohr; Kast; Ricca; De Lisi; Radicchi; Revol et al.; etc.*). Right facial paresis has been observed in a personal case of acute chronic myeloid leukemia. As already stated, involvement of the facial nerve may be the first clinical sign of the underlying disease. The suggestion of *Rouquès,* first made in 1946, that leukemia should be suspected in otherwise inexplicable double facial paralysis, is still valid (*Labauge et al.*).

Paralysis of the facial nerve is usually sudden and complete. Treatment may result in transient improvement but complete regression is rare. In a case reported by *Dameshek and Gunz,* right facial paralysis was the first sign of acute lymphocytic leukemia in a 43-year-old man. The condition showed no sign of improvement, in spite of the fact that treatment produced two complete clinical and hematological remissions totalling eight months. In addition, the terminal stage was heralded by paralysis of the hitherto unaffected left side of the face. In the case of chronic lymphatic leukemia reported by *Poppi and Morgante,* however, a picture of initial left followed by right facial paralysis regressed fairly quickly and completely under cortisone therapy.

Involvement of the acoustic nerve, leading to partial or sometimes total deafness (*Kast; Cooke; Scalori and Nobile; etc.*), or a Ménière syndrome (*Alt and Pineless*) is common. Unilateral or bilateral involvement of the common oculomotor nerve (*Trömner and Wohlwill; Garvey and Lawrence; Viets and Hunter; Massaroli: etc.*). the abducent, and the trigeminal nerve has also been reported. Trigeminal involvement may be followed by neuralgic pains in an area served by one of its branches (*Ricca; Trömner and Wohlwill; Williams et al.; etc.*), or by paresthesia.

Signs of damage to the other cranial nerves are less common, particularly in the case of the last ones, though here ascendent polyradiculoneuritis may occasionally be observed (*Mouriquand et al.*). Dysphonia probably caused by involvement of the recurrent laryngeal nerve was reported by *Lugaresi et al.,* while paralysis of the tongue resulting from damage to the hypoglossal nerve has been reported by *Eisenlohr* and by *De Lisi.* In a case of hemocytoblastic leukemia *Poppi and Morgante* observed right hypoglossal paralysis with hypotrophy of the right half of the tongue as the first clinical sign of hemopathy. This was followed by right lower facial nerve deficiency with loss of taste, and by signs of serious bilateral cochleovestibular lesions. Simple atrophy of the optic nerve was noted in aleukemic leukemia by *Gareis.*

Involvement of the cranial nerves is one of the typical signs of a cranial site in chloroma. Deafness, facial paralysis, and oculomotor involvement may be observed also. Neuralgia of the face or damage to the 11th and 12th pair is less common. Damage to the optic nerve and intracranial hypertension are occasional late signs.

Cranial nerve involvement led to a complex symptomatology in a personal case of chloroma in a 13-year-old girl (*d'Eramo and Del Duca*). The clinical picture showed the widespread extent of the leukemia: typical chloromatous parosteal infiltration of the skullcap with radiological evidence of osteolysis was accompanied by bone pain and osteolytic lesions at the distal end of the right radius, the pelvis, the upper third of the femurs, and the proximal diaphysis of the tibia on both sides. Radiological visualization of an undoubtedly leukemic infiltration of the cecum was matched by the clinical finding of a mass the size of an orange. The neurological symptomatology included paralysis of both the lateralis and superior rectus muscles, with convergent squint, central type right facial paralysis, and right hypoglossal paralysis unaccompanied by atrophy of the tongue. The picture was completed by slight bilateral exophthalmos, and examination of the fundus oculi showed retinal hemorrhage and bilateral edema of the optic disk. The presence of exophthalmos proved this latter sign to be due to compression resulting from chloromatous proliferation. CNS in contrast to peripheral involvement was shown by the centrality of the facial and hypoglossal paralysis and by the bilaterality of the eye paralysis picture. Multiple and circumscribed CNS changes involving the cortical centers of the right facial and hypoglossal nerves and the nuclei of origin of both oculomotor and abducent nerves (situated in the tegmentum of the cerebral peduncles and in the protuberance, respectively) were assumed in this case. The pupillary reflexes were unimpaired, indicating that the upper nuclei of the oculomotor nerves (concerned in the function of the internal ocular muscles) were undamaged.

In a second personal case of chloroma in a 12-year-old boy paralysis of the right rectus lateralis and superior were referable to peripheral involvement of the ocular nerves (probably caused by compression on the part of chloromatous tissue). The clinical picture included numerous adenopathies, very hard and painless swelling in the right frontal and in both parietal areas, slight exophthalmos and edema of the right upper eyelid. The patient complained of double vision. The pupillary reflexes were normal and examination of the fundus oculi was negative.

In comparison with involvement of the cranial nerves, that of the spinal nerves is less common. The most common manifestations include sciatic neuralgia (*Bernard et al.*[b]; *Revol et al.*) or the cauda equina syndrome (*Stepien; Bernard et al.*[b]; *Labauge et al.; Revol et al.* (the massive presacral tumor in this case has already been referred to); *etc.*).

We have also observed right sciatica in a 41-year-old man with long-standing splenomegaly and chronic myeloid leukemia diagnosed one year before. Radiography of the lumbosacral segment of the column and the pelvis showed a round patch of osteolysis about the size of a small bean in the right wing of the first sacral segment. This had clearly defined, uncondensed borders and was probably caused by leukemic infiltration (*d'Eramo and De Gaetano*). In another case (chronic lymphatic leukemia in a 46-year-old man), particularly severe left sciatic pain coincided with widespread hemorrhagic infiltration of the left buttock.

Isolated neuritis (*Moretti et al.*) and multiple neuritis (*Harris; Trömner and Wohlwill; Blaschy; Alajouanine et al.; Maggia and Grandesso; etc.*) are uncommon. Guillain-Barré type syndromes (*Alajouanine et al.; Boillin; Revol et al.; etc.*) or Landry type paralysis (*Mouriquand et al.; Lorenz de Haas*) are occasionally reported. The prognosis for the latter form is poor (*Critchley and Greenfield*).

Polyradiculoneuritis was noted by *Martinetti and Mazza* in a case of aleukemic leukosis with an extremely aplastic marrow picture, while two other cases presented demyelinizing leukoencephalopathy and lumbo-sacral peridural infiltration, respectively. In all three patients (part of a series of 52 cases of leukemia) the nerve symptom was the first sign of the underlying disease.

Cranial nerve involvement in ascending polyradiculoneuritis may occasionally mimic myopathy (*Revol et al.*), while associations between Aran-Duchenne type progressive muscular atrophy and lymphatic and myeloid leukemia, respectively, were reported as long ago as 1934 (*Sega*) and 1936 (*Micheli*). In *Sega*'s case leukemia was diagnosed ten months after the gradual onset of the muscular disease, and the writer himself had been led to deny any effective cause-and-effect relationship between them. Necropsy showed changes, caused by nodular leukemic infiltration, in both the white substance and the anterior and posterior columns of the gray substance along the whole length of the spinal cord, extravasation, and perivasal infiltration. In *Micheli*'s case, however, signs of both leukemia and muscle disease (bilateral hypotrophy of the thenar and hypothenar eminences, interosseous muscle atrophy, and hypotrophy of the scalene) all formed part of the initial picture. In this case, too, doubt was expressed concerning the existence of a true relationship between the muscular disease, particularly because of its clear-cut picture, and the leukemia (*Andreani et al.*). Necropsy was not carried out.

In reference to more recent times (1961), note the myopathic picture observed by *Privitera and Fiorini* in a case of lymphatic leukemia in a 17-year-old boy. Signs included hypotrophy of the small muscles of the hand, of the main muscles of the arm and forearm, of the serratus muscles, with winged scapula, and of the main muscles of the lower limbs. Rapid fibrillation was observed in the proximal segments of the upper limbs and the muscles of the scapular ring. Weakness in proportion to the degree of muscular atrophy was noted, as was increased fatigability. Upper and lower extremity osteoperiosteal and tendinous reflexes were lively at first, but gradually became weaker until they disappeared, and objective sensibility disturbances were observed. Anatomical evidence is lacking in this case.

Serious and particularly extensive involvement of the peripheral nerves and meninges was observed by *Baker and Oliver* in a 28-year-old man with acute myeloblastic leukemia. This picture appeared during a dramatic clinical and hematological remission induced by cortisones and antimetabolites. Aggravating headache with vomiting was the first sign, followed two months later by asthenia of the lower limbs and, in the third month, by flaccid paraparesis with absence of the deep reflexes. Slight asthenia of the arms (normal reflexes), peripheral type left facial paresis, and absence of left corneal reflex were also noted. The later signs included convulsions, damage to the left oculomotor nerves and bilateral papillary edema. The CSF displayed increased protein and diminished glucose values, with mononucleate cells ($884/mm^3$) presenting the same characteristics as sternal marrow blasts. The neurological symptom picture alternated between treatment-induced improvement and recurrence until the death of the patient, ten months after the appearance of the first signs. The terminal picture was one of acute generalization of the underlying disease with purpura, infiltration of the skin and subcutaneous tissue, and left pleural effusion. Immature white cells were not observed in the peripheral blood until shortly before death. The necropsy and histological data showed leukemic infiltration of several organs. This was particularly noticeable in the leptomeninx (base of the brain, around the cerebellum, and around the whole length of the spinal cord, which was completely encircled by infiltration). Many spinal nerve roots were also surrounded.

After an initial episode of priapism, a 30-year-old man with myeloid leukemia of nine months' standing observed by *Ott and Rabinowicz* presented a right lower extremity peripheral nerve syndrome, with thigh and leg amyotrophy, paralysis of the toes, paresis of the foot and weakness of the leg, depressed patellar reflex and no ankle and sole reflexes, reduced superficial sensibility in the common peroneal nerve and 5th lumbar root districts, and abnormal deep foot sensibility. Acrocyanosis was present in both feet, particularly the right. The psychological picture included a certain degree of feebleness of mind coupled with an indifferent and euphoric attitude. The anatomical and histological data showed various CNS, spinal nerve root, and sciatic nerve changes: demyelinization, hemorrhage, edema and fibrosis, thrombosis, and leukemic infiltration.

In a case of lymphatic leukemia of four years' standing in a 60-year-old woman observed by *Ulrich and Muller*, the terminal picture of polyneuropathy and meningeal symptoms led to death within a few months. Necropsy disclosed extensive peripheral nerve infiltration with myelin and axon destruction.

As stated, peripheral nerve compression (e.g. the sciatic nerve, *Klein and Steinhaus*) may be a feature of paravertebral chloroma. In a case of cervical chloroma observed by *Rouquès,* compression of the brachial plexus was followed by paraplegia caused by an epidural chloromatous nodule.

The complexity of the neurological picture and its pathogenetic interpretation are of interest in a case of chloroma reported by *Olmer et al.* During cortisone and antimetabolite-induced improvement of a promyelocytic blood picture in acute leukemia, bilateral paralysis of the 2nd branch of the 5th and left paralysis of the 3rd, 7th, 8th, 9th, 10th, and 12th cranial nerves (Garcin's syndrome) were observed, together with upper and lower extremity polyneuritis. Involvement of the 2nd branch of the right 5th cranial nerve was attributed to a chloromatous tumor in the right maxillary sinus, while the remaining nerve symptoms were attributed to a toxic pathogenesis (release of neurotoxic leukocyte ferments as a result of cytolysis treatment?). About 40 days later, gradual regression to total disappearance of the neurological picture was accompanied by marked improvement of the patient's general condition. After about three months, a distinct Horner's syndrome appeared during fresh appearance of the acute form of the underlying disease, while the terminal picture included paralysis of the limbs.

Herpes zoster appears to be more common in the leukemic patient than in the general population (*Gelfand*). Occipitofacial (*Tapie and Cassar*), dorsal and thoracic (*Quattrin et al.*), or dorsal and abdominal (*Wohlwill; Fischel*) sites have been observed in myeloid, basophilic, and acute leukemia, respectively. Generalized varicelliform herpes in lymphatic leukemia has been reported by *Frank L., Abrate and Baiotti, Lehmann, Duverne et al., Budner, Sbano and Andreassi.*

Leukemic infiltration of the herpes-invaded skin district has been observed by *Jadassohn* and by *Carlesimo et al.* (lymphatic leukemia), while the sequelae of herpes were accompanied by leukemic skin changes in the case of lymphatic leukemia reported by *Marchini and Grignani.*

Associations of herpes zoster and other diseases have been reported by *Giannini et al.* (varicella, in chronic lymphatic leukemia), *Gelfand* (varicella and parotitis, in chronic leukemia), and *Quattrin et al.* (impetigo, in basophilic leukemia). It should be noted that herpes zoster and varicella are now thought to be two different manifestations of the same virus (*Farrant and O'Connor; Weller and Stoddard*).

Bernard et al.[a] report the appearance of herpes zoster in a period of clinical remission of leukemia.

Facial herpes was noted in a personal case of acute chronic myeloid leukemia in a 9-year-old boy. In a case of acute leukemia in a 72-year-old man (kindly supplied by *Frugoni*), total body spread of herpes was noted. This case formed the subject of a thesis in clinical dermatology presented to the University of Padua by *Marigonda* in 1930. In some areas, the vesicles were isolated, while elsewhere their confluence formed large patches. Their content was clear in some cases and hemorrhagic in others. Necrosis, including areas of true skin gangrene, was a feature of the case. Immature white cells were observed in the CSF, though clinical signs of meningeal involvement were not present.

A pathogenic explanation for this association between herpes and leukemia has been offered by *Craver and Haagensen.* These workers postulate the widespread diffusion of a neurotropic virus, which infects a large part of the normal population and damages the afferent nerve when it is involved in leukemic infiltration.

However, diminished resistance to infection brought about in several ways by the underlying disease certainly is active in the association.

Herpes is more common in chronic leukemia, particularly the lymphatic forms, and is rarely reported for the acute form (in addition to the cases already cited, see those of *Keidan and Mainwaring, Mauro and Prato, and Introzzi*). The short course of the acute form may be a partial explanation (*Panelli et al.*). The association seems more common in the adult.

In a personal case of chronic myeloid leukemia a cerebral type carotid sinus syndrome was observed with notable swelling of the lateral cervical lymph glands in a 48-year-old man. Syncope occurred when the patient raised his head or turned it to the right. Partial loss of consciousness, with vertigo, pallor, tachypnea, and palpitations, was then observed.

The diagnosis of nerve changes in leukemia may be particularly difficult when the neurological picture is the first sign. Cell counts should be taken, combined if necessary with sternal puncture, in all cases of neurological damage when the etiology is not clear. If the findings are normal, the examination should nevertheless be repeated periodically so that the first sign of pathological change may be observed in good time.

The CSF is particularly indicative. The presence of immature cells may serve to attach a leukemic label to an apparently primary meningeal symptomatology or confirm such a determination by excluding inflammation when the underlying disease has already been diagnosed. Alternatively, a clinically silent meningeal involvement may be demonstrated in this way.

Even where leukemia has been established, differential diagnosis must consider the possibility of inflammation as an explanation for meningeal signs. In acute leukemia, in particular, viral, bacterial, or mycotic infection may result in both meningeal and CNS involvement. This may be caused by weakened body defenses as a result of granulocytopenia or hypogammaglobulinemia (*Aita*[a]; *Dreyfus; Nauciel and Lapresle; Zanussi*), dystrophic or deficiency tissue changes caused by the heavy use of antibiotics or by body factors as yet incompletely understood, and followed by pathogenic action on the part of saprophytes and mycetes, and proneness to infection as a result of the immunodepressive action of antimetabolites and cortisone.

The incidence of infection has been stressed by several workers (*Williams et al.; Goudemand et al.; Pierce*[b]; *Chini; Phair et al.*) and must always be kept in mind in the differential diagnosis of neuroleukemia. *Aita*[b], for example, asserts that about 25% of acute leukemia patients die as a result of septicemia. Recent contributions to this subject include those of *Symmers; Melli; Schneider; Burgess and De Gruchy; Dalton et al.; Finklestein et al.*, etc. *Symmers* refers to a case studied both clinically and postmortem, reported in *Drug-induced Diseases* (*Meyler and Peck*), in which seven episodes of infection of different origin were observed.

Some workers have suggested that a virus attacks both the nervous system and the hemopoietic organs, whose changes lead in turn to leukemia. This possibility is, of course, part of the wider question of the etiology of leukemia.

Some nerve changes in leukemia are not related directly to the basic disease and, though rarely observed, must be considered in differential diagnosis. These are changes of an aspecific, paraneoplastic type (the so-called "aspecific neuropathies" of *Labauge et al.*). Here there are no signs of infiltration or hemorrhage but of demyelinization. Changes of this type may be the cause of polyneuritis in leukemia (*Privitera and Fiorini; Olmer et al.*). Extensive demyelinization of the encephalon has been noted in chronic lymphatic leukemia (*Åström et al.*, two cases; *Cavanagh et al.*, one case; *Sibley and Weisberger*, one case). Similar alterations have been reported by *Martinetti and Mazza* and *Dolman et al.* These cases, together with those observed in other systemic blood diseases, are grouped under the heading "progressive multifocal leukoencephalopathy."

Intracranial hemorrhage in leukemia is most commonly observed in subjects of middle age, for whom no reason other than the underlying disease can be suggested. The clinical picture is often one of frank anemia and widespread hemorrhagic diathesis. Where the neurological episode is the first clinical sign of leukemia, these findings are of diagnostic assistance (*Scalabrino*) and invite hematological investigation. In some cases, however, other pathogenic factors may be at work and clinical diagnosis of the nature of the hemorrhage must resort to anatomic and histologic examinations (*Rossi*).

Retinal hemorrhage may also be noted. Its association with intracranial hemorrhage, however, is inconstant (*Wells and Silver*) and it must not be taken as a sure sign of the hemorrhagic origin of a neurological syndrome.

Retinal hemorrhages may be observed in as many as 70% of acute leukemia patients (*Bonnet; Borgeson and Wagener; etc.*). All types of involvement of the fundus oculi have been reported. One particularly common form is described as "spindle," "canoe," or "*en navette*" hemorrhage. This has a brilliant white center and is thought to be the result of leukocyte accumulation (*Murakami; Stock*).

Serious retinal involvement was noted in a personal case of chronic myeloid leukemia of six months' standing in a 25-year-old woman with an onset picture of violent headaches occurring almost every day. The later appearance of a scotoma in the right visual field led to examination of the fundus oculi. In the right eye, the optic disk appeared hyperemic, indistinct, and raised, while the veins were very congested and tortuous, and wine-red oval hemorrhage in the macula was accompanied by other retinal hemorrhages. In the left eye, the veins were turgid and tortuous, and there were roundish hemorrhages near the macula.

Involvement of the nervous system in leukemia may pose other diagnostic problems. In the case of convulsion, prior epilepsy may be suspected. Both cortisone and leukemic infiltration of the infundibulum and tuber may be equally responsible for polyphagia and obesity. Cortisone also may produce spinal cord and nerve-root symptoms (secondary to treatment-induced vertebral osteoporosis) or muscular changes (*Bernard et al.*[b]). Vincristine treatment for leukemia also may lead to peripheral nerve damage (*Evans et al.*[a]; *Moress et al.; Sandler et al.*); signs of neurotoxicity, even coma, were reported by *Slater et al.* High doses of L-asparaginase may cause mental confusion, depression, hallucinations, and coma (*Henderson, etc.*) or extrapyramidal manifestations (*Storti et al.*), while polyneuropathy may be the outcome of treatment with methylglyoxal-bis-guanylhydrazone (methyl-GAG).

Sometimes leukemia may develop in subjects with hereditary neurological abnormalities. In a group of four siblings, *Lampert* observed a

Louis-Bar syndrome in a 22-year-old girl and an association of this syndrome and acute lymphoblastic leukemia in her 3-year-old and 14-year-old brothers. The Louis-Bar syndrome is rare (101 cases by 1963) and is a recessive autosomal hereditary disease marked by progressive cerebellar ataxia and skin and conjunctival telangiectases, frequently accompanied by dysglobulinemia. Its association with leukemia poses interesting immunologic and genetic questions concerning the pathogenesis of this disease. An identical association has been reported by *Taleb et al.*

The appearance of neurological complications worsens the prognosis for leukemia. *Shaw et al.* note that the intrusion of meningeal changes shortens life expectancy, although only slightly, in the leukemic child, while *Hardisty and Norman* report 40% deaths in infantile acute leukemia within three months of diagnosis of the meningeal involvement. *Hyman et al.*[b] stress the value of early treatment. However, corrected meningeal forms are prone to relapse. *Gasser*, for example, observed five recurrences in the same patient.

The treatment of neuroleukemia is comprised in the treatment of the underlying disease. Intense cortisone treatment is advised in acute forms, together with antimetabolites such as 6-mercaptopurine or amethopterin (*Goudemand et al.*). *Wells and Silver* maintain that the neurological symptoms are more readily influenced by general antileukemia treatment than the hematological symptoms are. Blood antileukemic drug concentrations, however, are high by comparison with those in the nervous system as a result of the so-called hematoencephalic barrier. As already stated, this imbalance has been seen as a factor in the increased incidence of nerve complications in acute leukemia noted by many writers in recent years. Intrathecal injection of antimetabolites has been suggested particularly for intracranial hypertension and meningeal or meningocerebral infiltration (*Sansone; Gasser; Shanbrom et al.; Fanconi et al.; Labauge et al.; Stegagno et al.; etc.*). The results of such treatment have been analyzed by *Bernard et al.*[b] in 71 cases in the literature (since 1954) and 37 personal cases.

The clinical effect is most marked in cases of intracranial hypertension. A semicomatose, blind, and hydrocephalic patient observed by *Whiteside et al.* was able to read and carry on a conversation after 14 days of treatment. Partial regression of papillary edema and suture diastasis was also noted. Treatment led to the total regression of diastasis in one-third of the personal series of *Bernard et al.*[b]

Local encephalic syndromes are also benefited by intrathecal treatment. Remarkable regression is noted in cases of cranial nerve paralysis. In spinal cord and nerve-root changes, however, the results are less constant. CSF cell normalization is often spectacular, though protein levels fall slowly and never completely.

The treatment may sometimes be followed by partial or even complete regression of hematological signs (*Bernard et al.*[b]; *Hyman et al.*[a]). In most cases, however, the general clinical and blood picture remains unchanged in spite of the signs of nerve improvement.

Treatment-induced remission of a first neuromeningeal episode may be followed by one or more recurrences, with or without further hematological involvement. These further episodes may be equally subject to intrathecal therapy. Thus in a case reported by *Baker and Oliver,* a succession of neurological episodes was successfully treated with intrathecal methotrexate.

Intrathecal injection results in strong local concentration. There is also an appreciable passage of the drug into the blood, sometimes followed by the general improvement already mentioned. *Bernard et al.*[b] advise amethopterine on alternative days (first dose, 0.1 mg ± 0.05/kg; second dose, 0.2 mg ± 0.05/kg; subsequent doses, 0.3 mg ± 0.05/kg). The injections are continued until remission or the appearance of toxic signs. Six injections form an average cycle, twelve being the maximum. Local tolerance appears to be excellent.

Cytarabine, another antimetabolite, also has been used in the same way (*Landbeck and Eckler; Oehme and Meyer-Beeck*).

On rare occasions, hydrocortisone is administered intrathecally. Therapeutically useful liquor cortisone concentrations can be obtained by other routes as well.

Recent reports indicate that intrathecal administration of L-asparaginase is well tolerated by patients who have become methotrexate-resistant (*Bernard*). A rapid fall in cerebrospinal fluid leukemic cell values was observed, together with remission of clinical signs of meningeal involvement. This was of brief duration, however, despite the administration of maintenance therapy. *Bernard* also noted that L-asparaginase has a similar therapeutic effect when administered via a general route.

Good results have also been reported with 1,3-bis(2-chloroethyl)-1-nitrosourea (*Iriarte et al.*). This substance is administered intravenously and, being lipid soluble, is capable of crossing the hematoencephalic barrier (*Iriarte et al; Mathé; Landbeck and Eckler*). Hemorrhage due to thrombocytopenia may be observed, however.

CNS infiltration in leukemia is also treated with X-rays. At one time this was considered the best form of therapy (*Sullivan*[a,d]). Later work (*Sullivan et al.*), however, has shown that this does not give better results than intrathecal methotrexate in infantile meningeal leukemia.

Pierce[b] advises a total cranial dose of 400–2000 rads in 5–10 days, coupled with the suspension of specific medication. Transient alopecia is observed in all cases, while significant leukopenia is occasionally reported.

To obtain spinal fluid remission in infantile meningeal leukemia, *Sullivan et al.* recommend the irradiation of the entire cerebrospinal axis with a tumor dose of 1000 rads. When the subject is in marrow remission, radiation therapy is frequently accompanied by myelosuppression. These workers experimented with an association of 750–1000 rads (marrow remission cases) or 250–500 rads (marrow relapse cases) and two preirradiation and one postirradiation intrathecal methotrexate injections. Myelosuppression was observed in 50% of the marrow remission cases.

Cranial radiation and intrathecal methotrexate given early in remission of childhood acute lymphocytic leukemia, in addition to combination chemotherapy, seemed to reduce the incidence of nervous system relapse (*Aur et al.*). If administered to children at the time of initial diagnosis of acute leukemia, intrathecal methotrexate is considered useful in delaying the onset of CNS involvement in cases with elevated white blood cell values (*Melhorn et al.*).

Labauge et al. oppose the use of X-ray therapy in leukemic infiltration of the encephalon on the ground that the tissue is frequently edematous. They advise its use, however, in cases of cord compression due to infiltration.

Regression of an exophthalmos was brought about by a few days of X-ray therapy in a 12-month-old girl with promyelocytic acute leukemia observed by *Crombie*. This sign—the first symptom of the underlying disease—had followed a trauma in the orbital region. Autopsy showed infiltration of the orbit and this was most probably associated with a hemorrhagic pool at the time of injury.

Telecobalt therapy also is used in the treatment of CNS infiltration in leukemia.

Other forms of treatment include: intravenous injection of hypertonic glucose solutions and spinal puncture (this sometimes leads to regression) in intracranial hypertension; the administration of anticonvulsants in cases of convulsion; repeated spinal puncture and neurosurgery (decompressive windows or CSF derivation) in cases of hydrocephalus due to meningeal infiltration (*Hunt et al.*); laminectomy with resection of epidural leukemic tissue in cases of spinal cord compression.

Laminectomy, however, is often rendered unsuccessful by cord infiltration or irreversible degeneration of the spinal cord as a result of compression.

Transfusions are indicated particularly in the management of hemorrhage. In cases with low or nil blood fibrinogen values, activation of the fibrolinytic system by leukemia cell enzymes may be suspected and Trasylol may be considered as a possible remedy.

REFERENCES

Abrate, M. and Baiotti, G.: Considerazioni sull'associazione herpes zoster e leucemia linfatica cronica. Minerva med. 57:2918–2921 (1966).

Aita, J.A.: a) The neurologic manifestations of lymphoma, leukemia and myeloma (including polycythemia vera and macroglobulinemia). Nebraska med. J. 47:142–148 (1962). b) Neurologic manifestations of general diseases (C. Thomas, Springfield, Ill. 1964).

Ajuriaguerra, J. De; Lyon, G. and Colomb, D.: Syndrome d'hypertension intracrânienne au cours d'une leucose aiguë. Étude anatomo-clinique d'une observation. Acta neurol. belg. 59:1017–1032 (1959).

Alajouanine, T.; Thurel, R.; Castaigne, P. and Lhermitte, F.: Leucémie aiguë avec syndrome polynévritique et infiltration leucosique des nerfs. Rev. neurol. 81:249–261 (1949).

Allies, F.: Adipositas und Polyphagie bei Leukämie. Mschr. Kinderheilk. 106:237–239 (1958).

Alt, F. and Pineless, F.: Ein Fall von Morbus Ménière bedingt durch leukämische Erkrankung des Nervus acusticus. Wien. Klin. Wschr. 21:849–851 (1896).

Anderson, R. McD. and Taft, L. I.; The pathology of the central nervous system in childhood leukemia. Abstracts of papers 11th Congr. Int. Soc. of Haematology, Sydney 1966, p. 235 (V.C.N. Blight, Government Printer).

Andreani, F.; Sala, E. and Vercillo, L.: Su di un caso di leucemia acuta iniziato con paralisi periferica del facciale. Minerva med. 47:1816–1818 (1956).

Angio, G. G. D'; Evans, A.E. and Mitus, A.: roentgen therapy of certain complications of acute leukemia in childhood. Amer. J. Roentgenol. 82:541–553 (1959).

Åström, K. E.; Mancall, E. L. and Richardson, E. P.: Progressive multifocal leukoencephalopathy. A hitherto unrecognized complication of chronic lymphatic leukaemia and Hodgkin's disease. Brain 81:93–111 (1958).

Aur, R. J. A.; Simone, J.; Hustu, H. O.; Walters, Th.; Borella, L.; Pratt, Ch. and Pinkel, D.: Central nervous system therapy and combination chemotherapy of childhood lymphocytic leukemia. Blood 37:272–281 (1971).

Baker, G. P. and Oliver, R. A. M.: Neurological complications of acute leukaemia in remission. Lancet i:837–838 (1962).

Balestra, F. and Morandini, N.: Sindrome midollare trasversa come apparente prima manifestazione di leucemia acuta emocitoblastica. Minerva med. 53:1062–1065 (1962).

Barker, L. F.: Neutrophilic myelocytes in cerebrospinal fluid of a patient suffering from myeloid leukemia and their significance for the diagnosis of myeloleukemic infiltration of the leptomeninges. S. med. J. 14:437 (1921).

Bass, M. H.; Leukemia in children, with special reference to lesions in the nervous system. Amer. J. med. Sci. 162:647–654 (1921).

Bassol, J.: Leukaemic infiltration in the spinal canal as a cause of paraplegia. J. nerv. ment. Dis. 47:180–190 (1918).

Baudouin, A. and Parturier, G.: Sur les complications nerveuses des leucémies. Rev. neurol. 19:673–680 (1910).

BENDA: Leukämische Erkrankung des Zentralnervensystems. Klin. Wschr. 1898:228.

BERNARD, J. and SELIGMANN, M.: A study of 61 cases of leukemia treated with 6-mercaptopurine. Ann. N.Y. Acad. Sci. 60:385–401 (1954).

BERNARD, J.; BOIRON, M.; WEIL, M.; LEVY, J. P.; SELIGMANN, M. and NAJEAN, Y.: a) Étude de la rémission complète des leucémies aiguës (analyse de 300 observations). Nouv. Rev. franç. Hémat. 2:195–222 (1962).

BERNARD, J.; SELIGMANN, M.; TANZER, J.; LAPRESLE, J.; BOIRON, M. and NAJEAN, Y.: b) Les localisations neuro-méningées des leucémies aiguës et leur traitement par les injections intrarachidiennes d'améthoptérine. Nouv. Rev. franç. Hémat. 2:812–852 (1962).

BERNARD, J.: Personal commun. (1970).

BERNARD and TALAMON: in Revol *et al.*

BERTRAND. L.: Les leucoblastoses aleucémiques (Maloine, Paris 1946).

BIANCHI: in Bufano.

BLASCHY, R.: Polyneuritisähnliches Krankheitsbild bei Leukämie. Münch. med. Wschr. 76:2166–2167 (1929).

BOCKEL, R.; IMLER, M. and STHAL, J.: L'ammoniémie au cours des leucoses. Strasbourg méd. 15.309–315 (1964).

BOGGS, D. R.; WINTROBE, M. M. and CARTWRIGHT, G. E.: The acute leukemias. Analysis of 322 cases and review of literature. Medicine, Balt. 41:163–225 (1962).

BOILLIN, G.: Contribution à l'étude des manifestations neurologiques au cours des leucoses aiguës. Thèse Lyon (1960).

BONNET: in Labauge *et al.*

BORCHERS, H. G. and MITTELBACH, F.: Neurologische Störungen bei Blutkrankheiten. Internist, Berl. 2:105–117 (1961).

BORGESON, E. J. and WAGENER, H. P.: Changes in eye in leukemia. Amer. J. med. Sci. 177:663–676 (1929).

BRANDT, S.: Altérations leucémiques du système nerveux. Acta psychiat. neurol. 20:107–126 (1945).

BUDNER, S.: Generalized zoster in lymphatic leukemia and mycosis fungoides. Przegl. derm. 55:775–780 (1968).

BUFANO, M.: Le malattie neoplastiche dei tessuti emopoietici (Il Pensiero Scientifico, Rome 1963).

BURGESS, M. A. and DE GRUCHY, G. C.: Septicaemia in acute leukaemia. Med. J. Austr. 56:1113–1117 (1969).

BURNS: Observations on the surgical anatomy of the head and neck (Wardlaw & Cunninghame, Glasgow 1824).

BÜSING, C. W.: Rückenmarknekrose bei akutem Schub einer myeloischen Leukämie. Zbl. allg. Path. path. Anat. 99:123–125 (1959).

CAFARO, C.: Alterazioni del sistema nervoso centrale nelle leucemie acute. Policlinico, Sez. prat. 71:601–611 (1964).

CAMBIER, J.; LECHEVALIER, B. and LHUILLIER, M.: les complications neurologiques des hémopathies malignes. Rev. Prat., Paris 19:763–787 (1969).

CARLESIMO, O. A.; NINI, G. and BARDUAGNI, O.: Herpes zoster generalizzato in leucosi linfatica cronica. Riproduzione del quadro leucemico in sede di lesioni erpetiche. Minerva derm. 41:433–436 (1966).

CASOLINO: in Ninni and Rovello.

CASTAN, PH. and DEHING, J.: Coma révélateur d'une leucose aiguë chez un enfant, quinze jours après une vaccination perorale antipoliomyélitique. Étude antomoclinique et réflexions sur les lésions cérébrales des leucoses aiguës. Acta neurol. belg. 65:349–367 (1965).

CAVANAGH, J. B.; GREENBAUM, D.; MARSHALL, H. H. and RUBINSTEIN, L. J.: Cerebral demyelination associated with disorders of the reticulo endothelial system. Lancet, ii:524–529 (1959).

CAVAZZUTI, F.; MEZZELANI, P. and BELLATO, F.: Su due casi di leucosi acuta ad esordio clinico inconsueto. Minerva med. 60:976–980 (1969).

CHAES, L. B. and KALEMCIK, Z. N.: A case of chloroma of the spinal column. Vopr. Neurokhir., Moscow 25:59–61 (1961).

CHAPTAL, J.; JEAN, R.; PAGES, A.; IZARN, P.; BONNET, H.; EMBERGER, J. M. and AGHAI, E.: a) Complications neurologiques des leucoses aiguës de l'enfance. Montpellier méd. 57:299 (1960).

CHAPTAL, J.; JEAN, R.; PAGÈS, A.; BONNET, H.; EMBERGER, J. M.; MARTY, R. and OTHONIEL, J.: b) Méningite leucémique aiguë: étude clinique, hématologique et anatomique (une observation). Soc. Sci. méd. Biol., Montpellier (meeting 22 March 1963).

CHINI, V.: Leucemia paramieloblastica subacuta con sindrome del cono midollare, pleurite essudativa e infiltrato polmonare escavato. Policlinico, Sez. prat. 72:77–94 (1965).

CHRISTIAENS, L., and NUYTS, J. P.: Manifestation neurologique initiale d'une leucose aiguë chez un enfant de cinq ans. Lille méd. 8:515–518 (1963).

CONFINO, E.: Le chlorome de l'adulte. Thèse Montpellier (1963).

COOKE, J. V.: Acute leukemia in children. J. amer. med. Ass. 101:432–435 (1933).

CORNIL, L.: OLMER, D.; OLMER, J. and ALLIEZ, J.: Paralysie ascendante de Landry avec leucocytomyélie et syndrome de Froin au cours d'une leucémie myéloïde. Sang 6:114–120 (1932).

CORRIE, J. A.; COLEBATCH, J. H.; RICE, M. S. and EKERT, H.: Central nervous system infiltration in acute childhood leukaemia. Proc. austr. Ass. Neurol. 5:443–446 (1968).

CRAVER, L. F. and HAAGENSEN, C. D.: A note on the occurrence of herpes zoster in Hodgkin's disease, lymphosarcoma and the leukemias. Amer. J. Cancer 16:502–514 (1932).

CRITCHLEY, M. and GREENFIELD, J. G.: Spinal symptoms in chloroma and leukaemia. Brain 53:11–37 (1930).

CROIZAT, P.; DUCLOS, J.; BEYSSAC, J. and COURYON, J.: Cryptoleucémie aiguë à forme méningée. Lyon méd. 174:817 (1947).

CROMBIE, A. L.: Proptosis in leukemia. Brit. J. Ophthal. 51:101–104 (1967).

DALTON, H. P.; GERSZTEN, E.; ALLISON, M. J. and ESCOBAR, M. R.: Infections associated with leukemia and lymphoma. Virginia med. mthl. 96:221–223 (1969).

DAMESHEK, W.: Chronic lymphocytic leukemia—an accumulative disease of immunologically incompetent lymphocytes. Blood 29 (supplm.):566–584 (1967).

DAMESHEK, W. and GUNZ, F.: Leukemia (Grune & Stratton, New York-London 1964).

DEREYMAEKER, A.: Complications médullaries au cours d'une leucémie myéloïde aiguë. J. belge Neurol. Psychiat. 40:509 (1940).

DIAMOND, I. B.: Leukemic changes in brain; report of 14 cases. Arch. Neurol., Chicago 32:118–142 (1934).

DICKENMAN, R. C. and CHASON, J. L.: Alterations in the dorsal root ganglia and adjacent nerves in the leukemias, the lymphomas and multiple myeloma. Amer. J. Path. 34:349–361 (1958).

DOCK AND WARTHIN: in Ninni and Rovello.

DOLMAN, C. L.; FUERESZ, J. and MACKAY, B.: Progressive multifocal leukoencephalopathy. Two cases with electron microscopic and viral studies. Canad. med. Ass. J. 97:8–12 (1967).

DREYFUS, B.: Confrontations thérapeutiques. Nouv. Rev. franç. Hémat. 6:505–514 (1966).

DUVERNE, J.; BRIZARD, C. P.; MOUNIER, R. and VOLLE, H.: Zona généralisé et lymphose. À propos de deux observations dont une associée à une maladie de Paget osseuse. J. Méd., Lyon 48:187–193 (1967).

DUVOIR and PHILIPPE: Mort subite d'une enfant de 3 ans au cours d'une leucémie aiguë. Étude anatomo-pathologique d'hémorragies cérébrales d'un caractère particulier. Ann. Méd. lég. 6:24–29 (1926).

EISENLOHR, C.: Leucaemia lienalis, lymphatica et medullaris, mit multiplen Gehirnnervenlähmungen. Virchows Arch. path. Anat. 73:56 (1878).

ERAMO, N. D' and DEL DUCA, A.: Contributo allo studio del quadro oculare nel cloroma. Gaz. san., Milan 36:287–289 (1965).

ERAMO, N. D' and DE GAETANO, G.: Le alterazioni ossee nelle ematopie. S.E.U., Rome (1957).

ERAMO, N. D' and RABITTI, G.: Le manifestazioni neurologiche nelle leucemie. Boll. Soc. Med. Chir., Modena 67:147–157 (1967).

EVANS, A. E.; FARBER, S.; BRUNET, S. and MARIANO, P. J.: a) Vincristine in the treatment of acute leukemia in children. Cancer, Philad. 16:1302–1306 (1963).

EVANS, A. E.; GILBERT, E. S. and ZANDSTRA, R.: b) The increasing incidence of central nervous system leukemia in children. Children's cancer study group A. Cancer, Philad. 26:404–409 (1970).

FABIAN and NAEGLI: in Revol *et al.*

FANCONI, G.; GASSER, C. and HITZIG, W. H.: Leukämie und leukämoide Reaktionen im Kindesalter. In Heilmeyer and Hittmair, Handbuch der gesamten Hämatologic, vol. IV, pp. 198–235 (Urban & Schwarzenberg, Munich-Berlin 1963).

FARRANT, J. L. and O'CONNOR, J. L.: Elementary bodies of varicella and herpes zoster. Nature, Lond. 163:260–261 (1949).

FARREL, O.: Acute leukemia with hemorrhage. J. nerv. ment. Dis. 68:77 (1928).

FIALHO, F. and GOLLO, F. H.: Leucemia. Contribuição ao estudo de suas lesões viscerais. Rev. brasil. Cir. 35:217–224 (1958).

FIESSINGER AND MARIE: in Leidler and Russell.

FINKLESTEIN, J. Z.; WRIGHT, H. T. JR. and WARD, R.: Mixed viral infection: rubella and varicella in a patient with acute leukemia. J. Pediat. 75:306–308 (1969).

FISCHEL: in Ninni and Rovello.

FORKNER, C. E.: Clinical and pathologic differentiation of acute leukemias with special reference to acute monocytic leukemia. Arch. intern. Med. 53:1–34 (1934).

FRAENKEL: in Ninni and Rovello.

FRANK, L.: Generalized herpes zoster, encephalitis and lymphatic leukemia; case report. Arch. Derm., Chicago 64:192–194 (1951).

FRANK, T. J. F.: Leuchaemic retinitis: analysis of eye changes in 35 cases of leuchaemia, together with report of gross papilloedema in case of chronic myelogenous leuchaemia. Med. J. Austr. 1:364–369 (1935).

FRUGONI, C.: Di una particolare complicanza della leucemia mieloide (ematoma muscolare da mieloma intramuscolare). Riv. crit. Clin. med., Florence 9:533–546 (1908).

FULD, H.: Über die diagnostische Verwertbarkeit von Ammoniakbestimmungen im Blut. Klin. Wschr. 12:1364–1366 (1933).

GADRAT, J.; BOULARD, C.; MONNIER, J.; BERNARDET, P.; BOURSE, R. and PASTERNAC, A.: Tumeurs cutanées, croissance dysharmonique et accélérée, manifestations neurologiques, au cours d'une lymphoblastomatose aleucémique chez un garçon de 15 ans. J. Méd., Bordeaux 141:1269–1276 (1964).

GARCIN, R.; GRUNER, J. and TINEL, G.: Sur un cas de neurolymphomatose humaine; étude anatomo-clinique. Rev. neurol. 88:81–92 (1953).

GAREIS, R.: Einfache Optikusatrophie bei aleukämischer Lymphadenose. Klin. Mbl. Augenheilk. 130:659–666 (1957).

GARVEY, P. H. and LAWRENCE, J. S.: Facial diplegia in lymphatic leukemia. J. amer. med. Ass. 101:1941–1944 (1933).

GASSER, C.: Meningosis leucaemica. Schweiz. med. Wschr. 90:1193–1197 (1960).

GEITLIN: in Ninni and Rovello.

GELFAND, M. L.: Herpes zoster with varicelliform eruption and parotitis in chronic leukemia. J. amer. med. Ass. 145:560–561 (1951).

GÉLIN, G. and ROSAN, H.: Leucose aiguë avec leucoblastorachie et syndrome méningée. Rôle éventuel de la grossesse. Bull. Soc. méd. Hôp., Paris 67:633–636 (1951).

GERONIMI, C.; ABADA, M.; OULD, AOUDIA, J. P. *et al.*: Le début neurologique des leucémies aiguës. J. Méd. Maroc. 5:351 (1969).

GIANNINI, E.; ROSICA, V. and GALLO-CURCIO, C.: Erpes zoster e varicella in corso di leucemia linfatica cronica. Caso clinico. Gaz. int. Med. Chir. 70:1796–1805 (1966).

GILBERT, F. and RICE, E. C.: Neurologic manifestations of leukemia: report of three cases in children simulating acute bacterial meningitis. Pediatrics 19:801–809 (1957).

GIRARD, P.; CROUCE, M.; DUHAMEL and LEURIDAU: Syndrome méningée révélateur d'une leucose aiguë. J. Sci. méd., Lille 86:453–455 (1968).

GIRAUD, G.; LATOUR, H. and LÉVY, A.: a) Hémorragie du cône médullaire révélatrice d'une leucoblastose. Montpellier méd. 37/38:101–104 (1950).

GIRAUD, G.; CAZAL, P.; IZARN, P. and LÉVY, A.: b) Les thromboses leucémiques. Rapport XXX Congr. Franç. de Médecine, Algeria 1955 (Masson, Paris 1955).

GIROIRE, H.; CHARBONNEL, A.; VERCELLETTO and LEMOUROUX, P.: a) Sept observations de leucoses avec manifestations neurologiques. Gaz. méd. France 64:1551–1557 (1957).

GIROIRE, H.; CHARBONNEL, A.; KERNEIS, J. P. and LEMOUROUX, P.: b) À propos d'une exophtalmie maligne oedémateuse révélatrice d'une leucose. Presse méd. 67:817–820 (1959).

GOUDEMAND, M.; WATTEL, F.; WATTEL-WAREMBOURG, N. and DEHAENE, P.: À propos des manifestations neurologiques des leucoses aigues: 'la méningo-encéphalite leucosique à forme pseudo-tumorale'. Lille méd. 7:395–411 (1962).

GRIFONI, V.: Localizzazioni meningee della leucemia acuta. Notiz. Antiblastici, Milan 1:1–7 (1964).

GROCH, N.S.; SAYRE, G.P. and HECK, F. J.: Cerebral hemorrhage in leukemia. Arch. Neurol., Chicago 2:439–451 (1960).

HALFF, M.: Recherches sur l'ammoniémie; épreuve de l'ammoniémie provoquée. Strasbourg méd. 94:301–315 (1934).

HAMILTON, L. and ELION, G. B.: Fate of 6-mercaptopurine in man. Ann. N.Y. Acad. Sci. 60:304–314 (1954).

HARDISTY, R. M. and NORMAN, P. M.: Meningeal involvement in acute childhood leukaemia. Abstracts of papers 11th Congr. Int. Soc. of Haematology, Sydney 1966, p. 13 (V. C. N. Blight, Government Printer).

HARRIS, W.: A case of leukaemic polyneuritis. Lancet i: 122 (1921).

HATTA, T.: Proc. 33th Japanese Congr. of Intern. Med. (Tokyo, 1926).

HENDERSON, E. S.: Terapia della leucemia acuta. Aggiornamenti Emat., Rome 6:380–447 (1969).

HITZIG, W. H. and SIEBENMANN, R. E.: Scheinbare Schädelnahtsprengung bei Leukämie. Helv. paediat. Acta 10:590–601 (1955).

HORTON, B. T.: Nocturnal headache associated with chronic lymphatic leukemia. Med. Clin. N. Amer. 33:992–993 (1949).

HOWARD, J. P.; CEVIK, N. and MURPHY, M. L.: Cytosine arabinoside (NSC–63878) in acute leukemia in children. Cancer Chemother. Abstr. 50:287–291 (1966).

HOWARD, J. P.; ALBO, V. and NEWTON, W. A. JR.: Cytosine arabinoside. Results of a cooperative study in acute childhood leukemia. Cancer, Philad. 21:341–345 (1968).

HUNT, W.; BOURONCLE, B. and MEAGHER, J.: Neurologic complications of leukemias and lymphomas. J. Neurosurg. 16:135–151 (1959).

HUTINEL, J. and MARTIN, R.: Leucémie aiguë à forme d'hémogénie, mort brutale par complication cérébrale. Bull. Soc. Pédiat., Paris 27:327–331 (1929).

HYMAN, C. B. *et al.* a): Recognition of CNS involvement in acute leukemia in children and response to therapy. Proc. amer. Ass. Cancer Res. 3:330 (1962).

HYMAN, C. B.; BOGLE, J. M.; BRUBAKER, C. A.; WILLIAMS, K. and HAMMOND, D.: b) Central nervous system involvement by leukemia in children. I. Relationship to systemic leukemia and description in clinical and laboratory manifestations. Blood 25:1–12 (1965).

INTROZZI: in Panelli *et al.*

IRIARTE, P. V.; HANANIAN, G. and CORTNER, J. A.: Central nervous system leukemia and solid tumors of childhood. Treatment with 1,3–bis (2-chloroethyl)–1–nitrosourea (BCNU). Cancer, Philad. 19:1187–1194 (1966).

JADASSOHN: in Dameshek and Gunz.

JOSEPH, M. C. and LEVIN, S. E.: Leukaemia and diabetes insipidus; case report, with an unexpected effect of cortisone. Brit. med. J. i:1328–1331 (1956).

KAST, A.: Betiräge zur Pathologie der Leukämie. II Ueber Bulbärneervenlähmung bei Leukämie. Z. Klin. Med. 28:79 (1895).

KEIDAN, S. and MAINWARING, D.: Association of herpes zoster with leukemia and lymphoma in children. Clin. Pediat. 4:13–17 (1965).

KISSEL, P.; ARNOULD, G.; HARTEMANN, P. and DUREUX, M.: Tumeur épidurale à myéloblastes révélatrice d'une leucémie aiguë. Bull. Soc. méd. Hôp., Paris 69:881–886 (1953).

KLEIN, S. and STEINHAUS, J.: Ueber das Chlorom. Zbl. allg. Path. path. Anat. 15:49–51 (1904).

KOLKER, A. E.: Ocular manifestations of haematologic disease. In Brown and Moore, Progress in hematology, pp. 354–389 (W. Heinemann Med. Books, London 1966).

KOLOMOITSEVA, I. P. and MACHONKOVA, A. G.: Nervous system lesions in leukemias. Klin. Med., Moscow 36:67–71 (1958).

KRUMP, J. E.: Die Veränderungen des Hirnstrombildes bei malignen Hämoblastosen. V Kongr. europ. Gesellschaft f. Hämat., Freiburg i. Br. 1955, pp. 255–264 (Springer, Berlin-Göttingen-Heidelberg 1956).

KWAAN, H. C.; PIERRE, R. W. and LONG, D. L.: Meningeal involvement as first manifestation of acute myeloblastic transformation in chronic granulocytic leukemia. Blood 33:348–353 (1969).

LABAUGE, R.; IZARN, P. and CASTAN, P.: Les manifestations nerveuses des hémopathies. Rapport LXI Congr. Franç. de Psychiatrie et de Neurologie, Nancy 1963 (Masson, Paris 1963).

LAMPERT, F.: Akute lymphoblastische Leukämie bei Geschwistern mit Kleinhirnataxie (Louis-Bar Syndrom). Dtsch. med. Wschr. 94:217–220 (1969).

LANDBECK, G. and ECKLER, E.: Therapie der Leukamien. In Hertl and Landbeck, Leukamie bei Kindern (Thieme, Stuttgart 1969).

LANZA, G.: La istogenesi delle leucemie umane alla luce delle moderne conoscenze. Rass. clin.-scient. 35:201–207 (1959).

LARSEN, W. E. and MANNING, R. T.: Ammonia and leukemia. Observations on blood ammonia in leukemic patients. J. Kansas med. Soc. 62:302–304 (1961).

LASZLO, J.; LASZLO-KABALAY and GALL, M.: Altérations cérébrales au cours de la leucémie. Acta morph., Budapest 2:145–166 (1952).

LEACH, W. B.: Pathologic study of acute leukemia. II. A study of complications and cause of death. Ala. J. med. Sci. 2:243–248 (1965).

LÉCHELLE: in Labauge *et al.*

LEHMANN, H.: Zoster generalisatus varicellosus bei chronischer lymphatischer Lymphadenose. Derm. Wschr. 152:819–823 (1966).

LEIDLER, F. and RUSSEL, W. O.: Brain in leukemia: clinicopathologic study of 20 cases with review of literature. Arch. Path. 40:14–33 (1945).

LEREBOULLET: in Labauge *et al.*

LEVI, M. and ERAMO, N.D': Spiccata complicanza psichica (a tipo depressivo) e neurologica letale (emorragia cerebrale) in corso di leucemia mieloide cronica subacutizzata. Minerva med. giuliana 3:85–87 (1963).

LIEBREICH: in Ninni and Rovello.

LISI, L. DE: Sulle complicazioni nervose periferiche della leucemia. Riv. Neurol. 2:461 (1929).

LITTERAL, E. B. and MALAMUD, N.: Leukemia with predominant neurologic manifestations. Neurology, Minneap. 5:740–744 (1955).

LORENZ DE HAAS, A. M.: Syndrome de Landry dans un cas de leucémie. Rev. neurol. 85:306–310 (1951).

LOUIS-BAR, D.: Sur un syndrome progressif comprenant des téleangiectasies capillaires cutanées et conjonctivales symétriques, à disposition naevoïde et de troubles cérébelleux. Confin. neurol. 4:32–42 (1941).

LUCHERINI, T.: Considerazioni anatomo-cliniche sopra un caso di leucemia acuta. Haematologica 7:137–148 (1926).

LUGARESI, E.; TASSINARI, C. A. and GHEDINI, G.: Complicanze neurologiche nel corso di emopatie a carattere iper-displastico. Minerva med. giuliana 3:88–90 (1963).

MAGGIA, A. and GRANDESSO, R.: Sulle cosidette 'sindromi neuroleucemiche'. Acta med. patavina 23:454–469 (1963).

MARCHINI, E. and GRIGNANI, F.: Manifestazioni leucemiche cutanee insorte su esiti di herpes zoster in soggetto con leucemia linfatica. Rass. Derm. Sif. 18:61–69 (1965).

MARTINETTI, L. and MAZZA, L.: Manifestazioni neurologiche nell'emopatia leucemica. Progr. med., Naples 16:728–734 (1960).

MASQUIN, P. and TRELLES, J. O.: Précis d'anatomo-physiologie normale et pathologique du systeme nerveux central (Doin, Paris 1966).

MASSAROLI, P.: Di alcune complicazioni nervose nelle leucemie. Policlinico, Sez. med. 44:177–191 (1937).

MASTRANGELO, R.; ZUELZER, W. W.; ECKLUND, P. S. and THOMPSON, R. I.: Chromosomes in spinal fluid: evidence for metastatic origin of meningeal leukemia. Blood 35:227–235 (1970).

MATHÉ, G.: La chimiothérapie des cancers (leucémies, hématosarcomes, tumeurs solides); 2nd ed. (Expansion Scientifique Franç., Paris 1966).

MAURO, G. and PRATO, V.: L'erpes zoster nelle leucemie e nel linfogranuloma. Minerva med. 48:2954–2959 (1957).

MELHORN, D. K.; GROSS, S.; FISHER, B. J. and NEWMAN, A. J.: Studies on the use of "prophylactic" intrathecal amethopterin in childhood leukemia. Blood 36:55–60 (1970).

MELLI, G.: La leucemia linfatica cronica; in Corso superiore sulle malattie mielo-linfoproliferative, pp. 167–182 (C.E.A., Milan 1966).

MEYLER, L. and PECK, H. M.: Drug-induced diseases (Excerpta Medica Foundation, Amsterdam 1965).

MICHELI, F.: Leucemia mieloide subacuta in soggetto affetto da tremore ereditario e da atrofia muscolare tipo Aran-Duchenne. Minerva med. 27/I: 249–255 (1936).

MINNICK: in Revol *et al.*

MONGES, J.; OLMER, J. and GASGARD, E.: Leucémie lymphoïde avec ictère terminée par une hémorragie méningée. Sang 13:668–673 (1939).

MOORE, E. M.; THOMAS, L. B.; SHAW, R. K. and FREIREICH, E. J.: The central nervous system in acute leukemia: a postmortem study of 117 consecutive cases, with particular reference to homorrhage, leukemic infiltrates and meningeal leukemia. Arch. inter. med. 105:451–468 (1960).

MORESS, G. R.; D'AGOSTINO, A. N. and JARCHO, L. W.: Neuropathy in lymphoblastic leukemia treated with vincristine. Arch. Neurol., Chicago 16:377–384 (1967).

MORETTI, G.; STAEFFEN, J.; LORRAIN, J. and GAGGINI, R.: À propos d'une paralysie cubitale, manifestation clinique longtemps isolée et initiale d'une leucose subaiguë lymphoblastique. J. Méd., Bordeaux 136:836–840 (1959).

MOURIQUAND, G.; DAUVERGNE, M. and MONNET, P.: Syndrome neuro-oedémateux avec paralysie ascendante du type Landry au cours de l'évolution d'une crypto-leucémie. Lyon méd. 168:119–125 (1942).

MULLER: in Revol *et al.*

MURAKAMI: Ein Beitrag zu den Netzhautgefässveränderungen bei Leukämie. Klin. Mbl. Augenheilk. 1901:136

NAUCIEL, CH. and LAPRESLE, CL.: Les carences immunitaires. Rev. Prat., Paris 17:2567–2574 (1967).

NIES, B. A.; THOMAS, L. B. and FREIREICH, E. J.: Meningeal leukemia. A follow-up study. Cancer, Philad. 18:546–553 (1965).

NINNI, M. and ROVELLO, F.: Le localizzazioni extraemopoietiche della malattia leucemica (Ediz. Haematologica, Pavia 1953).

NONNE: in Revol *et al.*

OEHME, L. and MEYER-BEECK, D.: Terapia di attacco ed intervallore selle leucemie dei bambini e dei giovani. Med. tedesc. 6:180–184 (1970).

OLMER, J.; MOUREN, P.; CARCASSONE, Y. and GOSSET, A.: Chlorome avec manifestations neurologiques multiples, transitoirement améliorées par la thérapeutique. Marseille méd. 99:586–590 (1962).

OTT, TH. and RABINOWICZ, TH.: Étude clinique et anatomique d'un cas de neuropathie leucémique. Psychiat. Neurol. Neurochir. 64:158–175 (1961).

PANELLI, G.; MARIGO, S. and FERRERO, E: Istioleucemia insorta in còrso di grave herpes zoster disseminato. Haematologica 51:947–960 (1966).

PARKES WEBER, F.: Further rare diseases and debatable subjects (Staples Press, London 1949).

PETRONIO, V.; BONACCI, S.; MARIANI, B.; SANTERO, M. and SEZZI, M. L.; La leucemia eosinofila (considerazioni su un caso). Policlinico, Sez. prat. 75:248–258 (1968).

PHAIR, J. P.; ANDERSON, R. E. and NAMIKI, H.: The central nervous system in leukemia. Ann. intern. Med. 61:863–875 (1964).

PICARD, M.: Le complications médullaires des leucémies; Thèse Lyon (1941).

PIERCE, M. I.: a) Leukemia in children: treatment of 22 cases with 6-mercaptopurine. Ann. N. Y. Acad. Sci. 60:415–424 (1954). b) Neurologic complications in acute leukemia in children. Pediat. Clin. N. Amer. 9:425–442 (1962).

POLLI, E.: La leucemia (biologia e clinica) (Piccin, Padua 1967).

PONCHER, H. B.; WAISMAN, H. H.; RICHMOND, J. B.; HORAK, O. A. and LIMARZI, L. R.: Treatment of acute leukemia in children with and without folic acid antagonists. J. Pediat. 41:377–394 (1952).

POPPI, A. and MORGANTE, R.: Rari casi di leucosi ad esordio esclusivamente neurologico. Rif. med. 75:649–651 (1961).

PRIVITERA, A. and FIORINI, A.: Atrofia muscolare mielogena in decorso di linfoadenosi leucemica. Boll. Soc. Med. Chir., Cremona 15:93–100 (1961).

QUATTRIN, N.; DINI, E. and PALUMBO, E.: Leucemie basofile (Omnia Medica, Pisa 1959).

RADICCHI, M.: Diplegia facciale da leucemia acuta. Riv. Pat. nerv. ment. 72:646–648 (1951).

RAVETTA, A. and REZZONICO, S.: Su di un caso di leucemia mieloide con grave sindrome neurologica a localizzazione bulbo-protuberanziale. Recenti Progr. Med. 36:LV–LXX (1964).

REESE, H. and MIDDLETON, H. Y.: Mechanical compression of spinal cord by tumorous leukemic infiltration. J. amer. med. Ass. 98:212–217 (1932).

REVOL, L.: LACROIX, P. R. and CROIZAT, P.: Contribution à l'étude des manifestations neurologiques au cours des leucemies. J. Méd., Lyon 44:1007–1036 (1963).

REZZONICO, A. and REPETTO, S.: Comportamento dell'ammoniemia in corso di leucemia. Minerva med. 59:2365–2366 (1968).

RICCA, S.: Contributo allo studio delle alterazioni linfoadeniche del sistema nervoso. Riv. Pat. nerv. ment. 15:599 (1910).

RODRIGUEZ: in Leikin, S. L.: Leukemia: current concepts in therapy. Pediat. Clin. N. Amer. 9:753–768 (1962).

ROGER, H. and OLMER, H.: Les syndromes neuro-anémiques (Masson, Paris, 1936).

ROSENZWEIG, A. I. and KENDALL, J. W.: Diabetes insipidus as a complication of acute leukemia. Arch. intern. Med. 117:397–400 (1966).

ROSSI, R.: Tre casi di sindrome neuro-leucemica. Gaz. san., Milan 34:248–252 (1963).

ROTHMAN, A. R.; CARBONE, P. P.; RIESELBACH, R. and FREIREICH, E. J.: Paper electrophoresis of cerebrospinal fluid proteins in patients with meningeal leukemia. Cancer, Philad. 17:798–802 (1964).

ROUQUÈS, L.: Les complications nerveuses des leucémies. Ann. Méd. 47:152 (1946).

SANDLER, S. G.; TOBIN, W. and HENDERSON, E. S.: Vincristine-induced neuropathy. A clinical study of fifty leukemic patients. Neurology, Minneap. 19:367–374 (1969).

SANSONE, G.: La patomorfosi delle leucemie acute infantili curate: la adiposità tipo Frölich leucemica e la meningoleucemia. Minerva pediat. 6:463–471 (1954).

SBANO, E. and ANDREASSI, L.: Zoster generalizzato e leucemia linfatica cronica. Rass. Derm. Lif. 21:331–352 (1968).

SCALABRINO, R.: Leucemie acute ad impronta clinica esclusivamente o prevalentemente 'nervosa'. Boll. Soc. ital. Emat. 2:223–227 (1954).

SCALORI, G. and NOBILE, A.: Leucemia linfatica acuta con interessamento della tonsilla faringea, invasione della cavità cranica e compressione midollare da infiltrato epidurale. Riv. oto-neuro-oftal. 15:265–295 (1938).

SCHNEIDER, M.: Les infections bactériennes et fungiques au cours des leucémies aiguës. Sem. Hôp., Paris 43:438–439 (1967).

SCHULTZE: in Ninni and Rovello.

SCHWAB, B. and WEISS, S.: Neurologic aspect of leukemia. Amer. J. med. Sci. 189:766–778 (1935).

SEGA, A.: Sindromi neuroleucemiche. Su di un caso di atrofia muscolare progressiva di tipo Aran-Duchenne congiunto a leucemia linfatica cronica. Arch. Pat. Clin. med. 11:387 (1936).

SHANBROM, E.; MILLER, S. and FAIRBANKS, V. F.: Intrathecal administration of amethopterin in leukemia encephalopathy of young adults. New Engl. J. Med. 265:169–171 (1961).

SHAW, R. K.; MOORE, E. W.; FREIREICH, E. J. and THOMAS, L. B.: Meningeal leukemia. A syndrome resulting from increased intracranial pressure in patients with acute leukemia. Neurology, Minneap. 10:823–833 (1960).

SIBLEY, A. S. and WEISBERGER, A. S.: Demyelinating disease of the brain in chronic lymphatic leukemia. Occurrence of a case in the husband of a patient with multiple sclerosis. Arch. Neurol., Chicago 5:300–307 (1961).

SLATER, L. M.; WAINER, R. A. and SERPICK, A. A.: Vincristine neurotoxicity with hyponatremia. Cancer, Philad. 23:122–125 (1969).

SPITZ: Zur Kenntniss der Leukämischen Erkrankung des Zentralnerven-systems. Dtsch. Z. Nervenheilk. 19:467–481 (1901).

SPRIGGS, A.: Myeloid cells in cerebrospinal fluid. J. Neurol. Neurosurg. Psychiat. 21:305–307 (1958).

SPRIGGS, A. and BODDINGTON, M. M.: Leukaemic cells in cerebrospinal fluid. Brit. J. Haemat. 5:83 (1959).

STEFFEY, J. M.: The central nervous system manifestations of leukemia. A report of 6 cases with meningeal involvement. J. Pediat. 60:183–190 (1962).

STEGAGNO, G. A.; DIGILIO, G. and MULTARI, G.: Complicazioni neurologiche in corso di leucemia acuta nell'infanzia. Acta paediat. lat. 18:499–517 (1965).

STEPIEN: Méningopathie del la queue de cheval, d'origine leucémique. Rev. neurol. 1:821 (1929).

STOCK: Ueber Augenveränderung bei Leukämie und Pseudoleukämie. Klin. Mbl. Augenheilk. 1906:320.

STORTI: in Ravetta and Rezzonico.

STORTI, E.; FONTANA, G.; ASCARI, E. *et al.*: La L-asparaginasi nel trattamento delle leucosi acute. Minerva Med. 61:3635–3642 (1970).

SULLIVAN, M. P.: a) Intracranial complications of leukemia in children. Pediatrics 20:757–781 (1957). b) Leukemic infiltration of meninges and spinal nerve roots. Pediatrics 32:63–72 (1963).

SULLIVAN, M. P.; VIETTI, T. J.; FERNBACH, D. J.; GRIFFITH, K. M.; HADDY, T. B. and WATKINS, W. L.: Clinical investigations in the treatment of meningeal leukemia: radiation therapy regimens vs. conventional intrathecal Methotrexate. Blood 34:301–319 (1969).

SYMMERS, W. ST. C.: Infective complications of leukaemia, with special reference to the predisposing role of therapeutic measures. Abstracts of papers 11th Congr. Int. Soc. of Haematology, Sydney 1966, p. 234 (V. C. N. Blight, Government Printer).

TALAMON, J.: Leucémies aiguës avec manifestations neurologiques; Thèse Paris (1958).

TALEB, N.; THOMÉ, S.; GHOSTINE, S.; BARMADA, B. and NAHAS, S.: Association d'une ataxie-téleangiectasie avec une leucémie aiguë lymphoblastique. Presse méd. 77:345–347 (1969).

TAPIE, J. and CASSAR, A.: Sur deux cas de leucémie myéloïde avec complications nerveuses. Arch. Mal. Coeur 1919:218–226.

TARRO, E.: Lesioni encefaliche nelle leucemie. Pathologica 26:609–614 (1934).

THOMAS, L. B.: Pathology of leukemia in the brain and meninges: postmortem studies of patients with acute leukemia and of mice given inoculations of L 1210 leukemia. Cancer Res. 25:1555–1571 (1965).

TRÖMNER, E. and WOHLWILL, F.: Über Erkrankungen des Nervensystems, inbesondere der Hirnnerven bei Leukämie. Dtsch. Z. Nervenheilk. 100:233–259 (1927).

ULRICH, J. and MULLER, P.: Neurologische Komplikationen der Leukämien. Befall des peripheren Nervensystems und der Meningen bei einem Fall von chronischer lymphatischer Leukose. Schweiz. med. Wschr. 98:580–584 (1968).

VIETS, H. and HUNTER, F.: Lymphoblastomatous involvement of nervous system. Arch. Neurol., Chicago 29:1246–1262 (1933).

VLACH, V.; VITEK, J. and HOUBOVÁ, J.: The meningeal syndrome as an early sign of acute leukaemia in childhood. Cs. Neurol. 24:14–19 (1961).

WEIL, H.: Perakute Myeloblastenleukämie unter dem Bilde einer fieberhaften Querschnittsymelitis. Klin. Wschr. 18:547–548 (1939).

WELLER, T. H. and STODDARD, B. M.: Serial propagation in vitro of agents producing inclusion bodies derived from varicella and herpes zoster. Proc. Soc. exp. Biol., N.Y. 83:340–346 (1953).

WELLS, C. E. and SILVER, R. T.: The neurologic manifestations of the acute leukemias: a clinical study. Ann. intern. Med. 46:439–449 (1957).

WHITESIDE, J. A.; PHILIPS, F. S.; DARGEON, H. W. and BURCHENAL, J. H.: Intrathecal amethopterin in neurological manifestations of leukemia. Arch. intern. Med. 101:279–285 (1958).

WILLIAMS, H. M.; DIAMOND, H. D.; CRAVER, L. F. and PARSONS, H.: Neurological complications of lymphomas and leukemias (C. Thomas, Springfield, Ill. 1959).

WINKLER, W.: Über neurologische Symptome bei Leukämie mit einem Beitrag zur symptomatischen Aleukie. Z. ges. Neurol. Psychiat. 137:385–396 (1931).

WOHLWILL: in Ninni and Rovello.

ZANUSSI, C.: Carenza immunologica secondaria. Aspetti teorici e clinici. Minerva med. giuliana 7:95–108 (1967).

ZUELZER, W. W. and FLATZ, G.: Acute childhood leukemia: a ten-year study. Amer. J. Dis. Child. 100:886–907 (1960).

ZUNIN, C.: Un caso di leucemia acuta infantile ad inizio pseudoappendicitico; considerazioni cliniche ed anatomo-patologiche. Minerva pediat. 4:769–772 (1952).

Chapter VII

NEUROLOGICAL SYMPTOMS
IN LYMPHOSARCOMA

Nerve system involvement is not frequent in lymphosarcoma. In the series of 229 cases of lymphoreticular disease collected by *Hutchinson et al.*, neurological complications were present in 20% (45 cases: Hodgkin's disease, 32 cases; reticulosarcoma, 9; lymphosarcoma, 3; Brill-Symmers disease, 1).

Damage to the mediastinal nerve trunks, particularly the recurrent laryngeal nerve, in lymphosarcoma is a result of compression by lymphoglandular masses. The main trunk of the vagus is occasionally involved. *Corfini* reported a case with infiltration of the facial nerves, while *Kohut* and *Moore and Oda* have reported acute polyradiculoneuritis due to infiltration. *Lugaresi et al.* observed a case with monolateral cranial polyneuritis, associated with radiological signs of infiltration of the base of the cranium. Central nervous system infiltration and compression have also been reported. Cord compression is usually caused by epidural masses and is most commonly observed in the thoracic tract (*Aita*). Early intravenous administration of mechlorethamine, followed by radiation therapy, has given good results in such cases (*Williams, H.M., et al.*). Meningeal involvement, particularly in leukemic conversion cases, has been observed also (*Gendelman et al.*).

Herpes zoster, primarily on the chest, has been reported by *Rosenberg et al.* and by other writers. Rarely has involvement of the trigeminal district been noted (*Aita*).

In a personal case of lymphosarcoma of the small intestine in a 16-year-old boy (*d'Eramo and De Gaetano*), the abdominal onset was accompanied by right sciatic pain, which was improved by irradiation of the abdomen. A small mass was palpable in the left lower abdominal quadrant. There was considerable hypotonia of the right calf muscles, with slight pain hypoesthesia, though the tactile, thermic, and deep sensibilities were unimpaired. The right ankle and knee reflexes were very variable compared to those of the left leg. Skeletal radiography showed medium-sized areas of right iliac osteolysis with clear borders, touching each other at some points; alveolar osteolysis surrounded by clearly marked bone bridges in the ipsilateral supra-acetabular area and sacral wing; slight left iliac wing decalcification.

In a second personal case of superficial lymphoglandular (mainly inguinocrural) lymphosarcoma in a 58-year-old man, involvement of the cerebral trunk was demonstrated by: diplopia and palpebral ptosis resulting from partial paralysis of the right oculomotor nerve, with paresis of the levator palpebrae superioris and the rectus superior and medialis muscles; transmission bilateral hypoacusis, more marked on the left; right deviation, hemiatrophy, and trembling of the tongue caused by hemiparalysis. A slight rightward deviation of the gait could also be noted. Visual acuity was reduced and examination of the fundus oculi showed signs of a much earlier paramacular chorioretinitis.

"Progressive multifocal leukoencephalopathy" was noted by *Lloyd and Urich* in a case of lymphosarcoma clinically interpreted as Brill-Symmers disease. Other examples of leukoencephalopathy during lymphosarcoma have been reported by *Adams and Short* and by *Dolman et al.*

Demyelinization and softening of the spinal cord, in the form of necrotizing myelitis and in the absence of infiltration or compression, were observed by *Williams, R. A., et al.* in a case of lymphosarcoma. Paraneoplastic involvement of both the spinal and the cranial nerves in lymphosarcoma has been reported by *Gupta. Lugaresi et al.* also suggest a paraneoplastic origin for a multincuritis symptom picture with involvement of the right 6th, left 9th, and both 7th cranial nerves, as well as some spinal nerves, particularly the sciatics.

Association of a Louis-Bar syndrome and terminal lymphosarcomatosis was reported in two siblings by *Castaigne et al.*

A high incidence of nerve changes has been noted in Equatorial Africa in a form of lymphosarcoma described by some writers as "*Burkitt's* tumor." This is particularly frequent in young subjects and is characterized by the appearance of abdominal and maxillary masses (*Janota*). Paraplegia is the most common nerve sign. This is attributed to pressure exerted by retroperitoneal, vertebral, or epidural masses on arteries supplying the nerve structures or on the spinal cord. Infiltration, however, may occur in any area of the central nervous system, including the meninges, the hypophysis and its neighboring formations, the orbit, the cranial nerves, and the roots of the spinal nerves (*Janota*). In this writer's series of 26 cases, four presented paraplegia, while in seven others nerve involvement was demonstrated by convulsions or consciousness disturbances, with or without signs of cerebral site lesions. *Ziegler et al.* recently reported a series of 77 cases, 35% of which (46%) developed evidence of nervous system involvement, including paraplegia, cranial neuropathy, altered levels of consciousness, and presence of tumor cells in the CSF.

REFERENCES

ADAMS, J. H. and SHORT, I. A.: Progressive multifocal leucoencephalopathy. Scot. med. J. 10:195–202 (1965).

AITA, J. A.: The neurologic manifestations of lymphoma, leukemia and myeloma (including polycythemia vera and macroglobulinemia). Nebraska med. J. 47:142–148 (1962).

BURKITT, D.: A sarcoma involving the jaws in African children. Brit J. Surg. 46:218 (1958). A lymphoma syndrome in African children. Ann. roy. Coll. Surg. Engl. 30:211 (1962).

CASTAIGNE, P.; CAMBIER, I. et BRUNET, P.: Ataxie télanfiectasies, désordres immunitaires, lymphosarcomatose terminale chez deux frères. Presse méd. 77:347–348 (1969).

CORFINI, F.: Un caso di linfosarcoma a localizzazione rara. Haematologica 15:375–387 (1934).

DOLMAN, C. L.; FURESZ, J. and MACKAY, B.: Progressive multifocal leukoencephalopathy. Two cases with electron microscopic and viral studies. Canad. med. Ass. J. 97:8–12 (1967).

ERAMO D' and DeGAETANO: Le alterazioni osse nelle ematopie, S.E.U. Rome (1957).

GENDELMAN, S.; RIZZO, F. and MONES, R. J.: Central nervous system complications of leukemic conversion of the lymphomas. Cancer, Philad. 24:676–682 (1969).

GUPTA, S. P.: Neuropathy in lymphosarcoma. Case report. Indian J. med. Sci. 15:717–720 (1961).

HUTCHINSON, E. C.; LEONARD, B. J.; MAUDSLEY, C. and YATES, P. O.: Neurologic complication of reticuloses. Brain 81:75–92 (1958).

JANOTA, I.: Involvement of the nervous system in malignant lymphoma in Nigeria. Brit. J. Cancer 20:47–61 (1966).

KOHUT, H.: Unusual involvement of nervous system in generalized lymphoblastoma. J. nerv. ment. Dis. 103:9–20 (1946).

LLOYD, O. C. and URICH, H.: Acute disseminated demyelination of the brain associated with lymphosarcoma. Lancet ii: 529–530 (1959).

LUGARESI, E.; TASSINARI, C. A. and GHEDINI, G.: Complicanze neurologiche in corso di emopatie a carattere iper-displastico. Minerva med. giuliana 3:88–90 (1963).

MOORE, R. Y. and ODA, Y.: Malignant lymphoma with diffuse involvement of the peripheral nervous system. Neurology, Minneap. 12:186–192 (1962).

ROSENBERG, S. A.; DIAMOND, H. D. and CRAVER, L. F.: Lymphosarcoma: the effects of therapy and survival in 1,269 patients in a review of 30 years' experience. Ann. intern. Med. 53:877–897 (1960).

WILLIAMS, H. M.; DIAMOND, H. D.; CRAVER, L. F. and PARSONS, H.: Neurological complications of lymphomas and leukemias. (C. Thomas, Springfield, Ill. 1959).

WILLIAMS, R.A.; BILLINGS, J. J. and GRUCHY, G. C. DE: Acute myelitis complicating lymphosarcoma. Med. J. Austr. 49:128–133 (1962).

ZIEGLER, J. L.; BLUMING, A. Z.; MORROW, R. H.; FASS, L. and CARBONE, P. P.: Central nervous system involvement in Burkitt's lymphoina. Blood 36:718–728 (1970).

Chapter VIII

NEUROLOGICAL SYMPTOMS
IN HODGKIN'S DISEASE

The presence of neurological changes in Hodgkin's disease is no new observation. *Hodgkin* himself noted meningeal infiltration in a case of generalized granulomatosis. In 1870 *Murchison and Sanderson* gave the first detailed description of meningeal involvement, and in the same year *Goodhart* reported a case in which paraplegia followed spinal epidural infiltration. In 1875 *Hutchison* collected reports of the small number of cases then published and added a personal case with multiple site changes in the brain, spinal column, and lungs. A treatise published by *Gowers* in 1879 dealt with granulomatous changes in various organs, including the brain.

The subsequent literature has been more richly endowed and about 80 cases were reported between 1880 and 1955. In 1913 *Nonne* observed a patient who presented a spinal cord compression syndrome unaccompanied by clinical signs indicating Hodgkin's disease. This case was diagnosed intraoperatively by the discovery of a granulomatous neoformation in the vertebral cavities, and was the first known case in which a neurological complication was the first clinical sign of the underlying disease. A very similar case was reported by *Gertsmann* in 1915. Here paraplegia due to granulomatous pachymeningitis of the spinal cord was diagnosed at laminectomy.

The frequency of neurological complications in Hodgkin's disease has been assessed at 10% (*Dalla Volta and Patrizi; Labauge et al.*), though some workers have reported much higher percentages, e.g. 27.7% (10 out of 36 cases treated at the Montefiore Hospital in New York between 1914 and 1925) (*Ginsburg*) and 36% (*Sicard et al.*).

Thies et al., however, suggest that such high percentages are the result of a failure to distinguish between Hodgkin's disease and lymphosarcomatous forms or lymphatic leukemia. In their series (403 cases treated at the Freiburg University Medical Clinic between 1941 and 1959), neurological symptoms were observed in only 47 cases (11.6%). Of these

47 subjects, 23 were males and 24 females; 13 were under 30 years; 19 were between 30 and 50 years; and 15 were over 50 years old.

Nervous tissue infiltration is a rare anatomicopathological finding in Hodgkin's disease, since nerve lesions are usually caused by compression following epidural or osseal infiltration. Central nervous system (CNS) malacia is common and is the result of vascular occlusion caused by granulomatous tissue.

Frank cell polymorphism ("*bariolage cellulaire*") is a typical feature of granulomatous tissue. Reticular cell proliferation, including Sternberg-Reed cells (productive component), is accompanied by lymphocytes, granulocytes (particularly eosinophils), monocytes, and plasma cells (exudative component). In the lymph nodes, this tissue almost entirely replaces the normal parenchyma, following a first stage in which there is hyperplasia of lymphoid and histioreticular cells. Later, necrosis of the granulomatous tissue is replaced by fibrous or even hyaline tissue. The histological picture in other tissue and organs affected by the disease is the same.

Paragranuloma and Hodgkin's sarcoma (*Jackson and Parker*) are variant forms of Hodgkin's disease. In the former, the granulomatous tissue is poorly supplied with Sternberg-Reed cells and there is little fibrosis. In Hodgkin's sarcoma, there is intense reticular cell proliferation and mitotic activity.

The nervous system is not involved in paragranuloma according to *Labauge et al.*, though case no. 4 of the series of *Thies et al.* was of this type. *Sparling et al.* maintain that the brain and digestive tract are particularly vulnerable in Hodgkin's sarcoma. Of 25 cases of CNS involvement in the series of *Thies et al.*, however, 23 were histologically classified as typical granuloma, with one case each of Hodgkin's sarcoma (case no. 8) and paragranuloma (case no. 4).

Intracranial infiltration is rare and only about 30 cases were reported up to 1959 (*Labauge et al.*).

The usual picture is one of epidural infiltration, originating in the upper neck or peri- or retropharyngeal lymph nodes (*Sternberg; Lascelles and Burston*). Invasion is usually via the foramina in the base of the skull or more rarely (*Lascelles and Burston*) through the posterior wall of the sphenoid sinus. Infiltration then proceeds between the endocranium and the dura mater with the base of the skull as the site of choice. The external face of the dura mater is involved and this usually prevents further infiltration toward the brain (*Favre et al.*). Extensive epidural infiltration is not uncommon and may lead to serious compression of the brain. In some cases, the dura mater is massively involved (*Colrat; John and Nabarro*) and may be unable to prevent further infiltration. In the case reported by *Lascelles and Burston,* invasion of the whole of the posterior fossa was accompanied by involvement of the infundibulum, the trigeminal ganglion depression, and a temporal lobe.

Penetration of the brain may lead to reaction in the form of intense neuroglia proliferation (*Schmid*).

On rare occasions, epidural infiltration is secondary to granulomatous involvement of the cranial bone. In a case reported by *Fein and Newill,* granuloma spread from the frontal bone, sella turcica, and the lamina cribrosa to the dura mater, with occlusion of the superior sagittal sinus, and to the left frontal lobe, with extensive infiltration to the left ventricle; the gyrus cinguli was also involved.

Infiltration of the intracranial leptomeninges is rare. Crushing by granulomatous tissue causes alterations of the vessels (necrosis or infiltration of the vessel walls may be observed). The consequent reduction in blood supply leads to serious cerebral tissue damage (*Wepler; etc.*).

Granulomatous infiltration of the cerebral hemispheres is even less common. As already noted, the granuloma may spread to the brain (along the lymphatic spaces) from meningeal sites (granulomatous meningoencephalitis) or from bone sites. Since the primary sites are normally basal, the basal and lower lateral formations of the brain are usually involved. Complete destruction of the infundibulum and tuber have been reported (*von Hecker and Fischer; Sternberg; etc.*). The very rare cases which do not fall within this pathogenetic interpretation are attributed to blood-borne metastasis. Intracerebral sites attributable to hematogenic dissemination have been reported by *Ziegler, Ginsburg, Serebrjanik, Schöpe, Sparling et al., Thies et al., and Ljungdahl et al.* In *Ziegler's* case a granulomatous nodule was observed inside the frontal lobe. In that of *Serebrjanik,* a picture of true granulomatous encephalitis was formed by numerous small sites in the white matter, the basal ganglia, and the pons.

Hematogenic metastasization in Hodgkin's disease is explained as a result of wear of the vessel walls by the granulomatous tissue. The lumen is then penetrated and metastasizing emboli are formed.

Some workers (*Hallervorden; Schöpe; Sparling and Adams; Schricker and Smith*) recognize a primary Hodgkin's sarcoma of the brain, usually unaccompanied by extracranial diffusion.

Granuloma of the chiasma, optic nerves, infundibulum, and hypophysis unaccompanied by osteomeningeal changes, was classified as possibly primary in a case observed by *Storniello and Salvati.*

Both *Favre et al.* and *Thies et al.* have warned that the possible existence of primary granuloma of the nervous system is a deduction from what is essentially a clinical concept and cannot be demonstrated with certainty. *Labauge et al.* have noted that the onset of primary Hodgkin's sarcoma of the brain usually occurs at an advanced age (65 and 70 years in the cases of *Sparling and Adams*). In their opinion, this fact, together with the scarcity of necropsy date, militates against the classification of such sites as primary. They also point to the well-known frequency of clinically silent retroperitoneal adenopathies in Hodgkin's disease. They suggest, however, that there may be a close affinity between these granuloma forms and so-called primary CNS reticulosis (see appendix to Chapter XI).

It may be noted that in reticulosis of this type infiltration is mainly perivasal (see below), as in involvement of the central nervous system in systemic granulomatous disease (Hodgkin's disease, sarcoidosis) and in infectious granulomatosis (tuberculosis, toxoplasmosis) (*Rewcastle and Tom; Schmid*).

This question is, in any event, part of the larger and more complicated problem of the histogenesis of systemic blood diseases, to which reference has been made in connection with the origin of leukemic infiltration.

Spinal epidural infiltration is the anatomic sign of choice in granulomatosis of the nervous system: the alteration was present in 39 out of 45 literature cases collected by *Weil.*

Granulomatous tissue commonly looks like lard and at first sight appears to be part of the dura mater. The picture, therefore, is very similar to that of a pachymeningitis (*Goormaghtigh*). The neck and lumbar segments are the usual sites, and infiltration normally extends to the height of vertebra. In a case reported by *Bert,* however, the epidural space was invaded from the last cervical to the first lumbar vertebrae. *Askanazy*[a] observed a case in which infiltration was limited to a vertebral foramen.

Like an extradural tumor, infiltration compresses the cord, as well as the roots, the possibly infiltrated spinal ganglia, and the vessels. There is usually an area of maximum infiltration thickness responsible for major cord damage. As in the cranium, the dura mater normally forms an impassable barrier so that infiltration of the leptomeninx and the cord itself is extremely rare (case no. 8, *Thies et al.*).

The literature contains a unique case (*Urecchia and Goïa,* 1927) in which necropsy showed infiltration of the inner face of the dura mater and the pia mater in the lumbosacral segment of the spinal column. The funiculi posteriores of the cord and some nerve trunks of the cauda equina were also involved.

Epidural granulomatous infiltration normally originates in the paravertebral lymph nodes, commonly in the cervical and thoracic glands (less commonly in those behind the peritoneum), which means that the infiltration site is usually at the level of the cervical and dorsal segments of the cord. Access to the vertebral cavity is obtained via the foramina and the infiltration spreads along the neurolemma (*Bataini and Ennuyer*). The vertebrae are usually undamaged. Granulomatous spondylitis may also prove the departure point for the infiltration, which then penetrates the epidural space, encircling the posterior vertebral ligament. The entity was described for the first time by *Askanazy*[b,c] in 1912 and it is thought that the vertebrae may be involved by hematogenous dissemination. Primary granuloma of the skeleton is admitted by some writers (*Pellé and Massot; Kooreman and Haex; Romiti*) and denied by others (*Uehlinger; Craver and Copeland; Schinz*). Usually, however, the vertebrae are involved as a result of diffusion of the granuloma from neighboring adenopathies. When granulomatous spondylitis is present, the cord may be damaged both by subsequent compression on the part of crushed, fractured, or dislocated vertebral bodies and by epidural infiltration.

Some cases (including that of *Nonne*) suggest the possibility of primary granuloma in the epidural space. The data in the literature, however, are not conclusive (*Eugénis; Browder and de Veer; Verda*).

A further necropsy finding in Hodgkin's disease is that of peripheral nerve changes resulting from compression by adenopathies or granulomatous infiltration, or from infiltration itself.

Malacia or degeneration of nerve formations may be caused by occlusion of their supplying vessels.

Compression by granulomatous infiltration or by adenopathies may be responsible for such occlusion. A typical example is the compression exercised by laterovertebral adenopathies on vessels originating in the aorta and supplying the nerve roots. Laterocervical adenopathy has been observed as a cause of compression of the carotid arteries and hence of cerebral disturbances and changes. Occlusion may also be attributable to granulomatous proliferation within the lumen.

Cord malacia may lead to cavitary myelitis (*Walthard*). Edematous, necrotic or hemorrhagic malacotic sites may be observed in the brain. The fact that infiltration is usually basal indicates that the median paraventricular regions and the central gray nuclei are the sites of choice (*Winkelman et al.*).

It must also be remembered that degeneration of the central nervous system and necrosis may be the result of direct compression on nerve tissue.

Occasionally granulomatous infiltration of the basal meninges leads to hydrocephalus as a result of cerebrospinal fluid block (*Wepler; Schmid*).

Neurological symptomatologies are usually associated with the later stages of Hodgkin's disease. Unilateral involvement limited to one lymph node area is observed in the first stage of the disease; in the second stage, two or more areas may be affected. In the large series of *Thies et al.* the greatest frequency of nerve signs was in the third stage (generalization of the disease or the appearance of hepatosplenomegaly). *Williams et al.* state that nerve system involvement is a feature of the last quarter of the natural history of the disease. Early onset of nerve symptoms is unusual (one out of five cases according to *Froment et al.*). Nerve involvement as the presenting sign is even less common (see cases of *Nonne* and *Gertsmann; Walthard; Léger et al.; etc.*).

Signs of cerebral damage are very rare. Such damage is usually the result of compression caused by extradural infiltration rather than by infiltration of the brain itself. Two different clinical forms are observed: pseudotumoral and multifocal forms.

In the pseudotumoral form, the clinical picture is that of an endocranial tumor, resulting from gradual extension of the signs of cerebral site changes, followed by intracranial hypertension. Focal signs depend on the site of the lesion and may present as jacksonian type convulsion crises and/or deficit.

Convulsion as an expression of cerebral damage in Hodgkin's disease has been observed by several workers (*Colrat; Ginsburg; etc.*), though this sign may appear even in the absence of demonstrable cerebral change (*Belloni*).

The fact that infiltration is localized mainly at the base of the cranium explains certain clinical features: apparent posterior cerebral fossa syndromes; and relative frequency of diabetes insipidus (*Sternberg; Desbuquois; etc.*); serious cachexia and other signs of diencephalon and hypophysis damage, resulting from posthypophyseal, infundibulum, and tuber invasion.

Intracranial hypertension is not long absent from the clinical picture. It may be the result of several causes: cerebrospinal fluid (CSF) block, edematous reaction to neighboring infiltration, or, less commonly, intracranial hemorrhage. Massive cervicomediastinal adenopathy may interfere with the venous circulation occasionally and may result in cerebral edema.

Timely treatment may lead to the regression of cerebral change and to the prevention of further extension or the appearance of hypertension. In case no. 3 of the series of *Traldi and Artusi,* a 12-year-old boy with Hodgkin's disease of about four years' standing presented 5–6 hour periodic convulsion crises and an electroencephalographic picture of deep left frontal damage. Early intravenous treatment with 15 mg mechlorethamine followed by radiation of the left frontal region produced complete regression of the convulsions and an improved electroencephalographic picture.

In a case reported by *Thies et al.* (case no. 5) the clinical picture of Hodgkin's disease began with signs of cerebral damage very similar to those of pseudotumoral forms. The diagnosis was based on the necropsy data. In case no. 6 of the same series, cerebral damage was attributed to hemorrhage. Granulomatous infiltration and compression were excluded. The patient was a 49-year-old man with histologically demonstrated Hodgkin's disease. The terminal picture included paresis of the right arm, which was seen as a result of hemorrhage of the left middle cerebral artery. Frank thrombocytopenia was also observed.

In cases with symptoms of encephalic damage in several sites (multifocal forms), the semeiologic interpretation and diagnosis may be particularly difficult. On some occasions a single, massive and much extended granuloma may give rise to an apparently disseminated neurological symptom pattern, particularly if it is sited in the base of the cranium (*Labauge et al.*).

The cases reported by *Louis-Bar* and by *Fein and Newill* are good examples. In that of *Louis-Bar*, the first stage of the disease included initially flaccid, and later spastic, paraplegia, which regressed completely in a few months. Subsequently, intracranial hypertension was accompanied by paralysis of the right oculomotor and left facial nerves. The terminal picture was dominated by psychological disturbances very similar to those of Korsakoff syndromes and by signs of infundibulum and tuber involvement (diabetes insipidus, cachexia, loss of body hair, hunger crises, and shivering). These symptoms were explained by the discovery of a large intracranial mass.

Fein and Newill observed a 34-year-old man who had been treated for Hodgkin's disease for six years. Convulsion crises were followed by right ptosis, left hemiparesis, and paralysis of the right facial nerve. Later there were further convulsion episodes, the left deficit became spastic in nature, and there was right hemiplegia. Neurological remission lasting several months was followed by a renewal of the convulsion crises. Right hemiparesis and ptosis were observed shortly before death. Necropsy showed voluminous left frontal mass (more detailed reference has already been made to this finding), which had also invaded the corpus callosum and, in part, the right frontal lobe.

Electroencephalographic changes similar to those of essential epilepsy observed by *Krump* in 40 patients with Hodgkin's disease were attributed to toxic disturbances of the nerve cells.

Encephalic damage was personally observed in a 67-year-old man with histologically demonstrated Hodgkin's disease, and with a picture of the apparent onset of undulant fever which had lasted for several months a few years before. The final stage occurred after a long period of well-being. The patient's general condition deteriorated rapidly and undulant fever reappeared together with massive axillary lymph node enlargement. The terminal picture included jacksonian type convulsions involving the upper limbs, particularly on the left side, and stupor.

Spinal cord and nerve root damage is the most typical and most frequent sign of neurological involvement in Hodgkin's disease. In the series of *Williams et al.*, this condition was present in 75% of patients with nerve symptoms.

Three syndromes must be distinguished: cord compression syndromes, isolated radicular syndromes, and cord infiltration syndromes.

In cord compression syndromes, symptoms of paralysis are preceded by a pain stage. This usually lasts for some months, though it may range from weeks to years. The initial symptoms are slight and transient, since they probably represent neuralgia caused by compression of the peripheral nerve trunks. Later, however, the picture becomes typically radicular (*Froment et al.*), with tenacious fixed pain, unilateral at first and then bilateral, and aggravated by the slightest effort. Its distribution corresponds to the lymph node districts involved in the underlying disease. Intercostal and cervicobrachial neuralgia is common, while lumbar and sciatic pains are rare.

At this stage, objective examination may be most unrewarding. At most, localized rigidity of the spine may be observed and pain may be elicited by tapping a spinous apophysis.

Pain is followed by paraplegia, usually of a spastic nature, though flaccid forms are not infrequent (*Nayrac and Goudemand*; *Thies et al.*). The onset of paraplegia is rapid. A complete picture of paralysis appeared in less than a month in three out of four cases in the series of *Froment et al.* In some cases, indeed, a few days or even a few hours may be enough for the cord deficit to appear or even become complete. Instances of the slow development of paralysis, however, have been reported (*Belloni*), and paralysis may occur without preceding pains (*Williams et al.*).

A female patient observed by *Walthard* had been mountain climbing before being confined to bed by violent back pain. A day and half later, a clear syndrome of cord section was observed. Tetraplegia due to involvement of the cervical segment of the cord appeared overnight in a case observed by *Lemierre and Augier*. Vertebral fracture and dislocation was radiologically demonstrated postmortem. In a very similar case observed by *Williams et al.* the patient died suddenly while bending over, because of symptom-free granulomatous infiltration of the second cervical vertebra, followed by its spontaneous fracture and dislocation, and resultant immediate compression of the cord. *Labauge et al.* suggest that there is a strong probability that preexisting myelomalacia, a result of vasal obliteration, is also responsible in such cases.

Paralysis is usually accompanied by signs of pyramidal irritation, and sensibility and sphincter disturbances. In spite of the rapid development of the symptoms, the clinical picture is usually that of slow cord compression.

The neurological picture may take other forms. Mention has already been made of tetraplegia in the case of high cervical compression and the possibility of cord section following sudden compression. Where the cervical lesion is low, an association of upper limb peripheral and lower limb spastic paralysis may be observed. The initial phase of epidural involvement may present as a Brown-Séquard syndrome, with paralysis of one or both limbs on the side of the lesion and dissociated anesthesia involving some ipsilateral senses and their complementary contralateral senses.

Associations of upper limb peripheral paralysis and lower limb cord compression syndromes may be the expression of various neurological changes. In case no. 9 of the series of *Thies et al.* peripheral nerve involvement of the upper limbs, with ingravescent arm and small hand muscle atrophy, was due to infiltration of the brachial plexus. The granuloma was responsible also for cord compression due to collapse of the 7th cervical and 1st thoracic vertebrae, resulting in flaccid paraparesis of the lower limbs.

Spontaneous remission of cord compression symptoms is typical of Hodgkin's disease. Pain may regress for several months (*Goormaghtigh*) or more than one year (*Boidin*). Remissions of paralysis are less common and of shorter duration.

In addition to CSF examination and myelography (which may show marked meningeal block), radiological examination of the spinal column should also be done in cases of cord compression in Hodgkin's disease, particularly when cord symptoms open the clinical picture. Changes in the vertebral bodies may be observed by this means.

It should be noted, however, that only first-order or, with some techniques, second-order bone structure changes can be observed radiographically. Radiological visualization of vertebral osteoporosis, for example, will be dependent on a 50% or higher loss of bone substance (*Turano*). The possibility that radiography of the column will not give complete and timely warning of vertebral change must be therefore be

borne in mind. In 100 cases examined postmortem by *Schinz*, 65
presented histological signs of vertebral change, whereas radiological
signs of bone lesion had been reported for only 35. Repeated examinations are therefore advisable, together with stratigraphy if required.

The radiological picture of vertebral granulomatosis (*d'Eramo and
DeGaetano*) includes signs of osteoporosis and osteolysis (sometimes
accompanied by vertebral deformities: herring-bone appearance, crushing, cuneiform fracture, usually with the apex forward) or of eburnation. Usually several vertebrae are affected and the vertebral body is the
site of choice, while the transverse and spinous apophyses are rarely
involved (*Vazquez Piera and Kasdorf*). Osteolysis and osteosclerosis may be
observed in association. Collapse of a vertebral body may be accompanied by swellings of the supporting marginal bone, which bridge the
adjacent intervertebral discs. The interspaces are usually normal.

Lymphography is also useful in cord compression, since it will indicate
the deep abdominal adenopathies which point strongly to a diagnosis of
Hodgkin's disease.

A cord compression syndrome was observed in a personal case
(*d'Eramo and DeGaetano*) of primarily mediastinal Hodgkin's disease of
about six years' standing in a 32-year-old woman. The picture included
vertebral pain, kyphosis of the first dorsal vertebrae and paralysis of the
back, abdominal, and lower extremity musculature (the latter initially
flaccid (with areflexia) and later spastic). In the spastic stage, there was
hyperreflexia, with kneecap and foot clonus and bilateral Babinski's
reflex. The abdominal reflexes were absent. Tactile and pain sensibility
was virtually nil in the affected areas, while the thermal sense was
delayed. Examination of the cerebrospinal fluid showed frank albuminocytologic dissociation. Radiography of the spinal column showed
kyphosis with vertex at D3, with deformation and decalcification of the
right half, and particularly marked involvement of the articular apophyses.

Infiltration of the lumbosacral epidural space may produce serious
radicular involvement with the characteristics of a more or less typical
cauda equina syndrome, but without cord change (so-called "isolated
radicular syndromes"). In cases of higher epidural infiltration, signs of
cord lesion are usually a more or less rapid addition to the radicular
syndrome (*Cognazzo et al.*). This is not always so, however, as in cases
reported by *East and Lightwood* (Duchenne-Erb radicular paralysis),
Parkes Weber and *Bode* (scapular pain and amyotrophy of the upper
limbs), and *Askanazy*[a] (bilateral radicular paralysis with onset in two
stages, completely free of signs of cord change, probably because
radiotherapy was employed). Survival for 15 years from the appearance

of neurological signs was reported in a case of isolated radicular syndrome in the series of *Thies et al.* (case no. 11).

Radicular symptoms unaccompanied by other neurological signs were observed in a personal case of lumbar vertebrae eburnation in a 40-year-old man (*d'Eramo and DeGaetano*). The patient had complained of severe lumbar pain radiating for some days to the right flank. Radiography showed eburnation of the lumbar vertebrae with marginal osteophytes on the bodies and reduction of the L4–L5 space.

Granulomatous infiltration of the cord is rare. Clinical pictures of intramedullary lesion without signs of compression should suggest a possible diagnosis of myelomalacia due to vascular occlusion, or aspecific paraneoplastic cord changes (see appendix to the present chapter) as alternatives to cord infiltration. With regard to circulation disturbances laterovertebral adenopathies may compress cord-supplying vessels. In the case observed by *Urecchia and Goïa* (infiltration of the funiculi posteriores and some nerve trunks of the cauda equina, with irregular degeneration of Goll's and Burdach's columns) total flaccid paralysis with sphincter disturbances, but without pyramidal signs, developed within four weeks. *Labauge et al.* have noted, however, that radicular and cord infiltration was slight in this case, and that the patient's widespread meningeal granulomatosis may have been responsible for his nerve signs. A complex neurological picture recalling that of the Brown-Séquard syndrome was observed in a case of Hodgkin's disease reported by *Boudin et al.* This consisted of left thermoanalgesic dissociated hemianesthesia (from C2, later from C5, to L4), with left areflexia and right hyperreflexia. The absence of radiological evidence of spinal change and of signs of meningeal cavity block suggested a diagnosis of intramedullary granulomatous infiltration.

The possibility of cord granulomatosis was examined in cases reported by *Kissel et al.* and *Traldi and Artusi* (cases nos. 1 and 2). Necropsy was not done in these cases or in that of *Boudin et al.*

In case no. 1 of the series of *Traldi and Artusi*, neurological involvement produced the first sign of the underlying disease. This consisted of upper and lower limb distal extremity paresthesia, particularly on the right, later accompanied by subjective sensations of cold and sudden, fleeting pain. Objective examination revealed: bilateral tendency to fall, particularly to the right; bilateral flattening of the thenar and hypothenar eminences, particularly on the right, and atrophy of the interosseal muscles; increased lower limb deep reflexes and decreased cremasteric and abdominal reflexes; very slight lower limb tactile hypoesthesia, with thermal anesthesia on the lateral surface of the legs, particularly on the right; plantar heat and pain anesthesia on the head of the 1st metatarsus; apallesthesia, with unimpaired sense of position; loss of heat and pain sensibility, though not of tactile, right fourth and fifth finger sensibility. There were no radiological signs of spinal change or signs of meningeal cavity block. The fact that this syringomyelia type syndrome responded to irradiation of the cervical and dorsal segments of the spinal column suggested a diagnosis of cord infiltration at the cervical enlargement.

A clinical picture of peripheral neuropathy with diabetes insipidus and terminal hallucinations was attributed to cord granulomatosis by *Sohn et al.* Necropsy showed infiltration of the transparent septum, fornix, hypothalamus, optic chiasm, left 5th cranial nerve, and medulla oblongata.

Involvement of the peripheral nerves is most commonly the result of compression by adenopathies, usually unaccompanied by infiltration of the nerve trunks.

Cranial nerve involvement is rare (*Roger and Olmer*), though *Williams et al.* have reported 24 personal cases (not always accompanied by necropsy data) and suggest that the 3rd, 5th, and 7th pairs are the sites of choice. The involvement of several nerves may produce complex pictures, such as cerebellopontile angle syndrome (*King and Richardson; Metzger et al.*), multiple paralysis (*Coulonjou*), and Garcinlike syndromes (*Lafon et al.*).

In a case of Hodgkin's disease of two years' standing observed by *Labauge et al.* in a 47-year-old man, a right cervical adenopathy regressed under radiation treatment but reappeared with optic neuritis and right hemiparalysis involving all but the 1st, 2nd, and 4th cranial nerves. Regression was obtained with radiotherapy, except with respect to the 6th and 12th nerves. Three years later, headache and vertigo episodes were accompanied by the reappearance of the cranial paralysis picture, together with left 6th cranial nerve paresis. Radiography showed a large, irregular jugular foramen, while the lower lip of the optic canal had disappeared, leaving it in communication with the sphenoidal sinus. Vertebral angiography showed leftward and considerable anteroposterior displacement of the basilar artery. Further radiation treatment was not tolerated, and rapid, though partial, regression of the nerve symptoms was obtained with mechlorethamine.

In this case, the radiological evidence of foramen damage on the same side as the adenopathy and the cranial paralysis, coupled with the angiographical data, suggested the possible presence of a granulomatous expanding process in the posterior cranial fossa.

In case no. 7 of the series of *Thies et al.* the radiological changes of the base of the cranium were even more apparent and included destruction of the base and dorsum of the sella turcica. The neurological picture included right oculomotor paresis, with affective disturbances and intermittent confusion. The patient, aged 63 years, had originally presented, two years earlier, left laterocervical adenopathies, followed by mediastinal and axillary adenopathies. The onset of diplopia brought the case to the attention of the writers.

Cranial nerve involvement in Hodgkin's disease is usually the result of compression of endocranial granulomatous masses, which usually originate in cervical adenopathies or peri- or retropharyngeal granulomatous infiltration. In other cases compression of cranial nerves by cervical or mediastinal adenopathies may be responsible. Involvement of the vagus and its recurrent branch is particularly common and presents as intractable, persistent coughing or hoarseness, aphonia, or tachycardia. Multiple-site nerve compression has been observed by *Gralinger* in a case with a picture of left vocal cord paralysis undoubtedly due to mediastinal adenopathies, together with right facial and soft palate deficiency; necropsy was not performed.

As in the case of radicular and cord syndromes, involvement of the cranial nerves may sometimes be followed by spontaneous remission. The fact that different peripheral cranial symptoms may be observed in individual recurrence episodes indicates that the natural history of the neurological picture may vary considerably. In a case observed by *Roger and Olmer*, regressive involvement of the right 6th cranial nerve and of the left 11th cranial nerve was followed by transient peripheral left facial paralysis and hypoesthesia of the left 5th cranial nerve.

According to *Lascelles and Burston,* spontaneous remission of cranial nerve involvement may be explicable in terms of the regression of ischemic lesions secondary to vascular thrombosis or to transient edema of the nerve trunk. These workers observed ischemic lesion of the cavernous sinus segment of the left 3rd cranial nerve in a 36-year-old woman with Hodgkin's disease whose picture had included diabetes insipidus, headache, and speech and swallowing difficulties. As mentioned earlier, this patient also presented extensive infiltration of the base of the cranium, invading the whole of the posterior fossa, as well as the infundibulum, the trigeminal ganglion depression, and a temporal lobe.

An even more unusual neurological picture was observed by *Vidal and Anselme-Martin.* This included a left Avellis and a right Tapia syndrome.

There are also optic nerve changes. *Voisin* has reported unilateral optic neuritis accompanied by dehiscence of the external wall of the foramen, leading to a spear-point appearance. Bilateral optic atrophy (primarily on the left side) was observed by *Colrat;* necropsy was not done in this case, however.

In case no. 4 of the series of *Thies et al.,* serious generalized granulomatosis with involvement of the left trigeminal nerve and right ptosis were both preceded and accompanied by serious choroid and retinal changes, which made enucleation necessary in both eyes.

Cranial nerve involvement may be associated with a sphenoidal fissure syndrome also. *Paraf and Pennez* have reported a case in which paralysis of the oculomotor nerve was followed by that of the abducent nerve, together with corneal and nasal mucosa anesthesia. A negative radiographical finding suggested the presence of granulomatous nodules blocking the ligament of Zinn, and this was confirmed at necropsy. *Suckling* observed a case in which paralysis of the abducent nerve was the only sign of a granulomatous nodule in the sphenoidal fissure.

Involvement of the spinal nerves is very frequent in Hodgkin's disease (82 out of 302 cases in the series of *Williams et al.*). The differentiation of trunk and radicular pain is often difficult, as is true in the first period of the pain phase of cord compression syndromes.

Cervical, brachial, and sciatic pain patterns mirror the distribution and course of the nerve involved. Such pain is persistent, but less intense than that observed in cancer.

Sciatic pain is usually attributable to large retroperitoneal adenopathies which are sited in the abdomen or pelvic basin and compress the sacral plexus. Alternatively, it may be caused by granulomatous osteolysis of the ischium (*Labauge et al.*) or involvement of the reticuloendothelial elements of the nerve sheath in the underlying disease (*Di Guglielmo*).

Cicala stresses the fact that the clinical picture of Hodgkin's disease may open with signs of nerve pain and that these may appear even years before the typical signs of the hemopathy. In his opinion, this pattern is very common. Sensory and motor distress may involve one or more nerves, frequently in areas where the first signs of superficial lymph node swelling appear later. Pain is continuous, but typically undulant from the outset, with 2–3 hour peaks at set periods of the day (late afternoon, evening, early night). In cases where symptoms of pain are associated with undulant fever, these appear 24–48 hours before the fever cycle, increase in intensity with the increase in temperature, and regress 24–48 hours before remission of the fever itself. Where fever is continuous or continuous with remissions, pain is persistent, with peak periods usually 24–48 hours before the fever peaks.

Lugaresi et al. observed a case in which febrile polyneuritis was the first clinical sign of Hodgkin's disease. Diagnosis of the underlying blood disease was made eight months later on the appearance of laterocervical lympth node swellings, one of which was examined histologically.

In a personal case of Hodgkin's disease in a 63-year-old man with hepatosplenomegaly, anemia, and recurrent fever episodes of about six months' standing, the radiologically demonstrated appearance of mediastinal adenopathies was accompanied by persistent hiccups, undoubtedly caused by compression and irritation of the phrenic nerves. Histological signs of typical granulomatous changes in a superficial adenopathy in the right groin led to a diagnosis of Hodgkin's disease.

In another personal case (*d'Eramo and DeGaetano*), the onset of frank clinical signs of lymphogranulomatosis of about three months' standing was preceded, one year earlier, by lumbar and sacral pain and sciatica, followed by cervical pain and slight pain at the knees. Objective examination showed that pain could be elicited by pressure on the spinal column and the sacroiliac joints, particularly on the right. Radiography showed slight decalcification and osteolysis of the left iliac ala, together with osteolysis of the sacrum and of the posterior arch of the right 5th rib.

Involvement of the laterovertebral sympathetic system has sometimes been noted. This is due to adenopathy compression and appears in the form of a Horner's syndrome, sometimes associated with Raynaud type disturbances. Involvement of the brachial plexus may appear as Pancoast's syndrome picture (*Laus and Treves*).

Herpes zoster is more common in Hodgkin's disease than in other systemic hemopathies. The 34 cases collected by *Ravetta* in 1941 showed no marked sex frequency, though a large percentage of subjects were between 20 and 40 years of age. Other reported frequencies for this complication include: 13.04% (*Baldridge and Awe*); 5.3% (9 out of 170 cases) (*Kuentz*); 6% (13 out of 212 cases) (*Belloni*); 4% (16 out of 403 cases) (*Thies et al.*); 4.6% (*Heine*); 18.7% (*Molander and Pack*). According to *Klima and Gött,* herpes is the most frequent neurological disturbance in Hodgkin's disease.

Herpes was generalized in two cases of the series of *Thies et al.,* whereas intercostal (6 cases), brachial (4 cases), lumbar (2 cases), and crural (1 case) sites were observed in the series of 13 cases reported by *Belloni.* The disease is commonly localized in areas corresponding to the specific Hodgkin sites (*Belloni; Patrassi and Menozzi*). In a 23-year-old student observed by *Patrassi and Menozzi,* herpes was seen in the left intercostal region, while granulomatous involvement included the corresponding mediastinal areas, in addition to pulmonary and laterocervical sites.

Herpes is generally of late onset (*Belloni; Patrassi and Menozzi; Thies et al.*) and is usually of the simple type, cases with hemorrhage or gangrene being rare. Pain is usually slight and the condition may regress (*Sokal and Firat*).

Klima and Gött have reported a case of gangrenous herpes zoster localized in the distribution area of the first branch of the trigeminal nerve. Atrophy of the optic nerve and total ophthalmoplegia were later noted. Necropsy revealed basal granulomatous meningoencephalitis.

Herpes and varicella may be associated. According to *Sokal* and *Firat,* this association will be found in 8% of Hodgkin's disease cases. These workers have observed localized herpes, herpes followed by generalized varicella, and generalized varicella without herpes. The last two forms are accompanied by poor prognosis, with mean survival times of less than one year.

The most likely explanation for the association of herpes and Hodgkin's disease, an explanation which recalls the view of *Craver and Haagensen* concerning the association of herpes in leukemia, is that granulomatous involvement of the spinal ganglia or the nervous system, or alternatively simple irritation of the posterior ganglia by neighboring adenopathy or bone lesions, favors the implantation of the herpes virus. In Hodgkin's disease, therefore, the infection may be regarded as an attack virosis, probably hematogenous, and distributed in accordance with the localization of the granulomatosis sites (*Patrassi and Menozzi*). As noted in Chapter VI, however, diminished resistance to infection certainly contributes to the onset of herpes zoster in systemic blood diseases. It should also be remembered that many data now available suggest a similarity between the herpes and the varicella virus.

The symptom picture of granulomatous lesions of the central nervous system often includes clinical signs of meningeal involvement.

Cerebrospinal fluid lymphocyte values of 360/mm³ and in six cases followed by 15/mm³ were observed by *Serebrjanik* and *Louis-Bar,* respectively, while a value of 58/mm³ was noted during the paraplegic episode of the case reported by *Urecchia and Goïa.* Involvement of the meninges is most commonly evidenced by meningeal reaction.

In very rare cases, meningeal involvement may appear as granulomatous meningitis and assume both a clinically and anatomically dominant role.

Barker has described a case of Hodgkin's disease accompanied by acute meningoencephalitis.

Headache, vomiting, photophobia, and vertigo crises of one year's standing in a case reported by *Winkelman et al.* were considered functional in nature until the appearance of lymph node swellings. The terminal picture included left hemiplegia. Necropsy showed typical disseminated granulomatosis of the meninges with areas of cerebral softening without infiltration.

Epilepsy crises and an intracranial hypertension syndrome occurred six weeks before death in a patient with Hodgkin's disease of one year's standing reported by *Wepler*. Necropsy showed considerable widespread infiltration of the basal leptomeninges and a granulomatous site in the right cerebral hemisphere.

A similar case has been observed by *Schmid*. Here Hodgkin's disease was complicated by intracranial hypertension after four years. The CSF contained 43 lymphocytes/mm³ and 1.20 g ⁰/oo albumin; three weeks before death these values had risen to 385/mm³ and 3 g⁰/oo. Necropsy showed massive granulomatous infiltration of the basal meninges.

This patient, a 30-year-old woman, had also presented Hodgkin involvement of the last thoracic and the first three lumbar vertebrae leading to a cord compression syndrome three years after the first granulomatosis symptom. Lumbar herpes zoster was also present. Ingravescent sensorium disturbances were followed by the patient's death in deep coma. In addition to severe meningeal damage, necropsy revealed widespread lymph node and visceral diffusion of the granuloma (the spleen had a porphyroid appearance and there was infiltration of the inferior lobe of the right lung). In addition to signs of vertebral change, infiltration of the basilar part of the occipital bone was noted.

In a very interesting case reported by *Gillot et al.,* meningitis in a 6-year-old boy was at first referred to tuberculosis. The CSF values were 315 lymphocytes/mm³ and 1.80 g⁰/oo albumin. Six months later, a cervical adenopathy appeared, and biopsy led to the correct diagnosis. During the following three years—the patient was still living at the time of the publication of the paper—meningeal symptoms were constantly present, together with signs of intracranial hypertension and bilateral paralysis of the abducent nerve. Albuminocytologic dissociation was occasionally noted.

In case no. 3 of the series of *Thies et al.* the symptom picture included poor general condition, septic type fever, sensorium disturbances, and marked nuchal rigidity. Small, freely mobile lymph glands were palpated in the laterocervical region. There was no enlargement of the spleen or liver. The CSF was hypertensive and the albumin value was high. Biopsy of a laterocervical lymph node confirmed the diagnosis of Hodgkin's disease.

In an important case reported by *Matera et al.* the intraoperatively observed meningeal damage consisted of massive tumor-like granulomatous infiltration of the inner surface of the dura mater. This was located in the left frontal, parietal, and temporal regions and was crushing the brain. The clinical picture had the appearance of an intracranial neoplasia (signs of intracranial hypertension, with motor aphasia and right upper limb deficit). Ventriculography showed a rightward shift of the right cerebral ventricle. The albumin content of the CSF was only slightly increased (0.40 g%oo) and there was a positive globulin reaction.

Eosinophilic meningitis was observed by *Courtenay Evans and Mc-Elwain* in a case of Hodgkin's disease with infiltration of the central nervous parenchyma, optic nerve, and spinal cord.

An intracranial site simulating Cushing's pterional meningiomas was reported by *Koulouris et al.* The tumor was localized by scanning (see below) and angiography.

As already noted, nerve complications are usually observed in the later stages of Hodgkin's disease, with the result that their diagnosis is not difficult. In the absence of a clearly defined clinical picture of Hodgkin's disease, the diagnosis of early appearing neurological forms may be assisted by the observation of individual clinical signs indicative of Hodgkin's disease (fever unresponsive to antibiotics, skin pruritus, liver and spleen enlargement, etc.). The appearance of lymph node swelling and an indicative biopsy picture will, of course, be vitally important diagnostic signs. Bronchoscopy can be employed to obtain a cylinder of lymph node tissue from tracheobronchial adenopathies. A Schiessle needle is passed via the bronchoscope into the protrusions of the tracheal wall caused by the swelling and material is removed with an aspirating syringe (*Heilmeyer*) (fig. 8).

Lymphopenia, eosinophilia, and a negative skin reaction to tuberculin are significant findings. In the case of spinal syndromes, particular importance must be attached to radiological evidence of spinal column bone changes and the lymphographic and pneumoretroperitoneal demonstration of deep abdominal adenopathies. Granulomatosis should be mooted in every instance of a spinal syndrome of obscure etiology.

In some cases, however, the complete absence of clinical guides prevents assessment of the nature of the neurological changes and diagnosis may turn solely on the operative findings (*Nonne; Gertsmann; etc.*).

With regard to differential diagnosis, the presence of neurological symptoms in Hodgkin's disease may be no more than a purely casual association between granulomatosis and neurological changes of another kind. It is possible for both Hodgkin and etiologically distinct nerve signs to coexist in the same patient.

In case no. 10 of the series of *Thies et al.,* a cord compression syndrome attributable to Hodgkin's disease was associated with prior and independent epilepsy. At the time of admission, this had led to a crepuscular state, with the result that exact interpretation of the overall nerve picture was extremely difficult.

The possibility of infection of the nerve structures must also be borne in mind. This may be the result of the immunological deficiency (see below) proper to the underlying disease, or the result of cytostatic, cortisone, or X-ray therapy. Rapidly fatal tubercular meningitis may develop (*Milliez*). In a particularly serious case of Hodgkin's disease, reported by *Borchers and Mittelbach,* the spread of specific pulmonary infiltration to the meninges occurred during radiation treatment for mediastinal granulomatosis. Cerebral and meningeal cryptococcosis with a clinical picture of pseudotumoral meningoencephalitis has also been observed (*Debré et al.; Freeman*). The possibility of infection should, indeed, be examined in every case of granulomatosis accompanied by particularly frank meningeal symptoms, especially since granulomatous meningitis is rare. Its presence will be betrayed by aspecific liquor findings, the absence of CSF bacteria, and the lack of meningeal response to antibiotic therapy.

The possibility of aspecific paraneoplastic nervous system changes must also be considered.

Where radiation treatment has been employed for spinal lesions, irradiation myelopathy is a possible consequence (*Bonduelle et al.;*

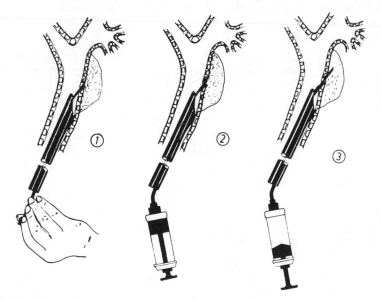

Fig. 8. Technique for the withdrawal of granulomatous tissue from tracheobronchial adenopathies: (*1*) introduction of the needle via the bronchoscope; (*2, 3*) puncture of a paratracheal lymph node (Fig. 5 in *Heilmeyer*).

Alajouanine et al.). This condition will appear as paralysis of the lower limbs. The motor deficit is often asymmetric and may be predominantly crural. Alternatively, a Brown-Séquard syndrome may be observed on the irradiation side. The anesthesia and irradiated areas may share the same upper boundary. In addition, there will be no evidence of spinal compression, that is, the manometric and myelographic findings will not indicate meningeal cavity block and albuminocytologic dissociation will not be observed.

Differential diagnosis must also assess the possibility of neurological signs secondary to treatment with vincaleucoblastine or vincrystine. The former may be followed by depression, hallucinations, and peripheral neuritis (*Keiser et al.; Vaitkevicius et al.; Gersanovich et al.*), while the latter is more frequently responsible for neurological complications, including pain and paralysis. Reversible alopecia may also be noted (*Anglesio*).

Diagnosis must also allow for the fact that the absence of alterations of the cranial bones does not exclude the presence of cerebral complications in Hodgkin's disease. These, in fact, are only rarely attributable to bone granulomatosis.

Cord compression syndromes must be distinguished from similar patterns in Pott's disease and cancer of the spine, in both of which paraplegia is commonly rapid in onset, as in Hodgkin's disease itself (*Froment et al.*). As already noted, the possibility of spontaneous symptom remission is typical of the radicular and cord syndromes observed in Hodgkin's disease.

The prognosis of Hodgkin's disease is worsened by the appearance of nerve complications, though early treatment may counterbalance this. Survivals of less than ten months were noted in three untreated patients in the series of *Thies et al.*, while 44 treated cases presented the following survival frequencies: 13 still alive at publication (in case no. 11 the neurological signs had appeared 15 years earlier); over 2 years, 3 cases; 1–2 years, 4 cases; 9–12 months, 7 cases; 6–9 months, 3 cases; 3–6 months, 1 case; 1–3 months, 3 cases; 1 month, 6 cases; unknown, 4 cases.

The association of cytostatic drugs and X-ray therapy is fundamental in the treatment of the neurological complications of Hodgkin's disease. Such treatment is particularly effective in cord compression syndromes where radiation must be begun early, in the radicular stage. X-ray treatment alone may lead to spectacular remission of both pain and paralysis, with sensory recovery usually in advance of recovery of motor function. In some cases, indeed, the radiosensitivity of cord compression syndromes may serve as a diagnostic guide to Hodgkin's disease (*Labauge et al.*). X-ray treatment produced considerable improvement in 66% of the 62 cases collected by *Williams et al.*

Mention may be made again of case no. 11 of the series of *Thies et al.* In this case granulomatosis of the upper lumbar segment of the spinal column had led to a clinical picture of radicular lesion. The patient, who received X-ray treatment, was still alive 15 years after onset of the neurological disturbances. In case no. 10 of the same series, combined cytostatic and X-ray treatment led to complete regression of a cord compression syndrome.

Cobalt therapy and cytostatics gave good results in a case of cord compression with serious vertebral change reported by *Labauge et al.* Complete sensory and motor recovery was obtained, though hyperreflexia of the lower limbs persisted. One year later the gait was completely normal and no sign of neurological damage remained.

However, radiation treatment is considered of little effect in intracranial infiltration (*Thies et al.*), though good results have been reported with telecobalt therapy (*Ascari et al.*).

It should also be remembered that the clinical signs of cerebral edema and, more particularly, intracranial hypertension may be aggravated by irradiation of the brain (*Labauge et al.*). Mechlorethamine has been found particularly effective in the treatment of cerebral sites (*Sokal and Glaser; Traldi and Artusi*). It should be noted, however, that blastomatous changes of the CNS are less responsive to cytostatic treatment than other body sites (*Borchers and Mittelbach*).

Ascari et al. also report the successful use of scintiscans to determine the site and extension of intracranial infiltration in two cases. The same technique was employed by *Gaelen and Lévitan* to demonstrate an intracranial granulomatous mass in a case of Hodgkin's disease. In this connection, the more recent paper by *Currie* and *Jardine* should be mentioned. Scanning can also be used with advantage in the investigation of spinal epidural granulomatous infiltration (*Fazio et al.*).

Large doses of cortisone may be effective in the management of nervous system changes in Hodgkin's disease.

A spectacular remission of nerve symptoms, coupled with partial normalization of the protein picture, was obtained by *Lugaresi et al.* with 300 mg hydrocortisone or 60 mg prednisolone per day in their case of polyneuritis.

In case no. 3 of the series of *Thies et al.* (granulomatous meningitis), the administration of cortisones and cyclophosphamide, was followed by defervescence, improvement of the sensory state, and regression of nuchal rigidity.

The notable effectiveness of X-ray therapy means that surgery is never mandatory in Hodgkin cord compression syndromes. (See also the recent paper by *Silverberg and Jacobs.*)

Surgical management, that is, resection, must, however, be considered in cases where the clinical picture is of intracranial neoplasia (*Matera et al.; Buckley and Warwick; etc.*).

The treatment of neurological changes in Hodgkin's disease must be begun as soon as possible to prevent the establishment of irreversible softening of the cord or brain.

As stated, long periods of remission may follow treatment of nerve signs in Hodgkin's disease. In a case of paraplegia due to epidural compression observed by *Anglesio and De Stefanis* the remission still continued four years after X-ray therapy. A continuing total absence of signs of nerve damage was noted in one case by *Schricker and Smith* three years after surgical resection and postoperative irradiation of a primary cerebral granuloma. Intermittent diplopia in the left lateral glance was the only sequela six years after resection of a Hodgkin tumor of the dura mater in a patient observed by *Williams et al.* Resection and postoperative irradiation of an intracerebral granuloma were followed by three years of well-being in a case observed by *Ljungdahl et al.*

More commonly, however, improvement is transient and recurrence (usually in situ) will be observed. This was the case in 17% of 52 patients observed by *Williams et al.* (50% within six months after the apparent cure, 50% within one year). In contrast to the ever-increasing radio-resistance of the underlying disease, a certain degree of radiosensitivity is displayed by neurological changes recurring after irradiation.

Treatment with gammaglobulins has been found useful in the management of herpes and varicella in Hodgkin's disease (*Sokal and Firat*). In these cases any treatment leading to further loss of immuno-logic status must be avoided. This is also true for associations of herpes and other systemic blood diseases.

Appendix. Para-Hodgkin neurologic syndromes

Aspecific, paraneoplastic nerve system signs are observed in Hodg-kin's disease more commonly than in other systemic hemopathies. These signs have also been called "para-Hodgkin syndromes" (*Gravelau et al.*). Such syndromes have various forms of clinical expression and normally arise in the course of an already diagnosed and treated case of Hodgkin's disease. Anatomical examination of the nerve structure will show demyelinization, without signs of compression on the part of granulomatous neoformations, infiltration, or softening or degeneration of vascular origin. The influence of radiation treatment is excluded by the history of the case and the anatomical and histological data.

The etiopathogenesis of paraneoplastic changes of the nerve system in the course of systemic blood diseases is still obscure. *Gravelau et al.* consider these conditions as processes "whose nature and mechanism are as yet a complete mystery." Several theories have been put forward. The presence of a neurotoxic factor has been suggested and the appearance of systemic anatomicoclinical features has been related to the susceptibility of the nerve structure to the noxa. In the case of leukemia, neurotoxic substances of this type might be released by the white cells during the cytolytic process induced by treatment, with the result that neurological symptoms appear at the same time as clinical and hematological improvement of the underlying disease (*Privitera and Fiorini; Olmer et al.; etc.*). Alternatively, in both leukemia and other systemic blood diseases, the proliferation of hematopoietic tissue might be an abnormal metabolic process resulting in the release of metabolites that are directly toxic to the nerve structures. Hemoblastic proliferation may also be responsible for the withdrawal of substances or enzymes that are indispensable to normal metabolism of the nerves. There is, indeed, an undeniable morphological similarity between paraneoplastic changes of the nerve system observed in systemic hemopathies and changes observed in pernicious anemia. It has been suggested also that a congenital or acquired metabolic abnormality of the body as a whole may be responsible for both the blood disease and the neurological syndrome.

The possibility of autoimmunological processes, or virus damage (*Waksman and Adams*) to the nerve structure favored by immunological deficiency, has been suggested. With respect to the nature of such a virus, some workers claim that both the blood disease and the neurological changes are attributable to a common virus. Note the findings of *Stochdorph,* reported by *Bodechtel et al.,* and those of *Dolman et al.* In electron microscope studies of cases of "progressive multifocal leukoencephalopathy," these workers noted presumably viral particles of the polyoma virus type in the oligodendroglial nuclei (see also *Morecki and Porro*). The high incidence of paraneoplastic nervous system changes in Hodgkin's disease lends force to the possibility that immunological factors may play a particular pathogenetic role in these morbid conditions. Hypoergia is a known feature of Hodgkin's disease and tends to be more apparent in the advanced stages. The immunological deficiency is attributable to a decrease in the number of small lymphocytes characteristic of the disease, though *Miller* thinks that the true explanation is that part of the cells are unable to carry out their function in the environment created by Hodgkin's disease. Other workers consider that the lymphoreticular tissue, the site of specific antibody synthesis under normal conditions, suffers a qualitative alteration in its function in Hodgkin's disease and produces antibodies that damage the host organism tissues.

German workers (*Oppenhein; etc.*), some as early as the nineteenth century, were the first to suggest the possibility of nonmetastatic changes in the nervous system in the course of visceral neoplasia. Since 1948, this view has been established in a number of observations (*Denny-Brown; Wyburn-Mason; Henson et al., etc.*). The question of aspecific neuropathies in systemic blood diseases was first examined in 1958 by *Åström et al.* These workers presented precise personal anatomical and clinical data and gave a different interpretation of the earlier cases. They also coined the term "progressive multifocal leukoencephalopathy" for the most serious of these forms.

Para-Hodgkin nerve diseases may be clinically divided into encephalic, cord, and peripheral syndromes.

Sixteen reports of encephalic syndromes may be seen in the literature (*Winkelman et al.; Bateman et al.; Christensen and Fog; Åström et al.; Cavanagh et al.; Dolman and Cairns; Gallai et al.; Kerneis and Durieux; Deep et al.; Castaigne et al.; Goldhammer and Braham; Morecki and Porro; Silingardi et al.*). These fall within the picture of "progressive multifocal leukoencephalopathy."

Usually the clinical symptoms are observed in subjects of about 50 years of age, though patients with lymphatic leukemia may be aged 70 years. The picture is one of widespread, but asymmetric, cerebral hemisphere damage. The onset is insidious and the course of the disease is subacute and progressive, usually unaccompanied by signs of intracranial hypertension (*Labauge et al.; Boudin*). The first symptoms may be focal (progressive hemiplegia, hemianesthesia, aphasia, hemianopsia, vision and gait disturbances) or indicative of more widespread cerebral involvement (change in behavior, apathy, mental confusion). Headache may be present sometimes and is a second-level sign. The various neurological disturbances worsen within the space of a few days or a few weeks. Focal signs are usually associated with confusion and progressive intellectual deterioration. In this stage, the patient is confused and uninterested, with major memory and language disturbances; agitation is rare. The reflexes are accented at first, but tend to become weak. Bilateral Babinski's reflex is common and sphincter disturbances may be noted. Vision disturbances include: diplopia, paralysis of the oculomotor muscles, blindness, deviation of the head and eyes, etc.

Remissions do not take place and the patient's condition gets more or less rapidly worse, passing from confusion and dementia to coma. Death usually occurs three to four months from the appearance of the first symptoms.

With the exception of the case reported by *Castaigne et al.*, convulsions have not been observed; decerebration has not been reported.

The electroencephalographic picture includes serious, widespread, though aspecific, changes which may be either anterior or both anterior and posterior.

Dermatomyositis was present in the case of leukoencephalopathy observed by *Deep et al.* These workers refer both the brain and the muscle signs to an autoimmunological mechanism secondary to the blood disease.

The anatomic findings display a process of cerebral demyelinization, which proceeds from small, often perivasal, islets, usually with indistinct borders, varying in diameter from the size of a pin's head to several millimeters. These are disseminated in the brain's white matter, but often show a preference for the subcortical zone. These sites tend to group together and thus, in most cases, are seen as large softening sites, sometimes with a gelatinous appearance. These changes are bilateral, though one side may be primarily affected. The cerebral trunk and the cerebellum are usually unimpaired.

Histological examination discloses a continuous series of myelin and cell lesions, apparently as successive stages of a single pathological process. The smallest changes consist of tiny perivasal microglial masses, unaccompanied by visible alteration of the myelin. Signs of demyelinization appear later. These form small islands, whose border is composed of numerous polymorphous microglial cells, proliferating astrocytes, and basophile nuclei. The nuclei are thick and rounded. They are of a very particular type and are probably derived from the oligodendroglia. Giant astrocytes, with multiple or bizarre nuclei, are observed in the middle of the more voluminous lesions, surrounded by numerous macrophages and with a background of fibrillar gliosis. Within the lesions, the axons are usually unimpaired, whereas their number is reduced in coalescent lesions. In subcortical lesions, the neurons are generally undamaged. As a rule, no inflammatory lesions are observed. Vasal changes are minimal (swelling of the endothelium, neoformation of capillaries) and thrombosis is never observed.

A clinical picture of progressive, widespread cerebral damage, originally diagnosed as virus encephalitis, was observed by *Kaufman* in a 61-year-old man with anatomicohistologically demonstrated Hodgkin's disease. The nerve system showed no signs of demyelinization, but the microscopic data showed widespread granulomatous infiltration of the cerebral meninges, the cerebral trunk, the cerebellum, the cord, and the dorsal roots of the spinal nerves. This case was also complicated by a typical Guillain-Barré syndrome and diabetes insipidus.

The clinical picture of para-Hodgkin cord syndromes is that of transverse myelitis. As can be seen from the extensive case material (*Allan and Blacklock; Shapiro; Aubry et al.; Beresford and Mac Letchie; Pakesch and Vinazzer; Hutchinson et al.*) these conditions seem typical of Hodgkin's disease itself, whereas they are particularly rare in ordinary neoplasia. The example observed by *Lhermitte* in cancer of the esophagus is the only case reported by *Gravelau et al.* The sexes are equally represented and the age of the patients ranges from 32 to 44 years.

Signs of cord involvement are usually noted one to seven years after the onset of the granulomatous disease. The neurological syndrome quickly takes shape, usually within a few days or a few weeks. In the case observed by *Hutchinson et al.,* on the other hand, two stages were observed, separated by a period of ten months, in which the symptom picture remained stationary. The most common initial signs are paresthesia and weakness of the lower limbs. This is followed by flaccid paraplegia, with areflexia and anesthesia, the upper limit of which is the mid-dorsal region. Lastly, sphincter disturbances are noted and eschar rapidly appears. Flaccid paraplegia may be preceded by a short period of spasticity (*Beresford and Mac Letchie*). Sensibility and sphincter disturbances may be absent (*Aubry et al.*). Both *Allan and Blacklock* and *Pakesch and Vinazzer* observed a gradual rise in the upper limit of sensibility disturbances accompanied, in the latter case, by respiratory paralysis. The CSF may show a slight increase in protein and cell content (0.80 g $^o/oo$ and 8/mm^3, *Hutchinson et al.*). Death occurs within 1–12 months.

The cord lesions are clearly segmentary and correspond to one or two vertebral bodies, though occasionally several sectors are involved and disseminated lesions are observed; in the case studied by *Pakesch and Vinazzer*, the cervical, dorsal, and lumbar segments were involved. The picture is one of necrotizing myelitis, though neither vascular nor tissue inflammation reactions are observed. The white matter is primarily involved: vacuolization, fragmentation myelin, on some occasions glial reaction (groups of microglial cells, astrocyte gliosis), and the presence of granular bodies may be observed. The axons are involved to a greater or lesser degree. The gray matter is also involved, particularly the motor cells of the anterior gray column. Considerable demyelinization of the funiculi is noted above and below the malacic area.

Para-Hodgkin peripheral neurological syndromes may be divided into sensory, motor, and combined sensory and motor forms. This classification must not be interpreted too strictly, however, since minor motor signs may be noted in the sensory forms.

These syndromes are usually observed in the course of an already diagnosed and treated granulomatosis, usually one to four years after its onset. In exceptional cases, they may form the initial sign of the hemopathy, as in a case of sensory neuropathy reported by *Gravelau et al.*, in which nerve disturbances appeared six months before the typical granulomatosis symptoms. The natural history progresses rapidly and death occurs within a few months.

The sensory forms recall the picture of neurological damage described by *Denny-Brown* in a case of bronchial carcinoma. The subjective symptom picture consists of paresthesia, dysesthesia, deep pain, a sense of visceral construction, and bizarre sensations (e.g. permanent feeling of sand in the hands in a case observed by *Morin*). The objective picture is dominated by deep sensibility disturbances; superficial sensibility disturbances are usually distal (involvement of the hands and feet is typical); ataxia may also be observed (*Gravelau et al.*), while areflexia or hyperreflexia is constant. The motor deficit is secondary but becomes more prominent as the neurological picture develops. In a case reported by *Mannès et al.* an anterior mediastinal tumor was the only Hodgkin site. Anatomical examination showed demyelinization of the posterior funiculi and spinal roots, the lateral funiculi being less commonly involved.

In the less common motor forms, progressive muscular deficiency is observed. This involves the limbs and appears as amyotrophy and total areflexia, without sensory symptoms. The picture is similar to that of motor involvement observed by *Henson et al.* in two cases of carcinoma of the breast and one of bronchial cancer. Anatomical examination shows massive alternation of the anterior gray column cells and the anterior spinal root fibers (*Morin*).

The combined sensory and motor forms produce a picture of serious polyradiculoneuritis. The clinical picture typically includes more or less complete flaccid tetraplegia and deep and superficial sensibility disturbances (*Allen and Mercer; Cameron et al.*). Respiratory, speech, and swallowing disturbances may be observed. The cerebrospinal fluid shows a positive reaction for globulin. In the case observed by *Cameron et al.* anatomical examination showed considerable demyelinization of the spinal roots, peripheral nerves, and spinal ganglia (particularly the proximal segment), together with changes in the anterior column cells. The same case presented slight polymorphous cellular infiltration of the spinal roots and nerves, though the writers did not attribute this to Hodgkin's disease. According to *Gravelau et al.*, the fact that infiltration was of modest extent indicates that it was not responsible for demyelinization.

The clinical diagnosis of "progressive multifocal leukoencephalopathy" in Hodgkin's disease is based on the appearance of a serious and rapidly ingravescent widespread cerebral damage syndrome, usually unaccompanied by signs of intracranial hypertension, in a subject with a long history of Hodgkin's disease which had already been treated. Differential diagnosis with respect to specific Hodgkin brain changes is difficult, and *Rewcastle and Tom* advise cerebral biopsy in such cases. Diagnosis will be further complicated if, as in the exceptional case observed by *Bateman et al.*, the cerebral change occurs before the underlying disease. Here the mental, visual, and motor disturbances of the very similar clinical picture of Schilder's disease may further complicate the diagnostic problem. The case reported by *Bateman et al.*, in fact, was initially interpreted as Schilder's disease.

Para-Hodgkin transverse myelitis must be distinguished from cord infiltration and the more common compression syndromes, since radiotherapy is ineffective in myelomalacia. Normal liquor manometric data and myelographic findings are a fundamental diagnostic indicator of the para-Hodgkin cord syndrome.

REFERENCES

ALAJOUANINE, T.; CASTAIGNE, P. and GRAVELAU, J.: Un cas de myélopathie cervicale post-radiothérapique. Bull. Soc. méd. Hôp., Paris 75:239–243 (1959).

ANGLESIO, E.: The treatment of Hodgkin's disease (Springer, Berlin-Heidelberg-New York 1969).

ANGLESIO, E. and STEFANIS DE: Un caso di linfogranuloma maligno con paraplegia guarito da 4 anni. G. Accad. Med., Turin 1945:1.

ASCARI, E.; MUSSINI, C. and FERRARI, G.: Sulle localizzazioni endocraniche del linfogranuloma maligno. Minerva med. 59:3083–3091 (1968).

ASKANAZY, M.: a) C.R. Soc. Méd. Genève 10:2 (1921. b) Lymphogranulom des Knochenmarks. Zbl. allg. Path. path. Anat. 31:557–558 (1920–1921). c) Lymphogranulomatose. J. Méd., Paris 51:170 (1931).

BALDRIDGE, C. W. and AWE, C. D.: Lymphoma; study of 150 cases. Arch. intern. Med. 45:161–190 (1930).

BARKER: in Whisnant et al.

BATAINI AND ENNUYER: in Klima and Gött.

BELLONI, F.: Studio clinico-statistico sul granuloma maligno fatto su 212 casi (Ediz. Haematologica, Pavia 1957).

BERT: in Goormaghtigh.

BOIDIN: in Labauge et al.

BONDUELLE, M.; BONYGUES, P. and EL RAMI, A.: Myélopathie cervicale post-radiothérapique. Rev. neurol. 99:310–313 (1958).

BORCHERS, H. G. and MITTELBACH, F.: Neurologische Störungen bei Blutkrankheiten. Internist, Berl. 2:105–117 (1961).

BOUDIN, G.; CASTAIGNE, P. and LEMÉNAGER: Les manifestations neurologiques de la maladie de Hodgkin; déductions sur les voies nerveuses sensitives par où chemine le prurit. Sem. Hôp., Paris 26:3455–3459 (1950).

BROWDER, J. and VEER, A. DE: Lymphomatoid diseases involving spinal epidural space; pathologic and therapeutic consideration. Arch. Neurol., Chicago 41:328–347 (1939).

BUCKLEY, T. F. and WARWICK, F.: Surgical management of intracranial Hodgkin's disease. J. Neurol. Neurosurg. Psychiat. 31:612–615 (1968).

CICALA, P.: Contributo alla sintomatologia nervosa del morbo di Hodgkin. Progr. Med., Naples 10:449–454 (1954).

COGNAZZO, A.; BRIGNOLIO, F. and GIVOGRE, P.: Manifestazioni neurologiche midollari in corso di linfogranuloma maligno. Min. med. 61:2027–2033 (1970).

COLRAT, A.: L'anémie éosinophilique prurigène (lymphogranulomatose); Thèse Lyon (1921).

COULONJOU, R.: Paralysie de plusieurs nerf craniens au cours d'une maladie de Hodgkin. Bull. Soc. méd. Hôp., Paris 59:253–254 (1943).

COURTENAY EVANS, R. J. and McELWAIN, T. J.: Eosinophilic meningitis in Hodgkin's disease. Brit. J. clin. Pract. 23:382–384 (1969).

CRAVER, L. F. and HAAGENSEN, C. D.: A note on the occurrence of herpes zoster in Hodgkin's disease, lymphosarcoma and the leukemias. Amer. J. Cancer 16:502–514 (1932).

CRAVER, L. F. and COPELAND, M. M.: Changes in bone in Hodgkin's granuloma. Arch. Surg. 28:1062–1086 (1034).

CURRIE, S. and JARDINE, G. W. H.: Intracranial Hodgkin's disease shown by radioisotope scan. J. Neurol. Neurosurg. Psychiat. 32:313–316 (1969).

DALLA VOLTA, A. and PATRIZI, C.: Linfogranulomatosi maligna (Vallardi, Milan 1929).

DEBRÉ, R.; LAMY, M.; NICK, J.; GRUMBACH and NORMAND, E.: Développement d'une méningite à 'torula histolytica' chez un enfant de douze ans, atteint de lymphogranulomatose maligne. Bull. Acad. nat. Méd. 130:443–449 (1946).

DESBUQUOIS, M. G.: Sur un cas de lymphogranulomatose maligne compliquée de diabète insipide. Bull. Soc. méd. Hôp., Paris 51:1355–1362 (1935).

EAST, C. F. T. and LIGHTWOOD, R. C.: Compression paraplegia in lymphadenoma. Lancet ii:807–809 (1927).

ERAMO, N. D': Le manifestazioni neurologiche nella malattia di Hodgkin. Policlinico, Sez. prat. 73:1269–1275 (1966).

ERAMO, N. D' and DE GAETANO: Le alterazioni osse nelle emopatie. S.E.U. Rome (1957).

EUGÉNIS, C.: Les manifestations cérébro-médullaires de l'adénic éosinophilique prurigène; Thèse Lyon (1929).

FAVRE, M.; DECHAUME J. and CROIZAT, P.: Les formes nerveuses de la granulomatose maligne. Étude anatomo-clinique, J. Méd., Lyon 12:757–766 (1931).

FAZIO, C.; AGNOLI, A.; BAVA, G. L.; BOZZAO, L. and FIESCHI, C.: La scintigrafia midollare. Tecnica con iniezione endovenosa di 99 mTc. Minerva med. 59:3459–3465 (1968).

FEIN, S. B. and NEWILL, V. A.: Cerebral Hodgkin's disease; case report of Hodgkin's granuloma with cerebral invasion. Amer. J. Med.,17:291–294 (1954).

FREEMAN: in Labauge et al.

FROMENT, J.; CROIZAT, P. and MASSON, R.: Des compressions radiculo-médullaires dans la granulomatose maligne. J. Méd., Lyon 19:71–86 (1938).

GAELEN, L. H. and LÉVITAN, S.: Solitary intracranial metastasis by Hodgkin's disease. Arch. intern. Med. 120:740–745 (1967).

GERSANOVICH, M. H.; DANOVA, L. A.; LABKOWSKY, B. M. ET AL.: Treatment of generalized lymphogranulomatosis and reticuloendothelioma with vinblastin. Ther. hung. 17:61–70 (1969).

GERTSMANN, J.: Beiträge zur Pathologie des Rückenmarks. Zur Frage der Meningitis serosa und serofibrosa circumscripta spinalis. Z. ges. Neurol. Psychiat. 29:97–167 (1915).

GILLOT, F.; SENDRA, L.; MARCHIONI, J. and ATTALI, A.: Maladie de Hodgkin à forme méningée. Pédiatrie 15:697–702 (1960).

GINSBURG, S.: Hodgkin's disease with predominant localisation in the nervous system. Arch. intern. Med. 39:571 (1927).

GOODHART: in Thies et al.

GOORMAGHTIGH, N.: Les complications nerveuses médullaires du lymphogranulome. Le Cancer 9:13–33 (1932).

GOWERS, W. R.: In Reynold, System of medicine, Philadelphia 5:306 (1879).

GRALINGER, J.: Lymphogranulomatose avec localisations nerveuses. Rev. méd., Liège 12:152–153 (1957).

GUGLIELMO, G. DI: Linfogranuloma maligno. In Lezioni di clinica medica e conferenze (ESI, Napoli 1949).

HALLERVORDEN. In Bumke, Handbuch der Geisteskrankheiten, Berlin 11:1063 (1930).

HECKER, H.VON and FISCHER, W.: Zur Kenntnis der Lymphogranulomatose. Dtsch. med. Wschr. 48:482–484 (1922).

HEILMEYER, L.: Nuovi problemi di diagnosi e terapia nel linfogranuloma. Fisiopatologia e clinica del sistema reticolo istiocitario (Atti delle Giornate Mediche Triestine), Trieste 1965, pp. 37–69 (Ediz. Scuola Med. Osped. Trieste, 1966). Recenti progressi nella diagnosi e terapia della linfogranulomatosi. Recenti Progr. Med. 39:439–464 (1965).

HEINE, K. M.: Zoster bei Leukose und Lymphogranulomatose. Münch. med. Wschr. 107:1038–1041 (1965).

HODGKIN, T.: On some morbid appearances of the absorbent glands and spleen. Trans. med. Soc. Lond. 17:68–114 (1832).

HUTCHISON, R.: Some disorders of the blood and blood-forming organs in early life. Lancet i:1402–1410 (1904).

JACKSON, H. JR. and PARKER, F. JR.: Hodgkin's disease; pathology. New Engl. J. Med. 231: 35–44 (1944). Hodgkin's disease; symptoms and course. New Engl. J. Med. 231: 639–646 (1944).

JOHN, H. T. and NABARRO, J. D. N.: Intracranial manifestations of malignant lymphoma. Brit. J. Cancer 9: 386–400 (1955).

KEISER, G.; BRUNNER, K. and MARTZ, G.: Klinische Erfahrungen mit VLB (Velbé), einem neuen Cystostaticum. Schweiz. med. Wschr. 92:486–493 (1962).

KING AND RICHARDSON: in Whisnant et al.

KISSEL, P.; ARNOULD, G. and HARTEMANN, P.: Lésions de la moelle épinière dans la maladie de Hodgkin. Rev. méd., Nancy 80:101–108 (1955).

KLIMA, R. and GÖTT, E.: Lymphogranulomatose. In Heilmeyer and Hittmair, Handbuch der gesamten Hämatologie, vol. V/I, pp. 122–158 (Urban & Schwarzenberg, Munich-Berlin 1964).

KOOREMAN, P. J. and HAEZ, A. J. CH.: Hodgkin's disease of the skeleton. Acta med. scand. 115:177–196 (1943).

KOULORIS, S.; LANG, E. R. and FOX, J. I.: Intracranial Hodgkins disease simulating pterional meningioma. Report of a case. Med. Ann. D.C. 38:86–87 (1969).

KRUMP, J. E.: Die Veränderungen des Hirnstrombildes bei malignen Hämoblastosen. V Kongr. europ. Gesellschaft f. Hämat., Freiburg i. Br. 1955, pp. 255–264 (Springer, Berlin-Göttingen-Heidelberg 1956).

KUENTZ, M.: Ètude statistique, clinique et thérapeutique de la granulomatose maligne. À propos de 170 observations; Thèse Lyon (1955).

LABAUGE, R.; IZARN, P. and CASTAN, P.: Les manifestations nerveuses des hémopathies. Rapport LXI Congr. Franç. de Psychiatrie et de Neurologie, Nancy 1963 (Masson, Paris 1963).

LAFON, R.; PAGÈS, P.; CAZABAN, R.; LABAUGE, R. and ABRIC, J.: Syndrome de Garcin incomplète d'origine hodgkinienne. Rev. Oto-Neuro-Ophtal. 28:230–231 (1956).

LASCELLES, R. S. and BURSTON, J.: Hodgkin's disease. Disease presenting with symptoms of cranial nerve involvement. Arch. Neurol., Chicago 7:359–364 (1962).

LAUS, S. and TREVES, B.: Sindrome di Pancoast-Tobias da linfogranuloma maligno. Rif. med. 75:718–719 (1961).

LÉJER H.; POUYANNE, H.; LÉMAN, P.; CHAUVERGNE, J.; VITAL, CL.; HOERNI, B. and VALLAT, J. M.: Maladie de Hodgkin révélée par une localisation intracranienne. Bordeaux méd. 3:113–118 (1970).

LEMIERRE, A. and AUGIER, P.: Localisations vertebrales au cours d'une lymphogranulomatose maligne. Luxation de la colonne cervicale avec brusque compression de la moelle.
Ann. Anat. path. 8:916–922 (1931).
LJUNGDAHL, I.; STRANG, R. R. and TOVI, D.: Intracerebral Hodgkin's granuloma. Report
of a case and review of the literature. Neurochirurgia, Stg. 8:113–118 (1965).
LOUIS-BAR, D.: Sur les manifestations cérébrales de la lymphogranulomatose maligne et le
problème de l'encéphalite lymphogranulomateuse. J. belge Neurol. Psychiat. 47:703–
728 (1947).
LUGARESI, E.; TASSINARI, C. A. and GHEDINI, G.: Complicanze neurologiche in corso di
emopatie a carattere iper-displastico. Minerva med. giuliana 3:88–90 (1963).
MATERA, R.; CLAVIJO, J. and COHEN, J.: Hodgkinioma (localización meningocerebral a
forma tumoral de la enfermedad de Hodgkin). Rev. brasil. Cir. 42:221–230 (1961).
METZGER, D.; DANY, A.; THOMAS, C.; HOLDERBACH, L. and KEMPF, Y.: Syndrome
unilatéral de l'angle ponto-cérébelleux dans un cas de maladie de Hodgkin. Rev. Oto-
Neuro-Ophtal. 28:112–114 (1956).
MILLIEZ: in Labauge et al.
MOLANDER, D. W. and PACK, G. T. Hodgkin's disease (C. Thomas, Springfield, Ill. 1968).
MURCHISON, C. and SANDERSON, W.: Case of 'Lymphadenoma' of the lymphatic system,
liver, lungs, heart and dura mater. Trans. Path. Soc. Lond. 21: 372 (1870).
NAYRAC, P. and GOUDEMAND, M.: Les complications nerveuses de la maladie de Hodgkin.
Rev. Prat., Paris 7:1885–1889 (1957).
NONNE, M.: Weitere Erfahrungen zum Kapitel der Diagnose von komprimierenden
Rückenmarkstumoren. Dtsch. Z. Nervenheilk. 47/48:461 (1913).
PARAF and PENNEZ: in Labauge et al.
PARKES WEBER, F. and BODE, D.: A case of abdominal lymphogranulomatosis maligna
(Hodgkin's disease) with high blood eosinophilia and lymphogranulomatous infiltra-
tion of the epidural fat. Lancet ii:806–807 (1927).
PATRASSI, G. and MENOZZI, L.: Il linfogranuloma maligno. Aspetti clinici insoliti. Gaz. san.,
Milan 31:83–92 (1960).
PELLÉ and MASSOT, H.: Un cas de granulomatose maligne à détermination vertébrale
primitive. (Forme pseudo-pottique de la maladie de Hodgkin). Bull. Soc. méd Hôp.,
Paris 55:372–378 (1939).
RAVETTA, M.: Erpes zoster nel decorso del linfogranuloma maligno. Haematologica
23:1303–1318 (1941).
REWCASTLE, N. B. and TOM, M. I.: Non-infectious granulomatous angiitis of the nervous
system associated with Hodgkin's disease. J. Neurol. Neurosurg. Psychiat. 25:51–58
(1962).
ROGER and OLMER: in Labauge et al.
ROMITI: in Balbi, M. and Bressi, D.: Localizzazioni scheletriche nel linfogranuloma
maligno. Radiologia 10:439–446 (1954).
SCHINZ, H. R.: Trattato di roentgendiagnostica; vol. II, p. 603 (Abruzzini, Rome 1952).
SCHMID, M.: Ein Fall von haematogener meningoencephaler Lymphogranulomatose.
Schweiz, Z. Path. Bakt. 20:769–775 (1957).
SCHÖPE, M.: Zur Frage 'Blastom-Encephalitis'. Arch. Psychiat. Nervenkr. 109:755–784
(1939).
SCHRICKER, J. L. and SMITH, D. E.: Primary intracerebral Hodgkin's disease. Cancer,
Philad. 8:629–633 (1955).
SEREBRJANIK, B.: Lymphogranulomatöse Meningo-Encephalitis und Polyradiculitis. Dtsch.
Z. Nervenheilk. 129:103–130 (1933).
SICARD, J. A.; COSTE; BELOT, J. and GASTAUT: Aspects radiographiques du cancer
vertébral. J. Radiol. Électrol. 9:353–382 (1925).
SILVERBERG, I. J. and JACOBS, E. M.: Treatment of spinal cord compression in Hodgkin's
disease. Cancer, Philad. 27:308–313 (1971).
SOHN, D.; VALENSI, Q. and MILLER, S. P.: Neurologic manifestations of Hodgkin's disease.
Intracerebral Hodgkin's granuloma. Arch. Neurol., Chicago 17:429:436 (1967).

SOKAL, J. E. and FIRAT, D.: Varicella-Zoster infection in Hodgkin's disease. Clinical and epidemiological aspects. Amer. J. Med. 39:452–463 (1965).

SOKAL, J. E. and GLASER, G. H.: Unusual neurologic syndrome in Hodgkin's disease. Ann. intern. Med. 44:1250-1259 (1956).

SPARLING, H. J. and ADAMS, R. D.: Primary Hodgkin's sarcoma of brain. Arch. Path. 42:338–344 (1946).

SPARLING, H. J.; ADAMS, R. D. and PARKER, F.: Involvement of nervous system by malignant lymphoma. Medicine, Balt. 26:285–332 (1947).

STERNBERG, C.: Die Lymphogranulomatose. Klin. Wschr. 4:529–534 (1925).

STORNIELLO, G. and SALVATI, F.: Rara localizzazione encefalica del linfogranuloma di Hodgkin. Riv. Anat. pat. Oncol. 24:457-475 (1963).

SUCKLING: in Labauge et al.

THIES, H.; KIEFER, H. und NOETZEL, H.: Die neurologischen Komplikationen bei maligner Lymphogranulomatose. Dtsch. med. Wschr. 86: 1908–1917 (1961). Die neurologischen Komplikationen bei maligner Lymphogranulomatose. Dtsch. med. Wschr. 86:1952–1956 (1961).

TRALDI, A. and ARTUSI, T.: Sulle localizzazioni nervose centrali della linfogranulomatosi maligna. Contributo clinico-terapeutico. Minerva med. 56:4348–4352 (1965).

TURANO: in Galli, G. and Capello, A.: Rilievi radiologici sullo scheletro in alcune emopatie. Minerva ortop. 6:542–544 (1955).

UEHLINGER, E.: Über Knochen-Lymphogranulomatose. Virchows Arch. path. Anat. 288:36–118 (1933).

URECCHIA, C. I. and GOÏA, I.: Contribution à l'étude de la lymphogranulomatose de la moelle. Presse méd. 35:179–181 (1927).

VAITKEVICIUS, V. K.; TALLEY, R. W.; TUCKER, J. L. JR. and BRENNAN, M. J.: Cytological and clinical observations during vincaleucoblastine therapy of disseminated cancer. Cancer, Philad. 15:296–306 (1962).

VAZQUEZ PIERA, L. A. and KASDORF, H.: Manifestaciones óseas de la linfogranulomatosis maligna. El Dia med. uruguayo 20, No. 240 (1953).

VERDA, D. J.: Malignant lymphomas of spinal epidural space. Surg. Clin. N. Amer. 24:1228–1224 (1944).

VIDAL and ANSELME-MARTIN: in Labauge et al.

VOISIN, M. J.: Atrophie optique d'origine canaliculaire au cours d'une maladie de Hodgkin, Rev. neurol. 81:749–751 (1949).

WALTHARD, K. M.: Rückenmarkserweichung bei Lymphogranulom im extraduralen spinalen Raum; Lymphogranulom des Uterus als Nebenbefund. Z. ges. Neurol. Psychiat. 97:1–19 (1925).

WEIL, A.: Spinal cord changes in lymphogranulomatosis. Arch. Neurol., Chicago 26:1009–1026 (1931).

WEPLER, W.: Über lymphogranulomatöse Meningoencephalitis. Virchows Arch. path. Anat. 323: 49-59 (1953).

WHISNANT, J. P.; SIEKERT, R. G. and SAYRE, G. P.: Neurologic manifestations of lymphomas. Med. Clin. N. Amer. 40:1151–1161 (1956).

WILLIAMS, H. M.; DIAMOND, H. D.; CRAVER, L. F. and PARSONS, H.: Neurological complications of lymphomas and leukemias (C. Thomas, Springfield, Ill. 1959).

WINKELMAN, N.W.; MATTHEW, T. and MOORE, T.: Lymphogranulomatosis (Hodgkin's disease) of the nervous system. Arch. Neurol., Chicago 45:304–318 (1941).

ZIEGLER, K.: Die Hodgkin'sche Krankheit (G. Fischer, Jena 1911).

Appendix. Para-Hodgkin neurologic syndromes

ALLAN, G. A. and BLACKLOCK, J. W. S.: Hodgkin's disease with paraplegia. Glasgow med. J. 103: 115–121 (1925).

ALLEN, I. M. and MERCER, J. O.: Spinal symptoms with lymphadenoma. J. Neurol. Psychopath. 17:1–15 (1936).

ÅSTRÖM. K. E.; MANCALL, E. L. and RICHARDSON, E. P.: Progressive multifocal leukoencephalopathy. A hitherto unrecognized complication of chronic lymphatic leukaemia and Hodgkin's disease. Brain 81:93–111 (1958).

AUBRY, LAFFARGUE and PORTIER: Myelose funiculaire à la période terminale d'une lymphogranulomatose maligne. Sang 19: 481–491 (1948).

BATEMAN, O. J.; SQUIRES, G. and THANNHAUSER, S. J.: Hodgkin's disease associated with Schilder's disease. Ann. intern. Med. 22:426–431 (1945).

BERESFORD, O. D. and MAC LETCHIE, N.C.B.: Hodgkin's disease; unusual case with spinal symptoms. Brit. med. J. ii:136–137 (1948).

BODECHTEL, G.; BORCHERS, H. G. and KOLLMANNSBERGER, A.: Enzephalopathie bei Blutkrankheiten. Dtsch. med. Wschr. 91:673–682 (1966).

BOUDIN, G.: Les syndromes neurologiques paranéoplasiques; in Les syndromes paranéoplasiques. Rapport XXXV Congr. Franç. de Médecine, Paris 1965, pp. 13–47 (Masson, Paris 1965).

CAMERON, D. C.; HOWELL, D. A. and HUTCHISON, J. L.: Acute peripheral neuropathy in Hodgkin's disease. Neurology, Minneap. 8:575–577 (1958).

CASTAIGNE, P.; BUGE, A.; ESCOUROLLE, R. and BERGER, B.: Leucoencéphalopathie multifocale progressive avec lésions corticales associées à un sarcome hodgkinien. Rev. neurol. 112:143–146 (1965).

CAVANAGH, J. B.; GREENBAUM, D.; MARSHALL, A. H. and RUBINSTEIN, L. J.: Cerebral demyelination associated with disorders of the reticuloendothelial system. Lancet ii: 524–529 (1959).

CHRISTENSEN, E. and FOG, M.: Case of Schilder's disease in adult with remarks to etiology and pathogenesis. Acta psychiat. scand. 30:141–154 (1955).

DEEP, W. D.; FRAUMENI, J. F.; TASHIMA, C. K. and McDIVITT, R.: Leukoencephalopathy and dermatomyositis in Hodgkin's disease. A case report. Arch intern. Med. 113: 635–640 (1964).

DENNY-BROWN, D.: Primary sensory neuropathy with muscular changes associated with carcinoma. J. Neurol. Neurosurg. Psychiat. 11:73-87 (1948).

DOLMAN, C. L. and CAIRNS, A. R. M.: Leukoencephalopathy associated with Hodgkin's disease. Neurology, Minneap. 11:349–353 (1961).

DOLMAN, C. L.; FURESZ, J. and MACKAY, B.: Progressive multifocal leukoencephalopathy. Two cases with electron microscopic and viral studies. Canad. med. Ass. J. 97:8–12 (1967).

GALLAI, M.; ECKHARDT, S. and AMBROZY, G.: A case of progressive multifocal leukoencephalopathy associated with Hodgkin's disease. Ideggyogy Szele 15:257–264 (1962).

GOLDHAMMER, Y. and BRAHAM, Y.: Neurological complications of Hodgkin's disease. Harefuah 72:50–52 (1967).

GRAVELAU, J.; POURQUET, P. and MORIN, M.: Manifestations neurologiques para-hodgkiniennes. Deux observations anatomo-cliniques. Sem Hôp., Paris 37:1500–1506 (1961).

HENSON, R. A.; RUSSELL, D. S. and WILKINSON, M.: Carcinomatous neuropathy and myopathy; a clincial and pathological study. Brain 77:82-121 (1954).

HUTCHINSON, E. C.; LEONARD, B. J.; MAUDSLEY, C. and YATES, P. O.: Neurologic complication of reticuloses. Brain 81:75–92 (1958).

KAUFMAN, G.: Hodgkin's disease involving the central system. Arch. Neurol., Chicago 13: 555–558 (1965).

KERNEIS, W. J. and DURIEUX, J.: Hodgkinian papillary cystadenolymphoma in the course of Hodgkin's disease with tuberculous antecedents and paraneoplastic terminal encephalic syndrome. Arch. Anat. Path. 10:99–104 (1962).

LABAUGE R.; IZARN, P.; and CASTAN, P.: Les manifestations nerveuses des hémopathies. Rapport LXI Congr. Franç de Psychiatrie et de Neurologie, Nancy 1963 (Masson, Paris 1963).

MANNÈS, P.; DERRIKS, R.; DELPORTE, F. and DEMEES, J.: Maladie de Hodgkin à forme de tumeur isolée du mediastin antérieur avec neuropathie sensitive de Denny-Brown. Lille méd. 10:111–115 (1965).

MILLER, D. G.: Hodgkin's disease, lymphosarcoma and chronic lymphocytic leukaemia. In Samter and Alexandre, Immunological diseases (Churchill, London 1965).

MORECKI, R. and PORRO, R. S.: Progressive multifocal leukoencephalopathy—Identification of virions in paraffin-embedded tissues. Arch. Neurol., Chicago 22:253–258 (1970).

MORIN: in Labauge et al.

OLMER, J.; MOUREN, P.; CARCASSONNE, Y. and GOSSET, A.: Chlorome avec manifestations neurologiques multiples, transitoirement améliorées par la thérapeutique. Marseille méd. 99:586–590 (1962).

OPPENHEIN: in Gravelau et al.

PAKESCH, F. and VINAZZER, H.: Zur Frage der spinalen Veränderungen bei Morbus Hodgkin. Wien Z. Nervenheilk. 4:204–209 (1952).

PRIVITERA, A. and FIORINI, W. A.: Atrofia muscolare mielogena in decorso de linfoadenosi leucemica. Boll. Soc. Med. Chir., Cremona 15:93–100 (1961).

REWCASTLE, N. B. and TOM, M. I.: loc. cit.

SHAPIRO, P. F.: Changes of spinal cord in Hodgkin's disease; report of two cases, with unusual skin manifestation in one. Arch. Neurol., Chicago 24:509–524 (1930).

SILINGARDI, V.; ASCARI, E. and PATRIGNANI, A.: A survey of the occurrence of neurological manifestations in 487 cases of Hodgkin's disease. Abstract, vol. XIII, Int. Congr. of Hematology, Munich 1970, p. 254 (Lehmanns, Munich 1970).

STOCHDORPH: in Bodechtel et al.

WAKSMAN, B. H. and ADAMS, R. D.: Infectious leukoencephalitis. A critical comparison of certain experimental and naturally-occurring viral leukoencephalitides with experimental allergic encephalomyelitis. J. Neuropath. exp. Neurol. 21:491–518 (1962).

WINKELMAN, N. W.; MATTHEW, T. and MOORE, T.: Lymphogranulomatosis (Hodgkin's disease) of the nervous system. Arch. Neurol., Chicago 45:304–318 (1941).

WYBURN-MASON, R.: Bronchial carcinoma presenting as polyneuritis. Lancet i: 203–206 (1948).

Chapter IX

NEUROLOGICAL SYMPTOMS IN SARCOIDOSIS

Sarcoidosis (Besnier-Boeck-Schaumann's disease) appears to have been first described as Mortimer's disease (from the name of the patient) by *Hutchinson* in 1869. Twenty years later, *Besnier* described a tuberculosis-like dermatosis which he called "lupus pernio" or "asphytic lupus." In 1897, *Boeck* reported a subcutaneous nodular infiltration syndrome and coined the term "sarcoids" for the nodules due to their similarity to sarcomas and leukemic infiltration. He later described sarcoid changes of the mucosa. In 1917 *Schaumann* demonstrated that Besnier's lupus pernio and Boeck's sarcoid were histologically indentical and stressed the fact that other organs besides the integument were involved. In 1919 he proposed the name "benign lymphogranulomatosis" to distinguish the disease from malignant granuloma. *Kuznitzky and Bittorf* had reported lung sites for the disease in 1915, while skeletal sites had been reported as early as 1902 by *Kienbock*; these were fully studied as "ostitis multiplex cystoides" by *Jüngling* in 1919. The first monograph on sarcoidosis is the exhaustive study of *Pautrier* (1940). More recent studies include those of *Löfgren, Turiaf, and Brun* (on intrathoracic sites of the disease), *Barièty and Poulet; Dragoni; Lebacq;* and *Hoppe.* Note also the recent works of *Daddi et al.* and *Miglioli* on pulmonary sarcoidosis.

The typical features of sarcoidosis have been described by the U.S. National Research Council as follows. Sarcoidosis is a systemic granulomatous affection whose etiology and pathogenesis are still unknown. The superficial and mediastinal lymph nodes, lungs, liver, spleen, skin, eyes, phalanges, and parotid glands are most commonly involved, though other organs and tissues may be affected. The *Kveim* test is often positive (local sarcoid nodules are observed from four to six weeks following intradermal injection of sarcoid tissue extracts). Tuberculin anergy is frequent. Other important laboratory data include increases in serum globulins and urinary excretion of calcium. The histological picture is characterized by the finding of epithelioid tubercules with little or no signs of necrosis. This finding, however, is not pathognomonic,

179

since it is observed in noncaseous tuberculosis, fungus infection, berylliosis, and local sarcoid reactions. Diagnosis will depend on the correlation of compatible clinical findings with a positive Kveim test or biopsy showing histological changes of the type described.

The epithelioid granuloma is composed of partially confluent nodules or tubercules consisting primarily of epithelioid cells of histiocyte origin, Langhans cells (with or without inclusions: asteroid bodies, Schaumann bodies) probably originating in the fusion of epithelioid cells (*Wanstrup and Christensen*), scattered lymphocytes, plasma cells, and peripheral layers of fibroblast. A crown of lymphocytes may be observed. As already mentioned, epithelioid granuloma is not pathognomonic for sarcoidosis, since it may be found in certain bacterial disease (brucellosis, leprosy) and in some cases of malignant granuloma, in addition to the diseases already mentioned. With respect to local sarcoid reactions, it should be remembered that they may occur in lymph nodes draining some form of malignant tumor.

After a time, necrosis may appear in the center of a sarcoid nodule. This is never caseous, but fibrinoid. This change was observed by *Ricker and Clark* in 100 of a series of 300 cases. Hyalinosis follows and progresses by sectors. However, the giant cells remain intact in the hyalinized areas for a long time. Lastly, widespread sclerosis of the nodule takes place as a result of thickening of the reticulum fibers. The epithelioid nodules also may be completely reabsorbed.

Early writers considered sarcoidosis to be a special form of tuberculosis. Gradually this view has been abandoned, though it is still supported by a number of writers, particularly in Germany (see the recent paper by *Kalkoff*). The alleged frequency of associations between sarcoidosis and tuberculosis is not borne out by the data in the literature. The simultaneous presence of tuberculosis has been established with certainty in only 3.1% of cases of the hemopathy (*Lebacq*). The pathogenic hypothesis most in favor today classifies sarcoidosis as an immunological disease occurring in subjects sensitive to an unidentified agent. The opinion that a single agent is responsible would seem to result from the fact that a positive Kveim test is virtually specific for sarcoidosis. This fact would at least suggest that a very limited number of pathogenic agents of similar structure are involved (*Lebacq*). As *Thibault* states, the identical Kveim test reaction observed by *Siltzbach* with American antigens in several countries in all five continents is a further indication that a single pathogenic agent is responsible. However, *Israel and Goldstein* have recently questioned the specificity of the Kveim-antigen reaction in the diagnosis of sarcoidosis.

Various features indicate the immunological nature of sarcoidosis. These include hyperglobulinemia, which may be responsible for deposits of a para-amyloid substance in the granulomatous tissue; signs of immunological deficiency, such as partial or complete tuberculin anergy and increased tolerance of homografts; the appearance of signs of allergy (erythema nodosum, uveitis, polyarthritis); the therapeutic effectiveness of cortisones.

Sarcoidosis is particularly common in the Negro. Most patients are aged between 20 and 40 years. In the case of acute forms, females are at greater risk.

Onset is often insidious and accompanied by vague symptoms. The disease is often discovered during clinical or radiographic examination carried out for other reasons. The initial symptom picture commonly includes lymph node swellings, weight loss, skin eruptions, coughing, and slight dyspnea. Slight temperature elevation may be noted, sometimes accompanied by serious asthenia.

The course of sarcoidosis is completely unpredictable. Spontaneous remission of even considerable manifestations may be noted and periods of stasis are sometimes very long. The picture may include regression and exacerbation, sometimes at long intervals, or an advance to later clinical stages.

The superficial and mediastinal lymph nodes and the lung parenchyma are the sites of choice (86% of the cases studied by *Lebacq*). A typical feature of lung involvement is the contrast observed between the mildness of the respiratory manifestation and the seriousness of the clinical findings. *Turiaf and Brun* have distinguished the following clinical and radiological forms of intrathoracic sarcoidosis: simple gangliomediastinal (without lung damage); mediastinopulmonary (with reticular type lung changes); pulmonary (reticulomiliary, macronodules, localized nodulo-infiltrating, widespread nodulo-infiltrating, localized coalescing, perihilar coalescing, mixed). Bronchial and pleural changes may be noted, particularly in the mediastinopulmonary form (*Schneider; Leitner*).

Localization in other organs is less common. In the series reported by *Lebacq*, liver involvement (41% of cases) followed lymph node and lung sites in order of frequency. Other localizations included: the skin (cutaneous sarcoids, erythema nodosum) (37%); eyes (23%); spleen (22%); heart (12%); joints (12%); nerves (11%); bones (5%); hypophysis (2%); parotid glands (2%); parotid glands and uvea (1%); muscles (1%); digestive system (1%).

Lacrimal sites have also been reported. This may be an isolated finding or may be associated with salivary gland damage (parotid and sublingual glands) (Mickulicz syndrome). Thyroid and renal involvement have also been observed.

As can be seen from the values given above, involvement of the nervous system was low in *Lebacq's* series. Similarly low frequencies were reported by *Gravesen* (7 out of 150 cases), *Ricker and Clark* (6 out of 300 cases) and *Löfgren* (2 out of 30 cases). *Goodson* is of the opinion that the nervous system is involved in from 1% to 5% of cases of sarcoidosis. His series of 63 cases (60 demonstrated by biopsy and three at necropsy) contained four instances of nerve damage and one of muscle damage. A proper assessment of the problem, however, must consider the possibility of clinically silent nerve changes. *Rudberg-Roos* examined the cerebrospinal fluid in 72 sarcoidosis patients without reference to the presence of nerve signs or symptoms. In 19 subjects liquor abnormalities were presented (increased protein and cell values), while only four of this group showed signs of nerve distress. Similarly, *Carstensen and Norvit* found abnormal liquor values in six out of 15 cases, only two of which presented neurological manifestations. It may be, therefore, that nerve structure damage is more common than the reported clinical series indicate.

Necropsy data are not more reliable, since they usually concern chronic cases and nerve changes linked to the initial phase of the disease can no longer be detected. *Ricker and Clark* found only three instances of cerebral change in a series of 22 necropsies; this may be compared with the three instances of neurological damage observed by *Askanazy* in 20 necropsies. Only 7.7% of 117 necropsy reports taken from the literature by *Branson and Park* referred to nerve system changes.

Nerve symptoms may open the clinical picture of sarcoidosis: this occurs in one out of four cases of neurological involvement according to *Garcin* and *Vic-Dupont et al.*

The leptomeninx is the site of choice, particularly at the base of the brain. Further expansion to the vessels may result in isolated or associated endarteritis, infiltration of the adventitia, rupture of the elastic membranes, thrombosis, or panarteritis (*Meyer et al.; Alajouanine et al.*[b]*; Garcin*). Vasal damage may be responsible for the intracerebral dissemination of sarcoid foci, particularly to the cerebral cortex (*Lenartowicz and Rothfeld; Alajouanine et al.*[b]), and is undoubtedly responsible for softening of the nervous system. The reported data seem to support the view of *Riser et al.*, that central nervous system (CNS) involvement in sarcoidosis should be considered true meningoangiitis.

Pictures of acute meningitis are rare. A fatal case was observed by *Naumann* in a 3-month-old child who presented acute convulsions and nuchal rigidity. Necropsy showed widespread meningeal sarcoidosis, with involvement of the leptomeninx, the falx cerebri, and the tentorium cerebelli. Subacute or chronic, pseudotumoral basal arachnoiditis is the most common clinical expression of meningeal involvement. Its course is similar to that observed in tuberculosis and Hodgkin's disease: slow development, essentially basal localization, and frequent signs of cerebral parenchyma damage. Involvement of the anterior area of the basal leptomeninx may be responsible for signs of liquor circulation block (possibly followed by hydrocephalus), coupled with damage to the hypophysis, infundibulum, and tuber, as well as ocular manifestations (*Simons and Merkel*). When the posterior area is involved, intracranial hypertension is the most important symptom, as was observed in a case of *Erickson et al*, in which necropsy revealed chronic adhesive arachnoiditis with hernia of the cerebellar tonsils. A similar picture, including the appearance over a period of two years of signs of hypothalamus involvement and bilateral papillary edema, was described by *Colover*. Surgery revealed adhesive meningitis blocking the foramina of the 4th ventricle. A posterior cranial fossa syndrome, with considerable tetraventricular hydrocephalus, was observed by *Garcin et al*. In this case, after an initial visceral stage, sarcoidosis in a 12-year-old girl was complicated by a symptom picture including vomiting, recurrent occipital headache, nuchal rigidity, disturbed static sense, horizontal nystagmus in the lateral glance, and signs of notable pyramidal damage (lower limb hyperreflexia and right Rossolimo's reflex). Puberal development was completely absent. The electroencephalogram (EEG) showed widespread, primarily right, cerebral changes. CSF protein values were high and there was considerable ventricular dilatation. Death occurred in less than one year, in spite of three neurosurgical derivations and cortisone therapy. Cortisone therapy, while effective in the visceral stage, was of no assistance in the treatment of the nerve signs. Necropsy showed distinct thickening of the intraventricular leptomeninges and infiltration of the choroid plexuses. Histological evidence of central nervous system involvement, including the typical, primarily perivasal, arrangement of the sarcoid infiltration in the brain sections, was obtained.

Meningeal damage leading to convulsion was observed in a case of lung and liver sarcoidosis by *Fazlullah* (case no. 1). There were no neurological signs of site lesions. The CSF protein value was increased.

Predominantly spinal arachnoiditis may be observed in some cases. In a typical picture reported by *Wood and Bream*, cord compression was accompanied by painful flaccid paraplegia and areflexia, together with a meningeal cavity block. Surgery showed that the otherwise normal cord was surrounded by thick arachnoidal sheaths of sarcoid type. Signs of cord compression were also observed by *Jefferson* in a case of sarcoid infiltration of the spinal leptomeninx.

Even when the meninges are not directly involved, the nerve signs of sarcoidosis are often accompanied by evidence of meningeal reaction. Out of the 118 cases collected by *Colover* 23 presented liquor changes. *Pennel* reports a frequency of liquor changes of 50%, while *Bernard* found liquor abnormalities in 25 out of 31 cases with nervous system involvement.

Dayras observed liquor cell values of 10–50/mm³ in 12 cases (50–100/mm³ in four cases and over 100/mm³ in three cases), while *Colover* has reported an all time high value of 162/mm³. Lymphocytes usually predominate. Increased CSF protein values seem to be constant (25 of the 31 cases in the series of *Dayras*). The usual value is about 1 g °/oo though values of 2 g are not uncommon (ten instances in the series of *Dayras*). Higher values are uncommon; 7.20 g °/oo (*Zahn and Weber*), 8 g °/oo (*Cares et al.*).

Very low glucose values (10–40 mg% ml) were observed in about half of the very few reported CSF determinations (*Pennel; Goodman et al.*). Apart from the possibility of cord block with its typical symptom picture, liquor pressure may be slightly increased. The colloidal gold reaction curve may show an abnormal pattern (*Goodman et al.*).

Involvement of the cranial nerves is closely related to that of the meninges. In a few cases, damage to these nerves may be a result of sarcoid adenopathies or glandular swelling (particularly of the parotids).

The facial nerve is frequently involved (in about 50% of cases with nerve signs according to *Labauge et al.*). *Matthews* is of the opinion that the most common neurological picture is that of paralysis of several cranial nerves, including the facial nerve in all cases, in acute or subacute sarcoidosis. In the 115 cases in the literature and three personal cases of *Colover* there were 36 monolateral and 22 bilateral instances of facial nerve paralysis.

Facial nerve paralysis may be accompanied also by uveoparotid involvement (*Heerfordt*'s disease). The original description of this disease by *Heerfordt* in 1909 was of an association of cranial and spinal nerve deficit, diabetes insipidus, and febrile uveoparotitis (so-called "uveo-parotid fever"). Ten years earlier, *Daireaus* had reported a case of "mumps neuritis," which was probably of a sarcoid nature. In 1923, in a paper entitled *Uveo-parotitic paralysis, Mac Bride* described a case of peripheral neuritis followed by uveoparotitis and paralysis of the 5th and 10th cranial nerves. Parotitis, Hodgkin's disease, and an unknown toxic agent were the suggested etiologies. Later instances of associations of polyneuritis and uveoparotitis have been treated as if they might have a tubercular origin. In 1937 *Waldenström* reported a case of uveoparotitis accompanied by signs attributable to damage of the cerebral trunk and cortex, the cerebellum, the meninges, and the peripheral nerves.

There is no clear nexus between paralysis of the facial nerve and the parotid alterations. Parotitis may occur a few days or a few months before or even after the facial nerve signs (*Goodson*). Compression of the nerve by the swollen gland has been postulated. In the absence of a visible gland enlargement, swelling in the stylomastoid foramen has been suggested. Loss of the sense of taste in 18% of facial paralysis cases (*Colover*), however, indicates a much more proximal localization for the lesion (*Goodson*).

Involvement of the facial nerve is usually sudden and without complications, though subsequent muscular spasms or contractures are occasionally observed. In the series of *Matthews*, however, this course was followed in four out of six cases.

Neuralgia symptoms may be evidence of facial nerve damage. In the first case reported by *Garcin*, paralysis of the right 12th cranial nerve was accompanied by neuralgia and signs of paralysis indicative of right facial nerve involvement and left suboccipital neuralgia. These symptoms formed the clinical overture of the underlying disease.

Involvement of the optic nerve was observed in 14% of the series of *Labauge et al.* This may be primary in exceptional cases (*Barbolini and Mastronardi*). *Colover* reported retinal changes in 16 of his series of 118 cases. Neuroretinitis and retrobulbar optic neuritis are the most frequent manifestations.

A case of sarcoidosis with arachnoiditis involving optic chiasm as its only clinical sign was reported by *Castorina et al.* It is known that this condition runs an intermittent course with sudden reduction of vision and concentric restriction of the visual field. Examination of the fundus oculi shows primary optic atrophy. The reported case was a 62-year-old housewife with gradual weakening of vision in the right eye (to the point of amaurosis) of about ten months' standing, and a similar symptom picture in the left eye of ten days' standing. Surgery showed the chiasm and optic nerves to be hyperemic and surrounded by arachnoid membranes. The patient died one year later in a road accident and the histological evidence was of lymphocyte infiltration of the leptomeninx at the gyrus cinguli and the gyri recti; perivasal sleeves consisting primarily of lymphocytes were observed in the corpus callosum, transparent septum, and the basal nuclei. Lymphocyte infiltration was noted also in the white matter below the right gyrus rectus. A section taken at the chiasm and optic nerves showed that the leptomeninx around the former was the site of nodular formations consisting of epithelioid and giant cells and lymphocytes. A section taken at the ashen tuber showed that the basal meninges and the floor of the 3rd ventricle were the sites of a nodular granuloma, whose individual nodules were composed of epithelioid and giant cells and accumulated lymphocytes. A large number of perivasal infiltrations were observed in the caudate and lenticular nuclei, the internal capsule, and the thalamus. The paraventricular nuclei of the hypothalamus were the sites of primarily interstitial lymphocyte infiltration. At the corpora mamillaria, infiltration of the leptomeninx and the brain was represented by a very small number of perivasal sleeves. A granuloma similar to that seen in the brain was observed in the posterior lobe of the hypophysis and in part of its anterior lobe.

Paralysis of the ocular nerves is common and often associated with disturbances of the intrinsic ocular muscle. Other ocular manifestations include uveal lesions, conjunctivites, keratoconjunctivitis sicca, inactive pain free dacryoadenitis, subacute (most common) or chronic iridocyclitis (*Lebacq*). These changes usually run a favorable course. An Argyll-Robertson-like pupil, not attributable to iritis, was observd in one case by *Matthews*. Exophthalmos due to infiltration of the orbit is not uncommon.

Ocular symptoms may be the only manifestation of the underlying disease, as in a case reported by *Alajouanine et al.*[a], in which sarcoidal infiltration had a tumor-like appearance. The picture included loss of visual acuity in the left eye, restriction of the field of vision and edema of the upper papillary border. The sarcoidal nature of a paraoptic tumor resected near the optic foramen was demonstrated histologically. One year later, a similar visual field picture observed in the right eye was improved by therapy. In this case, the ocular symptoms were isolated and correct clinical diagnosis was dependent on increased erythrocyte sedimentation rate and negative tuberculin test results.

Involvement of the other cranial nerves is less common. The series of *Colover* included 29 instances of swallowing disturbances, eight of involvement of the trigeminal nerve (facial or corneal anesthesia, pain in the trigeminal distribution district and, less commonly, bilateral paresis of the masseter muscle), seven of tongue paralysis and atrophy, two of anosmia, one of vocal cord paralysis, and one of musculus levator palati involvement.

Other workers have reported paresthesia and hyperesthesia attributable to trigeminal damage. Cochleovestibular deficiency (*Suchenwirth*) and total deafness (*Siltzbach and Greenberg*) may occur.

Associations of 9th, 10th, and 11th nerve paralysis may lead to a jugular foramen syndrome, as in a case observed by *Alajouanine et al.*[b], in which the neurological symptom picture appeared at the height of a clinical sarcoid condition.

In case no. 5 of the series of *Garcin*, involvement of the right 5th, 7th, 8th, 9th, 10th, and 11th cranial nerves was accompanied by left 11th and bilateral hypoglossus damage, right exophthalmos and bilateral blindness (of 14 years' standing in the left eye and two months' standing in the right eye). Examination revealed the presence of anterior and posterior uveitis together with sites of chorioretinitis along the venous walls. These were surrounded by inflammatory infiltration sleeves. Bone alterations were also observed. Bilateral submaxillary adenopathies appeared later and their histologic examination indicated a diagnosis of sarcoidosis. Cortisone therapy brought symptom improvement though blindness persisted.

In conclusion, then, it may be stated that the fundamental aspect of cranial nerve involvement in sarcoidosis is the presence of, usually multiple, successive or simultaneous deficiencies, whose development generally requires several years. Symptoms of paralysis are often both fluctuating and fleeting.

A typical example is case no. 1 of the series of *Garcin* in which a 50-year-old woman presented rapidly regressing attacks of right facial neuralgia. After six years the repeated episodes were accompanied by paralysis of the right 7th and 12th cranial nerves, lasting one year. About one year later, facial neuralgia was accompanied by diplopia, giddiness, and retrobulbar neuritis.

The fleeting nature of cranial nerve paralysis signs is also clearly shown in case no. 1 of the series of *Goodson*. A 32-year-old Negro woman complained of parotitis, left facial asthenia, weight loss, dysphagia, and dysarthria. Objective examination revealed left 7th, 9th, and 10th cranial nerve paralysis within a symptom picture of sarcoidosis. A neurological examination carried out three weeks later recorded partial paralysis of the 7th nerve only and this too regressed later.

Transience was a feature of all the cases of facial paralysis observed by *Silverstein et al.*

Damage to the hypothalamus and hypophysis is closely connected to damage to the meninges. The infundibulum and tuber seem to be initially involved (*Rickards and Barrets*). At a later stage the posterior hypophysis is involved via the peduncle. Specific infiltration may be seen in the intermediate part, the anterior hypophysis, and the walls of the 3rd ventricle also (*Schaumann; Raben et al.; etc.*).

Diabetes insipidus is the most frequent clinical symptom. This complication was the subject of the basic study by *Lesné et al.* (1935) and may be considered highly characteristic of encephalic sarcoidosis (20 of the 118 cases in the series of *Colover,* 20% of the series of *Jean-Girard* and 31.5% of that of *Dayras*). *Krauss* has reported a case in which this condition appeared 24 years before a clear picture of sarcoidosis. It varies in intensity from case to case and is often monosymptomatic. Its association with sometimes considerable glycosuria had been reported (*Riser et al.*).

Damage to the parotid gland may be the cause of intense thirst and may induce an erroneous diagnosis of primary polyuria (*Jean-Girard*).

Mixed hypothalamic and hypophyseal manifestations may be observed (amenorrhea, obesity, libido changes, etc.). In case no. 5 of the series of *Jefferson*, a 46-year-old man presented a picture of increasing obesity with polydipsia and polyuria, somnolence, loss of libido, sweating attacks, instability of character, and extremity tremor, terminating in fatal coma. Necropsy showed a mass which had spread from the floor of the 3rd ventricle to the anterior and middle cranial fossae, also involving the chiasm and the optic nerve. The hypophysis appeared unimpaired on gross examination. The tumor was shown to be sarcoid at histology.

Body and genital abnormalities (infantilism) are occasionally reported. An association of hypogonadism, obesity, and diabetes insipidus was reported by *Franceschetti and de Morsier.*

Invasion of the anterior lobe of the hypophysis must be considered exceptional. In a case observed by *Dérot et al.* massive infiltration of the hypophysis was responsible for terminal hypoglycemic coma.

In exceptional cases, an association of anterior hypopituitarism and diabetes insipidus may be observed. An endocrinological paradoxical association of this kind was present in a case of sarcoidosis reported by *Vic-Dupont et al.*, with a urine excretion of 14 liters per day. The signs of neurological damage in this case include: diplopia, recurrent headaches, and sensory disturbances. Two cases of sarcoidosis with diabetes insipidus and anterior hypopituitarism have been reported by *Lebacq.*

In two cases observed by *Bleisch and Robbins,* involvement of the hypophysis was not followed by any clinical manifestations.

A simple endocrinological symptomatology is rare in sarcoidosis, since such symptoms are usually associated with nerve and ocular signs, so much so, indeed, that an association of diabetes insipidus and ocular paralysis should always suggest the possibility of sarcoidosis.

Plair and Perry observed a case of hypothalamic-hypophyseal involvement with a picture of diabetes insipidus, reduced libido, hypothermia, vision disturbances, mental confusion, and convulsion episodes.

Although meningeal involvement may be followed by cerebral damage as a result of vasal alterations, direct invasion of the cerebral parenchyma may originate occasionally in the subarachnoidal space (*Goodson*).

The coalescence of sarcoid infiltrations in the brain may give rise to tumor-like formations. The clinical expression of cerebral sarcoidosis may take on a pseudotumoral or a multifocal form.

Pseudotumoral forms are not common. In a case observed by *Everts*, a sarcoid mass in the occipital lobe was accompanied by an intracranial hypertension syndrome, with hemianopsia, hemiparesis, and convulsions. In case no. 2 in the series of *Höök*, the clinical picture was marked by dementia, intracranial hypertension, and hemiplegia, followed later by coma. Surgery led to the discovery of a large granulomatous intraventricular mass involving the choroid plexuses and to a considerable improvement in the clinical picture.

In case no. 4 in the series of *Jefferson*, an intracranial sarcoid mass had been responsible for left lip corner convulsion crises over a period of four years. In case no. 6 a typical posterior cerebral fossa syndrome was referable to a granulomatous mass in the floor of the 4th ventricle.

Ventriculograms similar to those observed in cerebral neoplasia were noted by *Saltzman* in five cases of sarcoidosis.

In the case reported by *Goodman et al.* both the clinical and the radiological pictures indicated an expanding process localized in the anterior fossa. Surgery revealed a large pseudomeningioma in a subfrontal site, extending to the sinus sagittalis, the falx cerebri, and the left frontal lobe.

An interesting case was observed by *Thompson* in a 44-year-old Negro woman, who five years earlier had presented a clinical picture which included headache, left hemifacial paresthesia, asthenia, and vertigo, and was explained as slight ictus. Several months later, loss of weight and considerable decrease of muscular force were followed by episodes of nocturnal paroxystic dyspnea and outstanding effort dyspnea. Chest radiography showed infiltration of the base of the right lung, accompanied by pleural extravasation and paratracheal lymph node swelling. Hypoesthesia of the left cheek was demonstrated objectively. Glucose loading produced a diabetes type blood sugar curve. A two-month period of general improvement was followed by an episode of loss of consciousness with generalized, intermittent convulsions, primarily involving the left half of the face. This was followed by a second episode consisting of convulsions only. Cerebral angiography and pneumoencephalography gave normal findings. Thereafter convulsion episodes increased in frequency and led to terminal coma. Necropsy showed that the brain was adhering to the base of the cranium at the lower part of the left frontal lobe, while the left olfactory nerve was enclosed in a pale yellow tissue indistinctly bordering the cerebral cortex. Histological examination of the brain showed many isolated and coalescent follicles in the meninges and within the cerebral cortex, many of which had the appearance of active sarcoid lesions, while others were completely hyalinized. In other sections, the lesions were localized around the meningeal vessels, while others were found as solitary lesions within the cerebral parenchyma.

In the case reported by *Géraud et al.* the clinical picture was that of a tumor of the 3rd ventricle. Intraoperative biopsy of the thalamus was the basis for a diagnosis of sarcoidosis.

In the multifocal forms the clinical picture is determined by the various cerebral sites with the result that the symptom pattern is protean and often unclassifiable. It may include both motor and sensory signs, convulsion episodes, visual field changes, mental disturbances, and personality changes. On rare occasions, the basal nuclei are affected and a parkinsonian symptomatology is observed. *Jefferson* has reported supratentorial syndromes with signs of cerebellar damage (nystagmus, ataxia, dysarthria). Involvement of the cerebral peduncles may lead to clinical pictures simulating multiple sclerosis or angiomatous or gliomatous changes (*Jefferson*). A patient studied by *de Morsier et al.* presented a Korsakoff syndrome and flaccid tetraplegia. Necropsy showed widespread meningoencephalic infiltration with panangiitic lesions.

Reis and Rothfeld observed a 17-year-old girl with unilateral, followed by bilateral, blindness, papillary edema, optic atrophy, and exophthalmos. Right hemiataxia, pupillary signs, and pyramidal damage quickly followed. Sarcoidosis had also produced an unusual skin eruption and phalangeal lesions. A number of different changes were noted in the brain at autopsy: sarcoidal infiltration of the chiasm and optic nerves, involvement of the right gyrus rectus and the hypothalamus, malacic and granulomatous alterations of the left temporal lobe and basal ganglia, and involvement of the right caudate nucleus. Massive cerebellar lesions were also present.

An anatomically demonstrated case of cerebral damage due to multiple sarcoid tumors, with a symptom picture which included signs of hypothalamic involvement, was reported by *Robert*. An episode with the features of a decerebration syndrome was observed during hospitalization. Cerebral sarcoidosis was diagnosed from the results of intracranial needle puncture. Involvement of the lymph nodes was the only extracranial manifestation of the disease.

Camp and Frierson have reported a case of spinal cord and widespread brain damage in a 17-year-old Negro male. The neurological symptomatology developed over four years and began with headache and nervousness during sarcoidosis with a primarily lymph node clinical picture. The subsequent manifestations were variously influenced by treatment and covered a wide range: loss of memory, difficulty in studying, episodes of trunk pain, cramp-like sensations in the limbs, attacks of convulsion (the first followed by lethargy with loss of abdominal reflexes and anisocoria, though without change in the pupillary reflex in response to light), alteration of gait, left hyperreflexia, bilateral Babinski's reflex, euphoria and delirium episodes, urine incontinence, right ptosis, and outward rotation and hyperextension of the right lower extremity. The terminal picture included progressive sensorium damage, over and above the changes brought about by the first epilepsy episode, and serious integration deficit. The patient was somnolent, had difficulty in speaking, was quite unable to walk, and could not feed himself. Necropsy showed widespread nodular type sarcoid damage involving the whole of the meninges and the CNS, particularly the brain.

Primary sarcoidosis of the brain with the predominantly meningobasal localization and signs of widespread neurological damage was reported by *Di Biagio and Ederli.* The patient was a 44-year-old woman who presented a Korsakoff syndrome and a neurological picture consisting of static state and gait disturbances, various forms of nystagmus, hyperreflexia, and pathological reflexes.

The successful employment of hemispherectomy in the treatment of spastic hemiplegia and intractable epilepsy in a 13-year-old boy with widespread damage of the cerebral cortex is reported by *Pagni et al.*

Widespread vascular damage to the cerebral parenchyma may give rise to conspicuous cerebral edema and hence to a pseudotumoral syndrome instead of a multifocal syndrome (*Labauge et al.*).

In the case of circumscribed tumor-like sarcoid brain alterations, an apparently disseminated symptomatology may be observed. As *Chamberlain* has shown, however, intracranial hypertension and papillary edema are usually present.

Loken et al. have reported "progressive multifocal leukoencephalopathy" in sarcoidosis.

EEG evidence of general or local cerebral damage or epileptic foci may be obtained (*Suchenwirth*).

Cord and spinal nerve damage, excepting cord compression caused by primary meningeal damage—which has already been mentioned—is unusual in sarcoidosis. The case of cord sarcoidosis described by Reisner is the only instance of this form in the series of *Colover* (spontaneous improvement was observed).

Cord infiltration has been reported. This may be nodular and also may involve the meninges and nerve roots (*Simons and Merkel; Askanazy; Jefferson*). Cord atrophy has also been reported (*Askanazy*).

The clinical picture may include spastic paraplegia (*Pennel; Zeman*), amyotrophic lateral sclerosis with tetraplegia (as in the case of cord, brain, and muscle damage observed by *de Morsier et al.*), or chronic paraplegia (case no. 2 of the series of *Fazlullah*: myelographic evidence of meningeal cavity block, and surgical detection and removal of a medullary granulomatous mass). In a case observed by *Moldover* the cord alteration had resulted in bilateral D12 to L2 hyperalgesia, weakening of the cremasteric reflexes, impaired perineal sensitivity, and patellar and Achilles areflexia. The clinical history recorded trunk and right hip pain, difficulty in walking, impotence, and micturition disturbances. Urinary incontinence was also observed by *Chamberlain*.

Uvea and CNS inflammation was observed as an isolated manifestation of sarcoidosis for four years by *Kissel et al.* in a case in which various neurological signs had already been noted.

Clinically silent sarcoid infiltration of the spinal cord has been observed by *Erickson et al.*

Herrmann and Reckel have reported a case of partial transection of the spinal cord.

The clinical expression of spinal nerve involvement may include paresthesia, alternating sensations of hot and cold, or the appearance of radicular or trunk district, complete, or dissociated anesthesia areas, sometimes associated with the loss of one or more reflexes. Localized areas of paralysis may be referable to the deltoid, triceps, or serratus muscles. *Goodson* observed a 13-year-old boy with gait disturbances—the patient quickly became tired when walking—and calf pain. Clear neurological symptoms could not be elicited and bilateral damage of the peroneal nerves was postulated. *Jefferson* has reported an unusually rare polyneuritis picture, with involvement of the 7th cranial nerve. Spinal nerve involvement, demonstrated by the appearance of paresthesia, coupled with 2nd, 5th, 6th, 7th, and 8th cranial nerve damage, was reported by *Gupta and Katiyar*. Acute sarcoidosis (Löfgren's syndrome) coupled with polyneuritis has been noted by *Börner*. There have been reports of Guillain-Barré syndromes also (*Schott et al.; etc.*).

Spindle-like swellings of the median, cubital, and radial nerve trunks have been noted (*Mazza; Urban; Boeck*). The picture in the case reported by *Boeck* was very similar to that of leprosy.

Cascone has reported the appearance of herpes zoster in a case of pulmonary sarcoidosis.

Muscle damage may be striking and closely connected to nerve involvement in sarcoidosis. This condition was first noted by *Licharew* in 1908 and subsequent work has served to distinguish an amyotrophic form from a tumor-like form, in addition to clinically silent muscular infiltration detectable solely on biopsy (*Muratore et al.*; case no. 3 of the series of *Lafon et al.; Silverstein and Siltzbach; Vital et al.*). Muscle damage caused by sarcoidosis is more common than is generally believed (*Lebacq*). *Brain et al.* place sarcoidosis high on the list of acquired myopathies.

The amyotrophic forms present a picture of normally bilateral primary muscular atrophy, though unilateral or segmentary localizations may be observed. Atrophy is not a mirror of infiltration, but the functional deficiency is in proportion to the extent of the anatomic lesion. If paralysis is accompanied by areflexia, however, the probability of combined muscular and nervous localization must be considered. The spinal cord, the peripheral nerves, or the peripheral motor neuron alone may be involved (*Mazza*).

Atrophy is accompanied by muscle tenderness and in the advanced stages of the disease there appear hardness and loss of plasticity (*Snorrason's* fibrous myositis). Other symptoms of muscular sarcoidosis include muscle pain, sometimes generalized (*Çelikoğlu*), and muscle cramps. An extreme picture is reported by *Warburg*: atrophy, serious contractures, and radiological signs of calcification.

An interesting example of clinically primary muscular sarcoidosis has been reported by Lebacq. In this case the clinical picture included loss of weight and loss of upper extremity, scapular, and pelvic girdle muscle force. Biopsy led to the rejection of myasthenia and progressive muscular atrophy as diagnoses.

Myopathy was also the first clinical sign of sarcoidosis in a case published by *Andersson and Haga*. Four years elapsed from the appearance of muscle symptoms before acute iridocyclitis, hilar adenopathy, hypergammaglobulinemia, and hypercalciuria were observed. The Mantoux reaction was negative and muscle biopsy indicated sarcoidosis.

Tumorous forms are uncommon and sarcoid tumors in muscle are not usually observed. Such swellings are usually multiple and may be as large as a hen's egg (*Pautrier*) or may consist of much smaller nodules (*Goodson*). Localization at musculotendinous junctions has been reported (*Sundelin*).

Solitary muscle tumors are particularly rare. In case no. 2 of the series of *Lafon et al.*, a temporal swelling was the sole manifestation of sarcoidosis. Surgery showed an almond-shaped sarcoid growth within the belly of the temporal muscle. Loss of function is not common, though it may be observed if the sarcoid mass reaches a considerable size or if the nerve trunks are infiltrated.

An example of sarcoidosis-induced muscle pseudohypertrophy has been reported by *Russo and De Lieto Vollaro*. Biopsy showed epithelioid interstitial myositis.

Electromyography can do no more than exclude a nervous origin and diagnosis must be made on the basis of the histological data, coupled with the clinical picture (*Brain et al.; Lebacq; Jerusalem and Imbach*). Urinary creatin is offered by *Lebacq* as a good index of the activity of the disease. In his personal case, values were high (481 mg/24 hours), and very high levels have been reported by *Powell* (1053 mg/24 hours) and *Klotz et al.* (1495 mg/24 hours).

Sarcoidosis of the nervous system can be diagnosed with certainty only by biopsy following craniotomy or laminectomy. When histomorphological data are lacking, diagnosis may be considerably difficult, particularly when the nerve symptoms are the first sign of the disease and are unsupported by a wider clinical picture.

In cases where the neurological symptoms indicate the possibility of sarcoidosis, *Daniels'* method is to resect the lymph nodes commonly present in the prescalenic celluloadipose tissue, since these will display sarcoid alterations in the case of intrathoracic sarcoidosis. Evidence of clinically silent sarcoids can be obtained by muscle or hypochondriac organ biopsy. In the opinion of *Wurm*, liver biopsy gives positive results in about 60% of cases of sarcoidosis. Alternatively, bronchoscopy is used to obtain fragments of bronchial mucosa (*Friedman et al.; etc.*). Positive results will be obtained at the tracheal spur in about 50% of cases, according to *Turiaf*. Lastly, biopsy of the mediastinal lymph nodes may be done (*Carlens*). A *Kveim* test and tuberculin skin sensitivity test will be mandatory and a chest X-ray should be done to detect hilar adenopathies.

With respect to histological diagnosis the appearance of central necrosis in the sarcoid nodule may make differentiation from tuberculosis difficult. The features indicative of sarcoidosis are: fibrinoid as opposed to caseous necrosis; unimpaired reticular fibers rounding the epithelioid cells on silver impregnation; granulomatous tissue culture does not give rise to Koch bacilli and injection into the guinea pig produces no reaction.

From the clinical point of view, a Heerfordt's disease or a neurological picture consisting of uni- or bilateral facial paralysis, ocular signs, and meningeal reaction will be strongly indicative of sarcoidosis. Combined hypothalamus and hypophysis damage, however, is less significant and may be attributable to various etiologies.

In the differential diagnosis of meningeal and cerebromeningeal involvement in sarcoidosis a number of other forms must be considered: tuberculosis, Hodgkin's disease, mycosis, parasitosis, and cerebral abscess. The symptom picture of facial nerve paralysis coupled with parotitis may be imitated by degeneration of mixed tumor of the parotid gland. Pictures of pseudotumoral brain damage must be distinguished from those of true neoplasia. In cases of this kind, the final diagnosis often must be postponed until surgery or necropsy. Multifocal cerebral symptom patterns may be due also to multiple neoplastic metastases or hemorrhagic pachymeningitis. Cerebellar syndromes must be distinguished from those of cerebellar neoplasia or arachnoiditis with occlusion of the posterior fossa. In polyneuritic forms, diabetes, nodose panarteritis, porphyria, neoplastic infiltration, and leprosy may have to be considered. Lymphocytic meningitis, uveal and CNS inflammation, multiple sclerosis (*Hazeghi*), diphtheria, syringomyelia, and botulism are other diseases that may require differentiation.

The prognosis for CNS involvement in sarcoidosis is very poor, with death occurring in about 50% of cases after an average course of 2½–3 years. Meningeal forms and brain damage are the most serious in this respect. In contrast, peripheral forms tend to regress, though relapses are not uncommon. Unilateral blindness and total deafness are possible outcomes (*Siltzbach and Greenberg*).

In addition to symptomatic remedies, treatment is based on the administration of cortisones, though these are usually of little or no effect in cases of CNS involvement. *Labauge et al.* point out that intrathecal cortisone management has not yet been attempted. Brilliant results are, however, sometimes obtained (*Chamberlain; Moldover*). In the case observed by Moldover, total regression of the neurological manifestations was accompanied by a return of normal sexual activity. Peripheral forms, by contrast, usually benefit from cortisone therapy (*Arnould et al., etc.*) and remissions almost to the point of cure have been observed. Muscle alterations are also particularly responsive to cortisone.

In a case observed by *Brun*, a 55-year-old woman had presented progressive weakness over a three year period to the point of being unable to get out of a chair or to walk without support. The clinical picture was one of chronic polymyositis, with fibrosis and atrophy of the muscles, particularly those of the pelvic girdle, thighs, legs, and forearms. Left anterior tibial muscle biopsy showed roundish or long infiltration sites consisting of epithelioid cells, fibroblasts, and fibrocytes.

The perimeter of some of these sites displayed slight parvicellular infiltration, sometimes with rare giant cells. The surrounding muscle fibers showed all degrees of degeneration and atrophy. Cortisone therapy produced a rapid improvement within ten days, and after three months the patient was able to get out of a chair and carry out light domestic tasks.

A minimum treatment period of three months is required in acute forms. Chronic forms must be treated longer. Cortisones must be given as early as possible in all cases of nerve damage.

Chloroquine was used by *Fazlullah* in his case of cord involvement with chronic paraplegia. The patient was able to walk without assistance after treatment. A place may sometimes be found for the old practice of using calciferol though some workers advise against it (*Gatté*).

Surgical management is indicated in cases of intracranial hypertension due to basal meningeal or posterior fossa block, pseudotumoral pictures, or cord compression. In some cases (e.g. case no. 2 of the series of *Höök*) considerable improvement may be obtained.

REFERENCES

ALAJOUANINE, T.; FEREY, D.; HOUDART, R. and ARDOUIN, M.: a) Forme neuro-oculaire pure de la maladie de B.B.S. Amblyopie rapide par atteinte successive des deux nerfs optiques à un an de distance, Rev. neurol. 86:255–257 (1952).

ALAJOUANINE, T.; BERTRAND, I.; DEGOS, R.; CONTAMIN, R. and ESCOUROLLE, R.: b) Sarcoïdose ganglionnaire, cutanée et oculaire avec atteinte secondaire diffuse, périphérique et centrale du systeme nerveux. Rev. neurol. 99: 412–447 (1958).

ANDERSSON, R. and HAGA, T.: Kliniskt manifest muskelsarkoidos. Nord. Med. 74:1198–1199 (1965).

ARNOULD, G.; TRIDON, P.; PICARD, L.; WEBER, M. and FLOQUET, J.: Multinévrite au cours d'une maladie de Besnier-Boeck-Schaumann. Rev. neurol. 114:457–459 (1966).

ASKANAZY, C. L.: Sarcoidosis of the central nervous system. J. Neuropath. exp. Neurol. 11:392–400 (1952).

BARBOLINI, G. and MASTRONARDI, V.: Sarcoïdose primitive du nerf optique avec test à la métopirone très positif. Documentation anatomo-clinique. Poumon 23:453–465 (1967).

BARIÉTY, M. and POULET, J.: La sarcoïdose de Besnier-Boeck-Schaumann (Flammarion, Paris 1958).

BERNARD: in Labauge et al.

BESNIER, M. E.: Lupus pernio de la face; synovites fongueuses-tuberculeuses symétriques des extrémités supérieures. Ann. Derm. Syph., Paris 10:333 (1899).

BIAGIO, F. DI and EDERLI, A.: Sarcoidosi primitiva del sistema nervoso centrale. Policlinico, Sez. prat. 73:562–570 (1966).

BLEISCH, V. R. and ROBBINS, S. L.: Sarcoid-like granulomata of the pituitary gland. Arch. intern. Med. 89:877–892 (1952).

BOECK, C.: Multiple benign sarcoïd of the skin. J. cutan. genito-urin. Dis. 17:543 (1899). Nochmals zur Klinik und zur Stellung des 'benignen Miliarlupoid'. Arch. Derm. Syph., Berl. 121:707–741 (1916).

BÖRNER, E.: Sindrome di Löfgren (morbo di Boeck acuto) con polineurite. Med. tedesc. 5:127–129 (1969).

BRAIN, R.; RICHARDSON, A. T. and NEVIN, S.: Discussion on the acquired myopathies. Proc. roy. Soc. Med. 53:821–832 (1960).

BRANSON, J. H. and PARK, J. H.: Sarcoidosis. Hepatic involvement: presentation of a case with fatal liver involvement, including autopsy findings and review of the evidence for sarcoid involvement of the liver as found in the literature. Ann. intern. Med. 40:111–145 (1954).

BRUN, A.: Chronic polymyositis on the basis of sarcoidosis. Acta psychiat. scand. 36:515–523 (1961).

CAMP, W. A. and FRIERSON, J. G.: Sarcoidosis of the central nervous system. Arch. Neurol., Chicago 7:432–441 (1962).

CARES, R. M.; GORDON, B. S. and KREUGER E.: Boeck's sarcoid in chronic meningoencephalitis. J. Neuropath. exp. Neurol. 16: 544–554 (1957).

CARLENS, E.: Mediastinoscopy: a method for inspection and tissue biopsy in the superior mediastinum. Dis. Chest 36:343–352 (1959). Some aspects of mediastinoscopy. Rev méd. int. Photo Cinema Telev. 1:86–90 (1962). Méthodes biopsiques dans le cas de sarcoïdose intrathoracique. Bronches 13:630 (1963).

CARSTENSEN and NORVIT: in Bariéty and Poulet.

CASCONE, A.: Herpes zoster insorto in corso di sarcoidosi polmonare. Arch. Sci. Med. 126:369–373 (1969).

CASTORINA, G.; SILIPO, P. and PETIZIOL, A.: Aracnoidite ottico-chiasmatica e sarcoidosi cerebrale. Riv. Neurol. 32:125–141 (1962).

ÇELINOĞLU, S. I.: Türkiye' de sarkoidosis' in klinik özellikleri (24 vak' alik bir serinin incelenmesi). Türk Tip Cemiyeti Mecmuasi 34:748–764 (1968).

CHAMBERLAIN, M. A.: A case of sarcoidosis of the nervous system. Guy's Hosp. Rep. 111:25–32 (1962).

COLOVER, J.: Sarcoidosis with involvement of the nervous system. Brain 71:451–475 (1948).

DADDI, G. *et al.*: La sarcoidosi polmonare. Relaz. LXVI Congr. Soc. Ital. Med. Intern., Catania 1965 (Pozzi, Rome 1965).

DAIREAUS: in Goodson.

DANIELS, A. C.: Method of biopsy useful in diagnosing certain intrathoracic diseases. Dis. Chest 16:360–366 (1949).

DAYRAS, J. C.: Les atteintes du système nerveux central dans la sarcoïdose (à propos d'une observation anatomo-clinique); Thèse Paris (1957).

DEROT, M.; TCHOBROUTSKY, J. and ROUDIER, R.: Coma hypoglycémique mortel par hypopituitarisme secondaire à la localisation hypophysaire d'une sarcoïdose. Bull. Soc. méd. Hôp., Paris 75:225–230 (1959).

DRAGONI, G.: La malattia di Besnier-Boeck-Schaumann (Ediz. Minerva Medica, Turin 1961).

ERICKSON, T. C.; ODOM, G. L. and STERN, K.: Boeck's disease (sarcoid) of the central nervous system: report of a case with complete clinical and pathologic study. Arch. Neurol., Chicago 48:613–621 (1942).

EVERTS, W. H.: Sarcoidosis with brain tumor. Trans. amer. neurol. Ass. 72:128–130 (1947).

FAZLULLAH, S.: Sarcoidosis with involvement of the nervous system. Dis. Chest 41:685–688 (1962).

FRANCESCHETTI and MORSIER DE: in Colover.

FRIEDMAN, O. H.; BLAUGRUND, S. M. and SILTZBACH, L. E.: Biopsy of the bronchial wall as an aid in diagnosis of sarcoidosis. J. amer. med. Ass. 183:646–650 (1963).

GARCIN, R.; MARQUÉZY, R. A.; LAPRESLE, J.; BACH, CH. and DAYRAS, J. C.: Sur un cas de sarcoidose du système nerveux central. Étude anatomo-clinique. Presse méd. 65:1926–1930 (1957).

GARCIN, R.: Les atteintes neurologiques et musculaires dans la maladie de B.B.S. Psychiat. Neurol. Neurochir. 63:285–297 (1960).

GATTÉ: in Miglioli.

GÉRAUD, J.; RASCOL, A.; JORDA, J.; CAIZERGUES, P. and KAKKOUS, E.: La sarcoïdose cérébrale. À propos d'une observation anatomo-clinique. Rev. neurol. 112:85–89 (1965).

GOODMAN, S. S.; MURRAY, E. and MARGULIES, M. E.: Boeck's sarcoid simulating a brain tumor. Arch. Neurol., Chicago 81:419–423 (1959).

GOODSON, W. H.: Neurologic manifestations of sarcoidosis. S. med. J. 53:1111–1116 (1960).

GRAVESEN, P. B.: Lymphogranulomatosis benigna (Andelsbogtrykkeriet, Odense 1942).

GUPTA, N. and KATIYAR, B. C.: Neurological manifestations of sarcoidosis. J. indian med. Ass. 35:27–30 (1960).

HAZEGHI, P.: Les formes nerveuses de la sarcoïdose (maladie de Besnier-Boeck-Schaumann). Étude anatomo-clinique de deux cas. Schweiz. Arch. Neurol. Neurochir. Psychiat. 94:21–62 (1964).

HEERFORDT, C. F.: Ueber eine Febris uveo-parotidea subchronica an der Glandula Parotis und der Uvea des Auges lokalisiert und häufig mit Paresen cerebrospinaler Nerven kompliziert. Graefes Arch. Ophthal. 70:254 (1909).

HERRMANN, E. and RECKEL, K.: Die Sarkoïdose des Nervensystems und die Sarkoid-Myopathie. Internist, Berl. 10:385–388 (1969).

HÖÖK, O.: Sarcoidosis with involvement of the nervous system: report of nine cases. Arch. Neurol., Chicago 71:554–575 (1954).

HOPPE, R.: Sarkoidose (Schattauer, Stuttgart 1965).

HUTCHINSON, J.: Cases of Mortimer's malady (lupus vulgaris multiplex non ulcerous and non serpiginous). Arch. Surg., Chicago 9:307 (1898).

ISRAEL, H. L. and GOLDSTEIN, R. A.: Relation of Kviem-antigen reaction to lymphadenopathy. Study of sarcoidosis and other diseases. New Eng. J. Med. 284:345–349 (1971).

JEAN-GIRARD, CH.: Les formes neurologiques de la maladie de B.B.S.; Thèse Paris (1956).

JEFFERSON, M.: Nervous signs in sarcoidosis. Brit. med. J. ii:916–919 (1952). Sarcoidosis of the nervous system. Brain 80: 540–556 (1957). The nervous system in sarcoidosis. Postgrad. med. J. 34: 259–261 (1958).

JERUSALEM, F. and IMBACH, P.: granulomatöse, Myositis und Muskelsarkoidose. Klinische und bioptisch-histologische Diagnose. Dtsch. med. Wschr. 95:2184–2190 (1970).

JÜNGLING, O.: Ostitis tuberculosa multiplex cystica (eine eigenartige Form der Knochentuberkulose). Fortschr. Röntgenstr., vol. 28, pp. 375–383 (Hamburg 1919–1921).

KALKOFF, K. W.: Definition und Ätiologie der Sarkoidose. Dtsch. med. Wschr. 95:505–509 (1970).

KIENBOCK, R.: In Longcope, W. T. and Frieman, D. G. Study of sarcoidosis based on combined investigation of 160 cases including 30 autopsies from the Johns Hopkins Hospital and Massachusetts General Hospital. Medicine, Balt. 31:1–132 (1952).

KISSEL, P.; SCHMITT, J. and DUC, M.: Uvéo-névraxite, manifestation longtemps isolée de la maladie de Besnier-Boeck-Schumann. Rev. neurol. 114: 452–457 (1966).

KLOTZ, H. P.; RUBENS-DUVAL, A.; DESSE, G. and CHIMÈNES: La forme musculaire de la maladie de Besnier-Boeck-Schaumann. Rev. Rhum. 22:132–137 (1955).

KRAUSS: in Labauge et al.

KUZNITZKY, E. and BITTORF, A.: Boecksches Sarkoid mit Beteiligung innerer Organe. Münch. med. Wschr. 62:1349 (1915).

KVIEM, A.: En ny og specifik kutan-reaksjon ved Boeck's sarcoid. Nord. Med. 9:168–172 (1941).

LABAUGE, R.; IZARN, P. and CASTAN, P.: Les manifestations nerveuses des hémopathies. Rapport LXI Congr. Franç. de Psychiatrie et de Neurologie, Nancy 1963 (Masson, Paris 1963).

LAFON, R.; PAGÈS, P.; PASSOUANT, P.; LABAUGE, R.; MINVIELLE, J. and PAGÈS, A.: Localisations musculaires de la maladie de Besnier-Boeck-Schaumann. A propos de trois observations. Rev. neurol. 92:557–563 (1955).

LEBACQ, E.: La sarcoïdose de Besnier-Boeck-Schaumann (Arsica-Maloine, Bruxelles-Paris 1964).

LEITNER, J. S.: Der morbus B.B.S. (Schwabe, Basel 1949).

LENARTOWICZ, J. and ROTHFELD, J.: Ein Fall von Hautsarkoiden (Darier-Roussy) mit identischen Veränderungen im Gehirn und den inneren Organen. Arch. Derm. Syph., Berl. 161:504–519 (1930).

LESNE; LAUNAY and SEE: In Larcan and Picard, Manifestations neurologiques au cours des affections hematologiques. In Encyclopédie Médico-Chirurgicale, 17162 A 10 (Éditions Techniques, Paris 1966).

LICHAREW: in Labauge et al.

LÖFGREN, S.: Besnier-Boeck-Schaumann disease; clinical aspects. Nord. Med. 52:976–981 (1954).

LOKEN, A. C.; REFSUM, S. and JACOBSEN, W.: Progressive multifocal leucoencefalopathy in a case of sarcoïdosis; in Livre jubilaire de Ludo van Bogaert, p. 494 (Éditions Acta Med. Belg., 1962).

MAC BRIDE, H. J.: Uveo-parotitic paralysis. J. Neurol. Psychopath. 4:242–247 (1923).

MATTHEWS, W. B.: Sarcoidosis of the nervous system. Brit. med. J. i:267–270 (1959) Sarcoidosis of the nervous system. J. Neurol. Neurosurg. Psychiat. 28:23–29 (1965).

MAZZA, G.: Ueber das multiple benigne Sarkoïd der Haut. Arch. Derm. Syph., Berl. 91:57 (1908).

MEYER, J. S.; FOLEY, J. M. and CAMPAGNA-PINTO, D.: Granulomatous angiitis of the meninges in sarcoidosis. Arch. Neurol., Chicago 69:587–600 (1953).

MIGLIOLI, S.: La sarcoidosi dei polmoni (malattia di Besnier-Boeck-Schaumann) Brunelli, Bologna 1965).

MOLDOVER, A.: Sarcoidosis of the spinal cord. Report of a case with remission associated with cortisone therapy. Arch. intern. Med. 102:414–417 (1958).

MORSIER, G.DE; MAURICE, P. and MARTIN, F.: Besnier-Boeck diffus des muscles et lésions du système nerveux central (2 observations anatomo-cliniques). Acta neurol. belg. 54:34–51 (1954).

MURATORE, F.; VITERBO, F. and VULPIS, N.: Sarcoidosi o malattia di Besnier-Boeck-Schaumann. Medicina, Parma 3:503–574 (1953).

NAUMANN: in Colover.

PAGNI, C. A.; HAZEGHI, P. and WILDI, E.: Boeck's sarcoidosis revealed at hemispherectomy in a case of infantile encephalopathy with epilepsy. J. neurol. Sci. 3:76–89 (1966).

PAUTRIER, L. M.: Une nouvelle grande réticulo-endothéliose: la maladie de Besnier-Boeck-Schaumann (Masson, Paris 1940).

PENNEL, W.H.: Boeck's sarcoid with involvement of the central nervous system. Arch. Neurol., Chicago 66:728–737 (1951).

PLAIR, C. M. and PERRY, S.: Hypothalamic-pituitary sarcoidosis. A clinical and pathological entity: report of a case. Arch. Path. 74:527–535 (1962).

POWELL, L. W. JR.: Sarcoidosis of skeletal muscle; report of 6 cases and review of literature. Amer. J. clin. Path. 23:881–889 (1953).

RABEN, A. S.; LEVENSON, O. S. and LIVCLUNE, V. M.: Lesions of the nervous system in sarcoidosis (Besner-Boeck-Schaumann disease). Zhurn. Nevropat., Moscow 62:680–685 (1962).

REIS, W. and ROTHFELD, J.: Tuberkulide der Sehnerven als Komplikation von Hautsarkoiden vom Typus Darier-Roussy. Graefes Arch. Ophthal. 126:357–366 (1931).

REISNER, D.: Boeck's sarcoid and systemic sarcoidosis (Besnier-Boeck-Schaumann disease): study of 35 cases. Amer. Rev. Tuberc. 49:289–307 (1944).

RICKARDS and BARRETS: in Labauge et al.

RICKER, W. and'CLARK, M.: Sarcoidosis; a clinico-pathologic review of 300 cases, including 22 autopsies. Amer. J. clin. Path. 19:725–749 (1949).

RISER, M.; GAYRAL, L.; TURNIN, J. and STERN, H.: Formes neurologiques de la lymphogranulomatose bénigne. Toulouse méd. 60:609–618 (1959).

ROBERT, F.: Sarcoidosis of the central nervous system. Report of a case and review of the literature. Arch. Neurol., Chicago 7:442–449 (1962).

RUDBERG-ROOS, I.: The course and prognosis of sarcoidosis as observed in 296 cases. Acta tuberc. pneumol. scand. 41 (supplm. 52):1–42 (1962).

Russo, G. and Lieto Vollaro, P. De: L'interessamento muscolare nella malattia di Besnier-Boeck-Schaumann. Rif. med. 79:1327–1330 (1965).

Saltzman, G. F.: Roentgenological changes in cerebral sarcoidosis. Acta radiol., Stockh. 50:235–241 (1958).

Schaumann, J.: Études sur le lupus pernio et ses rapports avec les sarcoïdes et la tuberculose. Ann. Derm. Syph., Paris 6:357–373 (1916–1917). Notes on the histology of the medullary and osseous lesions in benign lymphogranuloma and especially on their relationship to the radiographic picture. Acta radiol., Stockh. 7:358 (1926). Étude anatomo-pathologique et histologique sur les localisations viscérales de la lymphogranulomatose bénigne. Bull. Soc. franç. Derm. Syph. 40:1167–1178 (1933). Lymphogranulomatosis benigna in the light of prolonged clincal observations and autopsy findings. Brit. J. Derm. 48:399–416 (1936). On the nature of certain peculiar corpuscles present in tissue of lymphogranulomatosis benigna. Acta med. scand. 106:239–253 (1941).

Schneider, P.: Die Boecksche Lungenerkrankung. Arch. klin. Chir. 260:523–531 (1948).

Schott, B.; Michel, D.; Lejeune, E.; Bouvier, M.; Vauzelle, J. L.; Girard, R.; Roumagoux, J.; Ramel, P. and Bouvier, S.: Polyradiculonévrites au cours de la maladie de Besnier-Boeck-Schaumann. J. Méd., Lyon 49:931–937 (1968).

Siltzbach, L. E.: Kveim test in sarcoidosis: study of 750 patients. J. amer. med. Ass. 178:476–482 (1961). Significance and specificity of the Kveim reaction. Acta med. scand. 176 (supplem. 425): 74–78 (1964). Il test di Kveim nella sarcoidosi. Simp. Int. Linfopatie non tumorali, Milan 1968. Gaz. san. Milan 39:385–390 (1968).

Siltzbach, L. E. and Greenberg, G. M.: Childhood sarcoidosis. A study of 18 patients. New Engl. J. Med. 279:1239–1245 (1968).

Silverstein, A.; Feuer, M. M. and Siltzbach, L. E.: Neurologic sarcoidosis. Study of 18 cases. Arch. Neurol., Chicago 12:1–11 (1965).

Silverstein, A. and Siltzbach, L. E.: Muscle involvement in sarcoidosis. Asymptomatic myositis and myopathy. Arch. Neurol., Chicago 21:235–242 (1969).

Simons and Merkel: in Colover.

Snorrason, E.: Myositis fibrosa progressiva in patient with lymphogranulomatosis benigna Boeck. Nord. Med. 36:2424–2425 (1947).

Suchenwirth, R.: Die Sarkoidose des Nervensystems. Münch. med. Wschr. 110:580–586 (1968).

Sundelin, F.: Tumeurs multiples disséminées dans les muscles des estrémités et rappelant la tuberculeuse par leur structure histologique. Acta med. scand. 62:442–460 (1925).

Thibault, P.: La sarcoïdose. Presse méd. 73:2925–2927 (1965).

Thompson, J. R.: Sarcoidosis of the central nervous system. Report of a case simulating intracranial neoplasm. Amer. J. Med. 31:977–980 (1961).

Turiaf, J. and Brun, J.: La sarcoïdose endothoracique de Besnier-Boeck-Schaumann (Expansion Scientifique Française, Paris 1955).

Urban, D.: Zur Kasuistik der Boeckschen Sarkoïde. Arch. Derm. Syph., Berl. 101:175 (1910).

Vic-Dupont; Margairaz, A. and Witchitz, S.: sarcoïdose du système nerveux central avec méningite chronique, hyperalbuminorachie et association diabète insipidehypopituitarisme antérieur. Bull. Soc. méd. Hôp., Paris 77:582–592 (1961).

Vital, A.; Vallot, J. M.; Bergouignon, M.; Arné, L. and Martin-Bruno, F.: Les localisations musculaires de la maladie de Besnier-Boeck-Schaumann. À propos de dix observations. Bordeaux méd. 3:925–946 (1970).

Waldenström, J.: Some observations on uveoparotitis and allied conditions with special reference to symptoms from the nervous system. Acta med. scand. 91:53–68 (1937).

Wanstrup, J. and Christensen, H. E.: Sarcoidosis. 1. Ultrastructural investigations on epitheloid cell granulomas. Acta path. microbiol. scand. 66:169–185 (1966).

Warburg, M.: Case of symmetrical muscular contractures due to sarcoidosis. J. Neuropath. exp. Neurol. 14:313–315 (1955).

Wood, E. H. and Bream, C. A.: Spinal sarcoidosis. Radiology 73:226–233 (1959).

WURM, K.; REINDELL, H. and DOLL, E.: Klinik und Ätiologie der Sarkoidose (Morbus Boeck); in Hoppe (loc. cit.), pp. 23–63.

WURM, K.: Diagnosi di laboratorio della sarcoidosi. Med. Tedesc. 2:319–320 (1966).

ZAHN and WEBER: in Labauge et al.

ZEMAN, W.: Über neuro-psychiatrische Syndrome beim Morbus Beznier-Boeck-Schaumann, Dtsch. med. Wschr. 76:1621–1622 (1951).

Chapter X

NEUROLOGICAL SYMPTOMS
IN MULTIPLE MYELOMA

(With an appendix on neurological manifestations
in cryoglobulinemia and Waldenström's disease)

The incidence of neurological complications in multiple myeloma is considered to be high. Some writers (*Geschickter and Copeland; Snapper et al.*) report frequencies of up to 40%.

Multiple myeloma (Kahler's disease) covers "a collection of different syndromes, whose common denominator is a primary disease, usually fatal and of unknown etiology, of the reticuloendothelial system characterized by atypical, disordered, invasive, and aimless proliferation of the plasma cells. Since the functioning bone marrow is almost constantly involved, often widespread skeletal lesions result. In the great majority of cases, a serious and as yet incompletely explained change in protein metabolism also plays a part " (*Di Guglielmo*, 1955).

Nerve system alterations are caused usually by compression of the nerves themselves and their vessels by infiltrates (*Silverstein and Doniger; etc.*); compression may be caused by amyloid masses also. The skeletal polarity of the disease explains why compression is so frequent. Because of the extensive contiguity of the spinal cord (with its vessels) and the vertebral column, and because of the massive diffusion of the vertebral changes, the radiculomedullary formations are particularly involved.

This is shown by the series of *Kirshbaum* (45% of cases with signs of radiculomedullary compression), *Geschickter and Copeland* (40%), and *Clarke, E.*[b] (20%). This last series includes 204 reported cases of radiculomedullary compression as well as 21 personal cases.

Lower, but still noteworthy, frequencies have been reported by *Kenny and Moloney* (14%), *Snapper et al.* (12.3%), *Serre et al.* (8.7%), *Magnus-Levy* (5%), and *Williams, H.M. et al.* (3.3%).

Seven instances of plasmacytoma were noted in 54 epidural tumors by

Shenkin et al., while 6% of 524 paraplegics observed over a period of 20 years at the Mayo Clinic presented epidural myelomatous infiltration (*Svien et al.*). Of 121 paraplegics reported by *Stratemeyer* 40% had an epidural tumor, 5% of a myelomatous nature. Plasmacytomas in three out of 102 cases of spinal compression were noted by *Tolosa et al.* *McKissock et al.* reported a plasmacytoma frequency of 4.4% in 545 cases of cord compression observed over 16 years.

Vertebral lesions and their respective nerve symptoms are not uncommon in plasma cell leukosis (leukemic myelomatosis).

However, cerebral alterations are very rare, as is infiltration of the spinal cord.

Cushing observed only four plasmacytomas in 2,000 intracranial tumors. *Bayrd and Heck* reported a total absence of brain damage in 83 multiple myeloma patients, and only three instances of cranial nerve paralysis and cerebral complication were observed in 97 cases by *Snapper et al.* The 172 cases observed by *Williams, H.M. et al.* included only four patients with cerebral involvement and two with cranial nerve paralysis.

In addition to paraneoplastic forms, other less common pathogenic factors may be responsible for neurological changes in multiple myeloma. These include dysglobulinemia, hemorrhage, anemia, and toxic conditions associated with renal insufficiency and hypercalcemia.

Hemorrhage in multiple myeloma is a consequence of the rich vascularization of the diseased tissue. In the terminal stage, however, it may be widespread as a result of thrombocytopenia secondary to massive bone marrow infiltration. Other causes include: damage to the vasal endothelia caused by hyperazotemia; hypoprothrombinemia and fibrinogenopenia resulting from liver damage (attributable, like kidney damage, to plasma cell infiltration and/or amyloidosis); and dysproteinemia (impaired hemostasis—leading to clotting defects—or infiltration of the meta-arteriolar and arteriolar walls) (*James et al.*). Dysproteinemia may have a capillarotoxic effect (the "malignant hemorrhagiparous dysglobulinemia" of *Bernard et al.*) or may damage the capillary enodthelial membrane, causing permeability alteration (*Bianchi et al.; Pende and Chiarioni*); dysproteinemia is undoubtedly a basic factor in the frequently observed "hemorrhagic overture" (*Azerad et al.*) of the disease (*Milliez and Mallarmé; André et al.; Pende and Chiarioni*).

Cerebral damage is rare and is usually referable to myelomatous localization in the bones of the base of the skull, since these are the regular site of intracranial neoformations. Only exceptionally do these neoformations originate in the dura mater (reported by *Armstrong et al.*), this being usually involved by way of extension from a neighboring bone site (*Piney and Riach; Davison and Balser; Sparling et al.*). Intraccrebral infiltration is also an exceptional finding (*French; Kramer; Labauge et al.*).

The body of the sphenoid and the apex of the petrous portion of the temporal bone are the usual points of origin. Early proliferation toward the sinus cavernosus and jugular foramen compresses and displaces the cranial nerves (particularly the 5th, 6th, and 8th) without infiltrating them. The dura mater usually prevents involvement of the brain and the further course of the process extends anteriorly toward the sphenoidal fissure and the orbital cavity and posteriorly toward the occipital fossa. The cerebral parenchyma is compressed and pushed back, normally without infiltration. Massive proliferation has been reported. Invasion of most of the posterior fossa with virtual destruction of the temporal and occipital bones was observed by *Cappell and Mathers*, while in case no. 20 of the series of *Sparling et al.* infiltration extended from the left half of the sphenoid to the left temporal bone, compressing and displacing the brain, cerebellum, and several nerve trunks.

Intracranial infiltration gives rise to a protean symptomatology. Headache is often prominent and may be the initial sign of intracranial involvement (*Morin et al.; Bodechtel et al.*). Frank hypertension pictures are reported (seven out of 40 cases—six at an early stage—found in the literature by *Clarke, E.*[a], in addition to one personal case) and may form the initial sign of the underlying disease (*Mahoudeau et al.*). In a case studied by *Bodechtel et al.* a large occipital plasmacytoma was responsible for frank edema of the optic disk and serious vision disturbances, fundus oculi hemorrhage, and diplopia, though the oculomotor muscles were unimpaired; the patient appeared confused, dazed, and somnolent.

Hypertension may be accompanied by signs of local cerebral damage, such as convulsions, hemiparesis, hemiplegia (*Mahoudeau et al.; Snapper et al.; Clarke, E.*[a]), or hemianopsia (*Clarke, E.*[a]). Convulsion crises are common; sometimes they are the initial signs of the hemopathy (*Denker and Brock*). They may multiply during its course and lead to terminal epilepsy (*Morin et al.*).

In the very rare cases of intracerebral infiltration reported by *French, Kramer,* and *Labauge et al., French* observed infiltration of the hypothalamus, clinically expressed as obstruction of the 3rd ventricle, though the data were not sufficient to show whether a solitary plasmacytoma or the encephalic localization of a generalized disease was at issue. In *Kramer's* case, the clinical overture included occipital headache and unsteadiness of gait before the underlying disease had been diagnosed. Later, jacksonian convulsion crises and confusion appeared and were followed by terminal coma. Necropsy resulted in the discovery of a soft, hemorrhagic mass occupying the cortex and subcortical area of the right temporal lobe. Histological examination showed this mass to be composed of plasma cells. Crushing of the vessels and anoxia of the nerve cells or dysproteinemia have been put forward as causes of the terminal coma. *Labauge et al.*, however, observed a case in which a symptom picture recalling that of intracranial tumor (recurrent frontal headache, slight dysarthria, and right lower facial paresis, which progressed to hemiparesis shortly before admission) was associated with asthenia, anorexia, and a slight rise in temperature. Confusion and psychomotor agitation appeared a few days after admission. The chest and head X-ray, fundus oculi, and electroencephalographic (EEG) data were normal, but ventriculography showed an expanding process in the left cerebral hemisphere. Surgery uncovered a diffused tumor in a left central site. This was mostly aspirated and histologically classified as a plasmacytoma. The patient died during the immediate postoperative period and necropsy was not done. This fact, coupled with the incompleteness of the clinical and radiological data, made it impossible to determine whether the diagnosis of solitary plasmacytoma was correct.

Paralysis of the cranial nerves is the dominant feature in the clinical picture of intracranial localizations in multiple myeloma.

The abductent nerve is involved most frequently (15 out of 24 cases in the literature and one personal case in the series of Clarke, E.[a]), sometimes bilaterally. The acoustic and trigeminal nerves are next in the order of frequency of involvement. Paralysis of the cranial nerves may be isolated; alternatively, paralysis of several nerves may cause complicated neurological pictures: cavernous sinus (*Delmas-Marsalet et al.*), sphenoid fissure, orbital apex, Gradenigo, and cerebellopontile angle (*Giraud et al.*[a]) syndromes. *Snapper et al.* observed unilateral 7th–12th cranial nerve damage in one case, accompanied by extensive cranial base osteolysis. Diagnosis rested on biopsy of a bluish swelling protruding from the external auditory meatus. The 3rd, 6th, 8th, 9th, and 12th cranial nerves were involved in the case reported by *Rovit and Fager*. The picture may resemble that of Garcin's syndrome (*Riser and Sorel; Calvet et al.*).

Delaney and Liaricos observed marked chorioretinal destruction in a patient who died of multiple myeloma. The clinical and histological evidence suggested that this lesion was an intraocular manifestation of the hemopathy.

Signs of extension of the infiltration to the hypophysis and diencephalon may form more or less early additions to the cranial nerve involvement picture. Diabetes insipidus was the opening sign in a case of multiple myeloma with considerable changes in the sella turcica observed by *Bach and Middleton.* Other instances of diabetes insipidus have been reported by *Aronsohn, Denker, and Brock,* and *Christophe and Divry.* In the case observed by *Christophe and Divry,* a 37-year-old woman presented a complex prediagnosis picture of hypothalamus and hypophysis involvement including amenorrhea, polyuria, polydipsia, irritability, and sleep disturbances, together with anisocoria. Necropsy showed infiltration of the lesser wing of the sphenoid bone and the sella turcica.

Clinically silent myelomatous infiltration of the posterior hypophysis was observed by *Coste et al.*[a]

Static sense and coordination disturbances are attributable to invasion of the posterior fossa.

For the sake of completeness, reference should also be made to the infrequent cases of meningeal involvement.

Infiltration of both the inner and outer surfaces of the dura mater is very rare, whether it be local, disseminated, or widespread, neighboring skeletal sites being the usual source of involvement. If bone lesions are absent, however, the possibility of primary dural infiltration must be borne in mind.

Unforeseen dural involvement detected at necropsy is occasionally reported (case no. 19 in the series of *Sparling et al.*). *Clarke, E.*[a] observed one patient who presented intracranial hypertension of one year's standing, with bilateral papillary edema and a spastic paralysis of the left upper limb. The intraoperative picture was of plasmacytomatous enlargement of the tentorium cerebelli, with repulsion of the right cerebral hemisphere. The parenchyma showed signs of softening, though there was no evidence of damage caused by infiltration. Necropsy indicated the solitary and hence primary nature of the dural infiltration.

Involvement of the arachnoid membrane was observed by *Morin et al.* in a 21-year-old male with a primarily neurological picture, including convulsion crises, recurrent headache, atypical gait disturbances, and signs of depression. Cerebrospinal fluid (CSF) cell values were increased (39/mm³ one year before death, but the contemporary protein value was normal (0.36 g °/oo). Death occurred during a convulsion crisis following a three-year course. Necropsy showed considerable infiltration of the arachnoid, while the cerebral parenchyma was unimpaired.

Clinically silent plasmacytoma of the rectum was detected via an acute meningitis syndrome in a case observed by *Vorreith.* Postmortem histologic examination showed infiltration of the pia mater, with small perivasal sites in some parts of the cerebral parenchyma and very small cerebellar sites.

Leptomeningeal infiltration also may be both clinically and biologically silent (case no. 2 of the series of *Barron et al.*).

In the case reported by *Mahoudeau et al.* the clinical overture of frank intracranial hypertension was followed by an intraoperative finding of a thick, subarachnoidal serous membrane lining the inner surface of the dura mater, giving rise to a typical "*en gelée*" appearance of the brain. Histologic examinations were not done and diagnosis was founded on a cervical biopsy carried out many years later.

An initial picture of meningitis with high fever was observed in a personal case of multiple myeloma in a 68-year-old woman. Necropsy showed widespread thickening of the leptomeninx of the vault of the brain, attributed histologically to plasmacyte infiltration, accompanied by serious anemia and disseminated myeloma of the skullcap and spinal column.

Localization in the orbit is rare and may consist of an original site in the orbital wall or the extension of the disease from the nasal cavities, facial sinuses, or the periocular tissues. Its clinical expression will be an orbital tumor or a sphenoidal fissure syndrome, or both. Compression of the frontal lobe may be observed, without invasion of the dura mater. *Pagès et al.* have reported an example of a solitary localization in the left orbit. *Lugaresi et al.* observed a patient with right exophthalmos, together with ingravescent headache and pathological fracture of the skullcap. In a case reported by *Bodechtel et al.*, proliferation of the orbit had produced left exophthalmos and doward displacement of the bulb.

Diagnosis of nerve alterations in multiple myeloma is discussed in connection with radiculomedullary damage. Here it need only be noted that intracranial infiltration must be differentiated from basal sarcoma and basal extensions of intracranial tumors.

Wherever possible, resection of intracranial plasmacytoma is the treatment of choice. Attention must be paid to the enhanced possibility of intraoperative hemorrhage arising from the considerable vascularization of the myelomatous tissue. X-ray induced remission of infiltration has been reported (*Snapper et al.*).

Mental changes in multiple myeloma may be attributable to hypercalcemia (*Merigan and Hayes; Polli; Snapper and Kahn*) and its consequent alteration of nerve cell membrane potential, or to hyperazotemia, which may lead to other nervous disturbances—convulsions, muscle and reflex abnormalities, etc. (*Silverstein and Doniger*).

An association of multiple myeloma and "progressive multifocal leukoencephalopathy" has been reported by *Bethlem et al.*

As stated, radiculomedullary damage in multiple myeloma is most commonly the result of osteoepidural infiltration.

This usually presents as a soft, friable, noncapsulated, gray-pink to raspberry or currant-colored red mass. The intensity of the redness may serve as an indication of its development potential. *Paillas et al.* observed a chloroma-like color in one case.

The dorsal segment of the column is the site of choice (134 dorsal compared to 33 cervical and 26 lumbar sites in the series of *Clarke, E.*[b]). Thoracic cord involvement was observed in 20 out of 27 cases of radiculomedullary compression reported by *Silverstein and Doniger*). This preference for the dorsal segment is related to the fact that the thoracic vertebrae are the site of choice (e.g. 14 out of 15 cases in the series of *Paillas et al.*) of the underlying disease.

Myelomatous tissue spreads to occupy part or all of the epidural space. When the entire epidural space is occupied, the dural sac is completely surrounded. The greatest thickness is observed near the vertebral bodies or the conjugate foramina. Infiltration may be limited to the length of its vertebra of origin or it may be much more extensive (D2–D9, case no. 13 of the series of *Clarke, E.*[b]; D4–D10, *Tolosa et al.*; L1–S1, *Verda*).

The cord and the spinal roots and their vessels are compressed, while the dura matter is hardly ever invaded: the myelomatous tissue usually adheres to its outer surface, from which, however, it may be more or less completely detached. Spontaneous intratumoral hemorrhage may be noted and may result in acutely aggravating spinal apoplexy (*Beck*).

Extraspinal invasion is usually directed rearward, mainly into the neck. Its route lies between the vertebral laminae and the spinous processes and reaches the muscle or even the subcutaneous layer. Forward invasion is rare: *Giraud et al.*[b] observed a case in which a fleshy, encapsulated red tumor on the anterior surface of the cervical segment was attached to the posterior wall of the pharynx. The body of C3 was filled with myelomatous tissue overflowing on to C2 and C4, the posterior portion of the disk betwen C3 and C4 had disappeared, and the cord was being strangled by the epidural spread of the tumor. The rarity of anterior expansion has been attributed to the solidity of the anterior vertebral ligament (*Bourdreaux*).

The posterior end of the ribs may be the initial site of epidural myelomatous infiltration (*Thomas et al.*): in this case, invasion takes place via the conjugate foramen, with early involvement of the transverse and articular processes and the pedicles.

Primary epidural infiltration has been postulated, though the reported observations are not fully conclusive (*Browder and de Veer; Verda; Tolosa et al.; etc.*). Their assertion of bone integrity as probative evidence, in fact, is open to question, since the limitations of radiography as a means of ascertaining the existence of skeletal lesions are well known. Operative exploration of the vertebrae, moreover, is far from easy and necropsy is the only dependable source of data.

Dalrymple's autopsy of the first recorded case of multiple myeloma (1848) is the historic landmark for the observation of skeletal changes. *Mac Intyre's* examination of multiple myeloma's anatomic and clinical features included a diagnosis of "mollities et fragilitas ossium." The skeletal changes observed were, in fact, considerable and involved the sternum, ribs, and spinal column; their consistency was reduced to such an extent that the bones could be sectioned with a knife.

Bone changes in multiple myeloma are particularly common (60% in the series of *Batts* and *Grosgurin;* 91.4% of the 55 cases of *Di Guglielmo*).

Such changes are secondary to proliferation and infiltration of the bone marrow and the high marrow content of the vertebrae makes them a favorite target. Anatomic examination shows the vertebrae to be friable and infiltrated by a reddish tissue responsible for thinning and destruction of the normal trabeculation. The vertebral body may retain its shape or be deformed as a result of crushing (leading to a biconcave lens or herring-bone appearance), subsidence to a greater or lesser degree, or fracture (wedge shape).

Various radiographic pictures correspond to these alterations. Widespread simple or hypertrophic osteoporosis, with axial or, less commonly, reticular trabeculation, has been described. If crushing or fracture is also present, this may be particularly extensive. Kyphosis or kyphoscoliosis is usually observed and the intervertebral disks are often swollen. Roundish areas of osteolysis also have been detected stratigraphically (*Bollini and Frassineti*) and eburnation of the vertebral bodies (known as "ivory vertebrae") also has been reported (*Biondetti; Labauge et al.*).

Spinal cord changes in multiple myeloma are essentially vascular in origin and infiltration is extremely rare. The main cause is compression of the marrow-supplying vessels by infiltrates. The picture may range from meningeal edema, often the result of venous obstruction, to necrotic softening, which may be extensive in severe cases. Direct compression from the epidural infiltrate, from vertebrae seriously damaged by infiltration, or from vertebral fragments may also be a cause of cord alterations.

The literature contains only one case of intradural plasmacytoma. A patient observed by *Sod and Wiener* presented myelomatous involvement of the inner surface of the dura mater, derived apparently from a spinal nerve root. The epidural space was completely free of infiltration and there were no radiographic signs of vertebral change.

Clinical symptoms of radicular and cord compression in multiple myeloma are usually observed in subjects of about 50 years of age; this is consistent with the mean age of appearance of the underlying disease (*Olmer et al.*).

However, cases involving much older or much younger subjects are not unknown. *Moeschlin* observed neurological signs in an 84-year-old man, while *Cosacesco* has collected eight instances of subjects under 30 years and a case reported by *Elisabalde and Lamblias* concerned a 5-year-old boy.

The fundamental symptoms are radicular pain and paraplegia.

The former are virtually constant (three out of four in the series of *Clarke, E.*[b] and 20 out of 22 in that of *McKissock et al.*) and appear at an early stage (*McKissock et al.; Paillas et al.*).

The onset of the symptoms is usually gradual and consists of dull, sometimes shooting pain, which is often attributed to simple causes such as arthrosis or earlier trauma, with the result that intervertebral disk distress or post-traumatic painful osteoporosis is incriminated. On rare occasions, the appearance of pain is both sudden and severe, as in a case reported by *Browder and de Veer* (onset during work; the initial diagnosis of pleuritis was rejected when paraplegia appeared some weeks later). Pain begins in the spine and may be aggravated by the slightest expenditure of effort. The interscapular region is the site of choice (*Clarke, E.*[b]) and pain in this area may raise a diagnostic suspicion in subjects in their fifties (*Paillas et al.*).

The later course is typically radicular, with either uni- or bilateral beltwise distribution.

As many as 86% of cases of multiple myeloma present pain due solely to skeletal involvement (*Bayrd and Heck*), usually of the spinal column.

The length of the preparaplegic pain period varies considerably and is thought to be longer in cases of solitary plasmacytoma (*Paillas et al.*). It may form the only clinical sign of the underlying disease for as long as a year. This fact, coupled with the tendency toward spontaneous regression and fresh onset of pain, makes diagnosis difficult or impossible in the absence of other signs.

In other cases, paraplegia is not preceded by radicular pain (6% and 7.3% in the series of *Svien et al.* and *Schneider and Mazabraud*, respectively).

Onset of paraplegia may be sudden (*Snyder and Wilhelm; Svien et al.; Giraud et al.*[b]; *Lugaresi et al.*). In the case observed by *Snyder and Wilhelm* complete flaccid paraplegia appeared without warning as the patient was rising. Sudden onset in the presence of the visiting physician was reported by *Giraud et al.*[b] in a case of cervical myeloma in a patient who had suffered from intractable cervical and scapular pain for a number of years and was seeking admission for its treatment. Pathologic fracture of a vertebra was followed by acute transverse cord lesion in the case reported by *Lugaresi et al.* As this case clearly shows, sudden onset is attributable primarily to vertebral collapse, possibly as a result of imperceptible trauma (*Erbslöh*), though an important part may also be played by myelomalacia.

It is, however, more common for a period of months (*Shenkin et al.*) or years (*Kissel et al.*) to elapse before complete motor deficit is reached.

Slow cord compression will be the picture in most cases. Spastic paraplegia is usually accompanied by sensory disturbances in the lower part of the body, and serious sphincter deficiency. Flaccid, or flaccid and spastic paralysis may be observed.

Where the onset of paraplegia is acute, the clinical picture may suggest cord section.

A Brown-Séquard syndrome may be noted (*Bay*).

Occasionally tetraplegia is reported in cervical plasmacytoma.

Epidural infiltration may be the cause of isolated sciatic radicular pain, or uni- (*Verda*) or bilateral (*Boulet et al.*) cauda equina syndromes. This is not common, though it may be noted that a cauda equina syndrome was observed by *Silverstein and Doniger* in five out of 27 cases of epidural infiltration.

Objective examination will show painful, elastic myelomatous swelling of the infiltrated vertebrae and palpation may be accompanied by faint crepitation as a result of collapse of the cortex and residual trabeculae. Spinal rigidity is a frequent finding. Pain following pressure applied to one or more apophyses at the upper limit of the area of anesthesia is equally common and must be taken as an indication for spinal radiography.

Radiological alterations have already been discussed. Widespread osteoporosis is virtually constant and may be associated with more serious changes involving one or more vertebrae. The observed skeletal damage does not necessarily mirror the extent of the radicular and cord symptomatology. Radiological techniques do not guarantee total detection of skeletal alterations and apparently normal pictures are not uncommon (e.g. seven out of 16 cases of vertebral plasmacytoma were without radiologic signs in the series of *Kissel et al.*).

Myelography and lumbar puncture will indicate the degree of compression and may reveal a Froin syndrome, though anatomic examination may sometimes show an absence of cord compression in spite of the clinical data (*Schott et al.*). However, lumbar puncture may be dangerous and sometimes leads to emergency surgery following its execution (*Clarke, E.*[b]). Also increased protein values do not necessarily indicate meningeal cavity block as they may be no more than an expression of meningeal involvement in a general state of dysprotein-emia.

CSF Bence-Jones proteins are occasionally observed.

Slightly increased CSF cell counts have been observed exceptionally in cases of epidural infiltration ($40/mm^3$ in case no. 1 and $16/mm^3$ in case no. 2 of the series of *Davison and Balser* and of *Pétridès,* respectively).

Where meningeal cavity block is not total, *McKissock et al.* advise the use of suboccipital myelography since this will permit visualization of both the upper and the lower limit of epidural infiltration with a single injection.

As in the less common case of cerebral complication, the diagnosis of radicular and cord compression syndromes is facilitated by their appearance when the underlying disease is already apparent. In some cases, however, both the pain and the motor component of the picture may be masked by manifestations of bone pain commonly observed in multiple myeloma and by terminal cachexia. In contrast, bone pain may be so intense and intractable as to suggest paraplegia dolorosa (*Gilbert-Dreyfus et al.*).

Neurological pictures are very often the initial sign of multiple myeloma (85% of the 204 cases of radicular and cord compression culled from the literature by *Clarke, E.*[b]). Diagnosis is then extremely difficult, though typically myelomatous radiologic signs of skeletal alteration, typical hyperdysproteinemia, Bence-Jones proteinuria, and bone marrow plasmacytosis will all serve as pointers.

Bone marrow puncture may have to be repeated to find the infiltrated area. Then puncture of the spinous apophyses of the diseased vertebrae (*Layani et al.*) or of paravertebral ossifluent masses (*Giraud et al.*[b]) may be useful.

In the initial pain stage of the radicular and cord compression syndromes, differential diagnosis must include consideration of vertebral arthrosis and post-traumatic diskopathy or painful osteoporosis. An initial diagnosis of Kümmell's disease was made in a case reported by *Coste et al.*[b] Visceral alterations (coronary insufficiency, biliary calculosis, appendicopathia) must be considered in cases of unilateral beltwise radicular type pain. Other diagnostic possibilities include: vertebral metastasis in cancer, Ewing's sarcoma (in the infrequent cases in which young subjects are involved), Guillain-Barré syndrome, and vertebral tuberculosis (paravertebral ossifluent masses or clinical and radiologic data suggesting Pott's disease; integrity of the intervertebral disk is usually the distinguishing feature of multiple myeloma). Radiologic evidence of trabeculation and cyst formation in a vertebral body suggested angioma or osteoclastoma in a case reported by *Layani et al.* and the true diagnosis was obtained by biopsy at the spinous apophysis of the diseased vertebra. The observation of eburnation does not warrant the rejection of multiple myeloma as a diagnosis.

Both cord and cerebral alterations, however, may be caused by intercurrent infection, which is the result of dysproteinemia, and hence an immunological deficiency, or of the use of antiproliferation treatment or cortisones. As in the case of Hodgkin's disease, concomitant cerebro-meningeal cryptococcosis may be observed (*Williams, H. M. et al.*). An instance of suppurative meningitis in myelomatosis observed by *Clarke, S. W.* was probably due to pneumococcus, since it responded to penicillin and sulfonamides and later to ampicillin, though the CSF was free of bacteria. Nerve alterations also may be the direct result of treatment in multiple myeloma: diseases caused by high doses of cortisone, radiation myelopathy (*Carson et al.*), trigeminal pain, hypoesthesia, or paresthesia following stilbamidine (*Snapper et al.; Silverstein and Doniger*), though this drug is rarely used today.

When, however, radicular and cord compression or the less common intracranial signs are the first manifestation of the underlying disease, diagnosis will usually be postponed to surgery and the attendant anatomic and histologic findings (*Snyder and Wilhelm; Alliez et al.; Svien et al.*). Neurosurgical management is urgent in some cases and there is no time for full clinical, radiological, and biological investigation.

Surgery (laminectomy with total or partial resection of the neoformation) followed by roentgenotherapy is the treatment of choice of radicular and cord compression and may lead to functional recovery in as many as 75% of cases.

X-rays alone may give good results (*Layani et al.; McKissock et al.*), including partial recalcification (*Snapper et al.*). However, surgery (which is not used in preterminal cases) is the usual prelude to radiation therapy, though it is not in itself sufficient to prevent recurrences (*Clarke, E.[b], Labauge et al.*). Radiation will be even more necessary where only partial resection or solely decompressive laminectomy is done.

Medical treatment (urethane, cortisones, stilbamidine, melphalan) is directed primarily to the relief of pain.

Instances of remission lasting for several years following combined surgical and radiation management have been reported. A patient observed by *Hagelstam* was in good condition and free from neurological disturbances six years after treatment, in spite of the presence of marrow plasmacytosis and a large vertebral site.

Particularly outstanding results have been noted in the treatment of solitary osteoepidural plasmacytoma, and regressions have lasted several years (*Donnelly and Grahn; etc.*). Other workers (*Paillas et al.; etc.*) have observed regressions for as long as 15 or 20 years, and it would not be improper to refer to some of these cases as truly cured.

Evaluation of treatment efficacy must include the possibility of spontaneous regression. Partial resection of a vertebral plasmacytoma for paraplegia was followed by the observation of total disappearance of infiltration and its replacement by fibrous and granulomatous tissue ten months later in a case reported by *Tremblay et al.*

In multiple myeloma, as in other systemic blood diseases, the observation of cord compression should be followed by the earliest possible treatment to prevent the onset of irreversible malacia.

Treatment may also be effective in the event of recurrence.

A neurological picture indicating funicular myelosis noted by *Baldassari et al.* in a case of multiple myeloma was greatly benefited by the administration of vitamin B_{12} and tranfusions for serious concomitant anemia.

It is uncertain whether multiple myeloma is responsible for direct peripheral nerve involvement: *Victor et al.*, for example, hold that peripheral signs must in all cases be considered aspecific paraneoplastic manifestations. Nevertheless, peripheral nerve infiltration has been reported. Numerous infiltrates (together with considerable demyelinization) observed postmortem in three cases by *Barron et al.* were held responsible for the *in vivo* symptomatology in two patients. This infiltration consisted of symmetric polyneuritis as the first clinical sign of the underlying disease, followed by progressive deterioration in one case, and apparent improvement, though accompanied by aggravation of the patient's general condition and death in cachexia and stupor, in the other. Infiltration of the sciatic nerve has been reported by *Brownell.*

Horner's syndrome was noted by *Snapper et al.* in a case of cervical plasmacytoma.

Herpes zoster has been noted by a number of workers (*Snapper et al.; Daneo; Greenstein and Cahn; Williams, H. M. et al.; Shanbrom et al.; etc.*). Ophthalmic herpes appeared three years before the appearance of the underlying disease in a case observed by *Di Guglielmo.* Two years earlier, this patient had presented cold-induced upper limb circulation disturbances, with acroasphyxia and left digital necrosis. Cryoglobulinemia was not observed. Blood viscosity values were high and increased as the temperature fell. Dysproteinemia proper to the underlying disease was suggested as responsible for both the herpes and the circulation disturbances. Generalized herpes was the initial clinical sign in a 77-year-old woman observed by *Thiers et al.* and an ulnar site has been reported by *Giovanelli et al.* Generalized gangrenous herpes, accompanied by serious neuralgia, was the main cause of death in a case reported by *Meiers and Gehrmann.*

The differential diagnosis of myelomatous and the more frequent aspecific forms of peripheral involvement is notoriously difficult and requires full evaluation of the clinical and more particularly the anatomic data. Four cases of uni- and bilateral carpal tunnel syndrome were clinically referred to myelomatous infiltration of the median nerve by *Grokoest and Demartini.* In one case, however, amyloid deposits were found intraoperatively in the forearm flexor tendon sheaths, and necropsy showed the median nerves to be free of such deposits, as well as of infiltration.

Identical amyloidosis-induced carpal tunnel syndromes have been published by *Grossman et al., Kyle and Bayrd, Blodgett et al., Munsat and Poussaint, Swinton et al.,* etc., while an association of the syndrome with macroglossia and amyloidosis of the finger tip skin and of the rectal mucosa has been reported by *Rittmeyer and Schlachetzki.* Compression of the brain (*Medoc et al.*), cord (*Pino; Williams, H. M. et al.; Roslund et al.*) and trigeminal ganglion (*Kyle and Bayrd*) by amyloid masses has also been reported.

Widespread bone pain and left sciatic neuralgia formed the clinical overture in a personal case of multiple myeloma in a 70-year-old man. Radiography (about one year later) showed typical skullcap, mandible, and trunk osteolysis and pointed to the correct diagnosis. A left Lasègue sign was also elicited. The sciatic picture was relieved by X-ray cycles on the pelvis.

Aspecific neuropathy localizations in the peripheral nerve system may be a result of myelomatous dysglobulinemia in addition to the etiopatho-genetic factors commonly held responsible for paraneoplastic neurologi-cal alterations in systemic blood diseases. *Michon et al.,* indeed, would place them in the group of dysglobulinemic neuropathies that includes some of the cerebral manifestations observed in multiple myeloma itself, the neurological alterations of Waldenström's disease and of the cryoglobulinemias.

Five aspecific cases of this type were noted by *Victor et al.* in 1958, following reports of isolated instances by *Davison and Balser, Scheinker, Kurnick and Yohalem, Estes and Millikan, Clarke, E.[c], Crow,* and *Kenny and Moloney.* Later observations have included those of *Borchers and Mittel-bach, Boudin et al., Ojea et al., Rohmer et al., Aguayo et al.,* and *Gupta and Prabhakar,* while *Silverstein and Doniger* (1964) observed nine cases and one example of carpal tunnel syndrome in 277 multiple myeloma patients studied at the Mount Sinai Hospital in New York. It cannot be claimed that aspecific nerve pictures are common, however.

Their presence is typically denoted by extensive spinal root and peripheral nerve degeneration in the absence of infiltration or compression (*Victor et al.*), expressed as segmentary demyelinization, sometimes accompanied by considerable neurolemma proliferation ("sclerosing interstitial neuritis"). Spinal ganglia involvement is uncommon and slight alterations of the anterior and posterior gray column cells may be classed as "ascending" in nature.

The aspecific, toxic multifunicular cord degeneration described by *Lindeboom and Mulder* has been attributed by other workers (*Schott et al., Labauge et al.*) to vascular damage, since the patient presented a typical epidural myeloma spinal compression syndrome (with meningeal block), in addition to an intramedullary necrosis cavity.

Clarke, E. considers these aspecific nerve pictures to be the expression of amyloid infiltration, though this hypothesis is as yet unsupported by data.

The fact that aspecific forms may be the only sign of the underlying disease for periods of months or even years makes diagnosis problematical, particularly when the laboratory data are inconclusive. In a case observed by *Boudin et al.* diagnosis could be arrived at only by CSF immunoelectrophoresis in the absence of pathological blood findings. More commonly, however, neurological signs are encountered within an identified blood picture, the long-standing nature of which is deduced from the fact that demyelinization is usually slow. Neuropathies accompanying solitary plasmacytoma have sometimes been reported (*Scheinker; Victor et al.; Rohmer et al.*).

Bilateral symmetrical sensory and motor involvement is usually the distinguishing feature of the clinical picture. Paresthesia and painful dysesthesia in the hands, and more particularly in the feet, normally testify to the presence of a neurological complication and are followed by deep sensibility alterations. Motor deficiency (amyotrophy and areflexia) simultaneously progresses from the lower to the upper extremities in most cases; distal symmetry is again the most common finding. *Boudin et al., Scheinker,* and *Rohmer et al.* have all observed examples of striking and rapidly ascendent pictures recalling polyradiculoneuritis and terminating in serious respiratory disturbances and involvement of the main air passages. These cases suggest retrograde degeneration of the cranial nerve nuclei in addition to the cord neurons, and even damage to the bulb and pons, as shown by clinical evidence. In the case reported by *Ojea et al.* the ascending nature of the affection was revealed by the appearance of respiratory disturbances caused by paresis of the intercostal muscles 11 and 8 months after the commencement of lower extremity sensory and motor abnormalities, respectively. The initial picture had also included polycythemia and it was not until this abated that the myelomatous nature of the disease became clear.

Increased CSF protein values are common (ranging from 0.5 to 3.4 g ⁰/oo in the series of *Victor et al.*), though their relation to the neurological picture has not been established (*Frantzen et al.*). Increases in cell levels are not common and the usual picture is of albuminocytologic dissociation without block. Protein alterations mirroring those observed in the blood will not necessarily be found on CSF electrophoresis. Bence-Jones protein is occasionally reported.

As stated, dysglobulinemia is considered responsible for a group of cerebral manifestations for which neither compression, infiltration, nor other causes independent of blood protein levels can be incriminated. Together with the neurological alterations of Waldenström's disease and the cryoglobulinemias, these form part of the so-called dysglobulinemic neuropathies (nerve manifestations in other types of dysglobulinemia are very rare).

The view that paraproteinemia is responsible for nerve damage would seem well founded and a relationship between blood paraprotein values and nerve signs has been shown by some workers (*Madonick and Solomon*). Increased CSF protein levels may be observed, however, in the complete absence of neurological involvement (*Degenhardt and Sheehan*); a comparable situation may be noted in the CSF hyperalbuminiosis of diabetes.

Thrombosis of the capillaries, including those supplying nerve tissues, is thought to occur in dysglobulinemia as a result of red cell conglomeration. Globulin precipitation in cryoglobulinemia is followed by the imprisonment of red cells in the semisolid protein precipitate and the same result may thus be assumed. An interesting case in point is that reported by *Hansen and Faber*. Careful plethysmographic and capillaroscopic studies *in vivo* demonstrated the formation of capillary-occluding protein microemboli in a patient with bilateral retinal thrombosis, cold-induced Raynaud-type symptoms and globulin precipitation at 37.5° C, followed by their dissolution on the application of heat. There can be no doubt that increased viscosity and its consequent deceleration of circulation and cell nutrition leads to severe damage to the delicate and complicated metabolic system of the nerve cell.

Toxic injury to nerve structures has also been attributed to paraproteins, in particular to blood and CSF Bence-Jones protein; conclusive data have yet to be advanced, however.

Thickening and collapse of capillary walls caused by protein or amyloid infiltration have been found histologically and constitute yet another mechanism which may result in nerve damage.

Protean symptomatologies have been attributed to dysglobulinemia-induced cerebral damage and their classification is difficult.

A distinction must be drawn between psychological manifestations and "paraproteinemic coma."

As long ago as 1937, *Davison and Balser* reported a case of depression syndrome, including hallucinations and a sense of persecution. The syndrome was clearly not referable to an observed dura mater myeloma-tous nodule. Signs of confusion, accompanied by paranoid reactions in two cases, were noted by *Snapper et al.* in 11 out of 97 multiple myeloma patients, whereas potentially responsible cerebral alterations were observed in only one of the seven necropsies performed. *Van Dommelen* reported what he called "kahlerian psychosis" (a paranoid form) in two out of 29 cases of multiple myeloma. The depression observed (*inter alia*) by *Morin et al.* in their case cannot be unreservedly attributed to dysproteinemia, since considerable infiltration of the arachnoidea and pia mater was also present. In another case reported by these workers, however, its incrimination rests on a more solid foundation, since the total regression of serious psychological disturbances in multiple myeloma of three years' standing appears to preclude their dependence on compression or infiltration. A patient studied by *Stankiewicz and Dymecki* presented confusion with serious anxiety, followed by depression and hallucinations. There were, however, various features of this case among which individual or collective responsibility for the syndrome might be sought (prior radiation treatment, postoperative onset, cranial and meningeal myelomas, considerable atherosclerosis of the vessels of the cerebral base). Persecutory delusion was reported by *Azzena et al.* This case was examined only clinically, though it may be noted that unilateral ptosis was the only symptom suggesting intracranial localization of the underlying disease.

The term "paraproteinemic coma" was coined by *Wuhrmann* (1956) with respect to coma observed in a typical case of multiple myeloma and attributed by him to considerable hyperproteinemia (15 g%) and CSF electrophoretic abnormalities unaccompanied by signs of abnormal renal or hepatic metabolism. The same conditions were observed by this worker in 12 cases of dysglobulinemia, four of which were marked by the onset of psychological manifestations immediately prior to coma. In nine of these cases necropsy was performed but since the writer does not mention the results, it may be assumed that cerebral alterations were slight or nonexistent.

Clinical data suggestive of paraproteinemic coma were noted by *Borchers and Mittelbach* in a case of multiple myeloma of nine years' standing in a patient who presented coma not attributable to renal, hepatic, cardiac, or pulmonary causes four days before death. The CSF data included increased albumin levels and mastic test curve changes.

Fatal coma was observed by *Kramer* in a case (mentioned earlier) with clear signs of protein dysmetabolism (increased blood and CSF levels [11.6 g% and 1.2 g%o] serum electrophoresis abnormalities, etc.) As already noted, myelomatous invasion of the right temporal lobe was also present and this would tend to diminish the importance of the part played by metabolic disturbances in the onset of coma. Since this worker, like *Wuhrmann* himself, considers paraproteinemic coma an expression of metabolic encephalopathy, however, he attaches particular significance to his observation of multiple hyaline thrombosis—leading to neuron anoxia—in the cerebral capillaries in this case.

Cortisones are the logical choice for the treatment of cerebral manifestations apparently attributable to dysglobulinemia, since they have been proved capable of securing partial or even total regression of protein disturbances in multiple myeloma. Their use in the management of paraneoplastic peripheral syndromes is also recommended, though herpes must be seen as a contraindication. The incrimination of intravasal red cell agglutination in supposedly dysglobulinemic nerve manifestations has led some workers (*Berlin*) to advise the administration of generous doses of vasodilatators (Priscol).

Appendix. Cryoglobulinemia, Waldenström's Disease

Both the central nervous system (CNS) and the peripheral nervous system may be involved in cyroglobulinemia.

CNS involvement was observed by *Hutchinson and Howell* in a picture which included massive extremity ischemia and anoxia with multiple gangrene. Aggravation was accompanied by particularly severe peripheral ischemia (frozen feet, facial cyanosis, etc.) and gradual loss of consciousness without signs of motor deficiency; regression was obtained with oxygen. Thrombocytosis (775,000/mm³) was a possible accomplice in the onset of both the ischemic and the neurological manifestations.

Cryoglobulinemia of such intensity that blood samples could be obtained only with heated syringes appeared in a case of multiple myeloma observed by *Marshall and Malone*. The terminal picture included coma, papillary edema, retinal hemorrhage, and venous turgor. Necropsy showed cerebral edema and small purpuric hemorrhage sites disseminated in the internal capsule and peduncles. Histological examination revealed that the small cerebral parenchyma vessels were surrounded by hemorrhagic extravasation and filled with (probably) protein hyaline and acidophile material.

High cerebral hemorrhage frequencies and examples of retinal hemorrhage may be found in *Dini et al.*'s cryoglobulinemia series.

The symptoms of peripheral damage are those of combined sensory and motor multineuritis triggered by low temperatures, and they appear in the form of episodes and intermittent regression. Spectacular summer regression may be observed.

A disseminated multineuritis picture with paresthesia of the extremities and extensor and lateral peroneal paresis in a lower limb has been reported by *Garcin et al.*[a] Radicular type superficial sensibility disturbances were also noted, but deep sensibility involvement was not observed.

Hand paresthesia with distal motor deficiency, rapidly progressing to amyotrophy, followed by deltoid, psoas, and leg muscle paralysis, formed part of the later picture in a case of cryoglobulinemia symptomatic of lymphosarcoma coupled with persistent Raynaud's syndrome reported by *Boudin et al.* Bilateral deafness was also noted.

In a case symptomatic of nodose periarteritis observed by *Garcin et al.*[d], distal numbness with 4th and 5th digit paresthesia was followed by calf cramp, involvement of the tibial compartments and hand extensores and interossei bilaterally, and, lastly, hypoesthesia of the last three digits.

An association of cryoglobulinemia and neuritis in the course of nodose periarteritis has been reported by *Buttler and Palmer* also.

Right facial anesthesia and multineuritis involving the left upper and both lower limbs (slight motor deficit, hypoesthesia as far as the root of the thighs, bilateral Achilles and unilateral patellar areflexia) were observed in a 30-year-old woman by *Labauge et al.* The patient was extremely sensitive to cold and a typical Raynaud's syndrome appeared later. Nodose periarteritis was excluded by muscle biopsies. Erythrocyte sedimentation rate dissociation (3 mm at 4°C and 37 mm at 37°C for the first hour) was typical of cryoglobulinemia.

Sensory and motor neuropathy pictures were noted by *Logothetis et al.*[b] in idiopathic cryoglobulinemia in a 39-year-old woman and in a case secondary to malignant lymphoma. The first patient also presented parotid and submaxillary gland swelling; cervical and inguinal adenopathies; lack of tearing; intermittent swelling of the fingers; chronic, recurrent ulcers on both legs; periodic purpuric eruptions, which developed into stocking-pattern, brownish spots on both legs, and which were associated with chills and fever.

Peripheral nerve involvement may consist of nothing more than cold-induced cramp or muscle pain.

Nerve complications are not common in cryoglobulinemia, particularly idiopathic forms.

Extremely serious asthenia and rapid exhaustion, together with a myasthenic type electromyograph picture, were observed in two idiopathic cases by *Quattrin et al.*

In addition to the blood picture, symptoms indicating pathological sensitivity to cold, Raynaud's syndrome, winter purpura, etc., will serve to incriminate cryoglobulinemia in the diagnosis of nerve signs.

With regard to differential diagnosis the aspecific neuropathies of multiple myeloma tend to be more symmetrical and regular in their distribution than those associated with cryoglobulinemia.

Differentiation of nerve pictures associated with ischemia and anoxia in the extremities in hemolytic anemia resulting from cold agglutinins may be obtained by immunological examination. In cryoglobulinemia, as in the other forms of dysglobulinemia, the absence of agglutinin responsibility can be demonstrated readily.

No effective treatment has yet been found for cryoglobulinemia. Peripheral vasodilatators may be administered and precautions against cold should be taken.

Waldenström first described macroglobulinemia (Waldenström's disease) as a clinical entity in 1944. Its nerve involvement pictures had already been the subject of study in 1936, however, when *Bing and Neel* reported CNS involvement in the course of some cases of "hyperglobulinemia" (Bing and Neel syndrome). Reexamination of their observations has since shown that they were associated with true macroglobulinemia (*Bichel et al.*).

The neurological pictures in this disease are certainly caused by CNS histiocyte-lymphoid infiltration; this is perivasal in arrangement and morphologically indistinguishable from that noted in other viscera. Nodular formations are rare, but their confluence and consequent tumor-like appearance have also been reported (*Edgar and Dutcher*).

Macroglobulinemia itself is also a cause of nerve damage. The question of pathogenesis has been discussed in connection with paraproteinemia of multiple myeloma. Here it may be noted that a para-aminosalicylic acid (PAS) -positive, acidophil substance, probably globulinic and perhaps identifiable in the macroglobulin, has been anatomically and histologically detected in nerve tissue. It has been observed in the obstructed lumen of small vessels and capillaries ("plasmatic thromboses" of *Rauber et al.*). Its presence in vessel exteriors is connected with endothelium alterations caused by anoxemia resulting from the circulation stasis that is brought about by increased blood viscosity (*Zollinger;*

Olmer et al.). PAS-staining inclusions of this substance inside nerve cells have also been reported (*Zollinger; Aarseth et al.*).

Nerve alterations may also be attributable to hemorrhage; the pathogenesis of the hemorrhage of multiple myeloma has already been discussed. In cryoglobulinemia, purpuric manifestations are caused by invasion of skin vessel walls by cold-precipitated cryoglobulins and/or their interference with the formation of thromboplastin, thrombin, and fibrin, resulting in poor coagulation. With regard to Waldenström's disease, it is thought that macroglobulins may adsorb clotting factors and coat the platelets in such a way as to render them inactive in the clotting process. Some workers (*MacKay et al.; Labauge et al.; Stefanini and Dameshek; Doumenc et al.; Izarn et al.*) have postulated interference with thrombin activity or infiltration and damage of the vessel walls. *Waldenström* has shown increased blood heparin values in some cases.

CNS alterations in Waldenström's disease are extremely diffuse. In one of the early observations of *Bing and Neel,* involvement of the encephalon, meninges, cord and spinal roots was equally intense. *Kakulas and Finlay-Jones* noted damage to the internal capsule, lentiform nucleus, hypothalamus, cerebral peduncles, pons, and cerebellum. Disseminated, multifocal symptomatologies are in keeping with such diffusion pictures.

Nerve manifestations may be expected in about 25% of cases (*Labauge et al.*). CNS involvement would appear more common (32 CNS, 14 peripheral pictures in the series of *Logothetis et al*[a]).

Onset may be any time from two months to two years after the commencement of the disease. The signs are most commonly very polymorphous and difficult to classify.

The literature contains a number of clinical examples of CNS involvement

The three early cases observed by *Bing and Neel* (1936), and *Bing, Neel, and Fog* (1937) concerned patients with both sensory and motor disturbances (paraparesis, pyramidal signs, and Babinski's reflex in one case). Necropsy showed plasma cell perivasal infiltration in the meninges and spinal cord.

A 62-year-old man with spastic hemiparesis, Babinski's reflex, and finger and toe torpor was observed by *Bichel et al.* (1950). The clinical picture also included epistaxis, loss of visual acuity, retinal hemorrhage, and adenopathies. The blood data indicated anemia, while the myelogram showed a high proportion of lymphoid cells. Hyperglobulinemia (7.5–11 g %) was noted and macroglobulins were observed in the ultracentrifuge. The CSF picture included globulins and increased lymphocyte values. Necropsy showed histiocyte-lymphoid infiltration of the bone marrow and nerve structures to the point of radiculomeningoencephal-opathy; basophile leukocytes were also present in the infiltrates.

Haas et al. later observed a case of rapidly regressing hemiplegia and aphasia accompanied by persecution delirium. *Mandema* reported pyramidal signs and meningeal damage. *Wanner and Siebenmann* noted paraplegia and coma; at the histological examination of the brain intratubal and perivasal invasion of the small cerebral vessels by a PAS-positive substance was found. A pyramidal syndrome and hemiparesis with hypertonia were observed by *Kappeler et al.,* while *Michon et al.* have reported left hemiplegia with prolonged coma.

Extrapyramidal manifestations have been described by *MacKay et al.* (notable Parkinson-type tremor) and *Kappeler et al.* (typical unilateral parkinsonian syndrome).

Tumor type, left temporal, and occipital symptoms followed by fatal cerebral trunk compression were noted by *Edgar and Dutcher* in a typical Waldenström's disease. Necropsy showed widespread brain damage, a histologically demonstrated lymphoplasmareticular left occipital lobe mass and nodular infiltration of the left frontal lobe.

Ventricular flooding and left thalamus hemorrhage have been reported by *Schaub* and *MacKay et al.,* respectively, while a meningeal hemorrhage episode was virtually the initial sign of the underlying disease in one of the two cases observed by *Bousser and Boivin.* Meningeal hemorrhage has already been noted by *Kanzow, Wanner, and Siebenmann,* and *Kappeler et al.*

Paraproteinemic coma was postulated in cases observed by *Wuhrmann*[b] and *Michon et al.*

Psychological disturbances were present in the case reported by *Haas et al.* and also were observed by *Kappeler et al.* in three out of 20 cases.

An example of spontaneous spinal epidural hematoma has been described by *Arseni et al.*

With regard to peripheral damage, it may be noted that cranial involvement usually concerns the 8th nerve. Frank deafness or lesser disturbances have been reported by *Bichel et al., Tischendorff and Hartmann, MacKay et al.,* and *Kappeler et al.* Vertigo and labyrinth deficiency were present in cases studied by *Fiere, MacKay et al.,* and *Kappeler et al.* Retrobulbar neuritis has been noted by *Bing and Neel* and optic atrophy by *Hagen* and *Haas et al.*

Spinal nerve involvement has been reported on a number of occasion intervals (*Garcin et al.*[b, c]); patellar areflexia (*Zlotnick*); paresthesia, slight motor deficiency deep sensibility disturbances, left lower extremity hyporeflexia (*Michon et al.*); polyneuritis (*Darnley; Ricci et al.;*

Azzena et al.); **Guillain-Barré** type syndrome (*Logothetis et al.*[a]). Spinal nerve involvement has also been observed by *Bodechtel et al.*

Lower extremity paresthesia and neuralgia were noted in a case of macroglobulinemia of 13 years' standing by *Aarseth et al.* Muscle asthenia and atrophy were later observed in the legs, whereas upper limb involvement was less evident. The picture was also rendered unusual by the presence of considerable hemolytic anemia, with reticulocytosis, high serum iron levels, and greatly diminished mean red cell life in the terminal stage. Necropsy showed widespread lymph node swellings and liver, spleen, and kidney enlargement. Microscopy revealed widespread lymphocyte and lymphoid cell proliferation, numerous plasma and mast cells, and considerable reticular cell proliferation in these organs, while similar infiltration was also noted in the meninges, around the brain and cord vessels, and in the sciatic nerves; swelling and degeneration of some sciatic nerve fibers was also apparent. Considerable cell loss was observed in the anterior gray columns. Quadricipital muscle degeneration, with fiber atrophy and frank nuclear pyknosis, was noted as well.

Serious symmetric sensory and motor polyneuropathy has been reported by *Gotham et al.*, together with electromyographic evidence of neuromuscular atrophy (increased conduction times). However, clear clinical signs of distal (hand interosseal and leg muscle) atrophy were present.

Lower limb nerve symptoms were observed in two cases by *Vital et al.* Peroneus brevis biopsy in one case showed histiocyte-lymphoid infiltration and dissociation of the muscle fibers. Perivasal infiltration with involvement of the vessel wall was noted, together with infiltration of the musculocutaneous nerve and enlargement of its endoneurium. Ultramicroscopy showed myelin fiber changes (lamellar Schwann cell cytoplasm, loss of typical periodicity, myelin sheath swelling, decreased axon size and amorphous appearance, as though compressed by the swollen sheath). At some points, these changes had reached a particularly advanced stage and an axon structure could no longer be made out. A similar musculocutaneous nerve biopsy picture was also noted in the second case.

Symmetric upper and lower limb sensory and motor polyneuropathy has been recorded as the initial sign of Waldenström's disease by *Saric et al.*

CSF changes are not constant and vary from case to case. Increased protein values were observed by *Layani et al.* in a case in which crushing of the vertebrae was also present. *Kanzow* has reported increased cell and albumin values in one case; in his opinion, macroglobulins are never present. Increased albumin levels and positive globulin reaction, though without macroglobulins, were noted in a case with cuneiform vertebra by *Michon et al.* and a similar positive reaction without macroglobulins has been observed by *Kappeler et al. MacKay et al.*, however, found both macro- and cryoglobulins in the liquor.

Fundus oculi changes ("fundus paraproteinemicus") may also be observed. Retinal hemorrhage is a frequent example of such changes and is more easily detected. Usually it is spread over the whole field in numerous sites. It may vary in appearance and size and may take the form of bands, blotches, streaks, or spots. Localization may be perivasal or unrelated to the vessels. The hemorrhages with a central white area observed in leukemia are rare (one case in the series of *Michon et al.*).

Increased blood viscosity may be responsible for alterations in the retinal veins, leading to turgor, dilatation, tortuosity, or irregular caliber ("pearl necklace," "string of sausages," etc.). An example may be found in the series of *Michon et al.* In other cases, simple annular restriction of limited extent and pale appearance may be observed. Thrombosis of the central vein has been reported also (*Waldenström; Ascenzi et al.; Fiere; Levrat et al.; etc.*).

Whitish exudates have been observed by *Korsten and Berneaud-Kötz, Kappeler et al.*, and *Michon et al.*, usually near the vessels. Noninflammatory, intra- and retroretinal exudation was histologically demonstrated by *Cagianut* in three cases, twice resulting in pronounced detachment at the posterior pole, while the membrane was thick and imbued with a strongly eosinophile homogeneous mass. This was also present in the lumen of the large vessels and its histochemical picture suggested a serum paraprotein origin. Slight hemorrhage and infiltration in the area of Schlemm's canal and the ciliary body completed the eye alteration picture.

The following alterations may be detected with a Baillart's ophthalmodynamometer: flattening of the venous trunks of the optic disk, arterial systole at this level, granulous venous current coinciding with increases in arterial pulse amplitude (the blood column is fragmented into numerous small red grains moving continuously toward the disk, and appearance of a granulous arterial current following increase of the instrument pressure. These manifestations have been fully studied by *Danis et al.* and *Paufique and Royer. Korsten and Berneaud-Kötz* consider them to be an expression of an early stage of the underlying disease. In a case reported by *Michon et al.* they were the only ophthalmological signs.

Papillary and peripapillary edema are rare and other exceptional findings include: arterial thrombosis (*Kappeler et al.*), microaneurysms (*Revol et al.*), and chorioretinitis caused by specific infiltration (*Kappeler et al.*).

Bilateral central retinal detachment involving the macular and paramacular areas, edema of the optic disks, and venous congestion were noted by *Stirpe* in two cases. Grayish exudates and hemorrhages were present over the whole of the retina, the latter being anterior to the retina when alongside the vessels and intraretinal when distant from them. In another case this worker observed papillary edema and venous congestion, together with old and recent hemorrhage sites disseminated over the posterior pole and near the disks.

As already stated, loss of visual acuity may be noted. This is usually referable to hemorrhage or infiltration. Amblyopia is rare (*Kappeler et al.*).

Histiocyte-lymphoid proliferation in Waldenström's disease may also be responsible for swelling of the lacrimal glands. A Sjögren syndrome may be noted (*Wuhrmann*[a]; *etc.*), sometimes accompanied by a Mickulicz syndrome (*Fankhauser et al.; MacKay et al.*). *Cagianut* has observed chronic iridocyclitis attributable to aqueous humor paraproteins and infiltration of the ciliary body, and, in another case, glaucoma resulting from exudation in the anterior chamber of the eye.

The diagnosis of Waldenström neurological manifestations presupposes recognition of the underlying syndrome. This in turn must be determined from both the laboratory and the clinical data. A finding of macroglobulinemia is not sufficient per se, since this may form part of other disease pictures.

The intervention of neurological complications is a discouraging prognostic sign. If cerebral hemorrhage is present, the fatal course of the disease, normally protracted (nine years in a case observed by *Olmer et al.*), may be accelerated.

Treatment of the disease embraces that of its neurological complications. Chemotherapeutic drugs and X-ray therapy have failed to give satisfactory results. Improvements have been observed with an association of stilbamidine and cortisones (*Labauge et al.*), though the frequent possibility of renal involvement means that caution must be exercised. *Olmer et al.* are of the opinion that cortisones are definitely useful and lead to improvements in general conditions, asthenia, and appetite, as well as regression of lymph node and spleen enlargement. They may also correct anemia and even dysproteinemia. *Di Guglielmo et al.,* in fact, have reported notable and lasting regression of organ enlargement, bone marrow infiltration, and protein alterations in two cases with massive doses followed by low-dose maintenance cycles. Other workers have obtained good results with chlorambucil (*Melli and Grifoni; Bayrd; Clatanoff and Meyer; Grifoni et al.; Wanebo and Clarkson*). Transient improvement has been reported following splenectomy aimed at reducing protein synthesis (*Long et al.*). Plasmapheresis leads to depletion of plasma proteins and hence a decrease in blood viscosity. It has therefore given good results in the treatment of neurological signs, retinal alterations, and hemorrhage (*Schwab and Fahey; Stefanini and Dameshek; Moulinier et al.*).

REFERENCES

AGUAYO, H.; THOMPSON D. W. and HUMPHREY, J. L.: Multiple myeloma with poly-enuropathy and osteosclerotic lesions. J. Neurol. Neurosurg. Psychiat. 27:562–566 (1964).

ALLIEZ, J.; BONNAL, J.; SERRATRICE, G. and BADIER BÉRARD: Compressions médullaires dans la maladie de Kahler. Rev. neurol. 89:376 (1953).

ANDRÉ, R.; DREYFUS, B.; JACOB, S. and LEY, G.: Sur les formes hémorragiques des myélomes. Rev. Hémat. 7:296–305 (1952).

ARMSTRONG, E. C.; FAULDS, J. S. and STEWART, M. J.: Two cases of multiple myeloma (plasmocytoma) with secondary deposits in dura mater. J. Path. Bact. 58:243–249 (1946).

ARONSOHN, H. G.: Zur pathologischen Anatomie und Symptomatologie der multiplen Myelome. Virchows Arch. path. Anat. 281:78–87 (1931).

AZERAD, E.; GRUPPER, CH. and CHAPUIS, G.: Myélome à plasmocytes vacuolés (cellules de Mott, troisième cas). Bull. Soc. méd. Hôp., Paris 66:97 (1950).

AZZENA, D.; GHIGLIOTTI, G.; ASTENGO, F.; COSTA, U. and MOLINELLI, G.: Manifestazioni neurologiche in corso di 'gammapatie monoclonali'. Rivista della letteratura e descrizione di 5 casi di mieloma multiplo e di 2 casi di macroglobulinemia di Waldenström con diverse compromissioni del sistema nervoso. Haematologica 52:999–1031 (1967).

BACH, M. J. and MIDDLETON, W. S.: Multiple myeloma and diabetes insipidus. J. amer. med. Ass. 97:306–308 (1931).

BALDASSARRI, R.; NICO, F. and SCOPPOLA, L.: Un caso di alfa-mieloma con plasmocitemia elevata ed insolita sindrome neuro-amenica. Policlinico, Sez. prat. 68:537–545 (1961).

BARRON, K. D.; ROWLAND, L. P. and ZIMMERMANN, H. M.: Neuropathy with malignant tumor metastases. J. nerv. ment. Dis. 131:10–31 (1960).

BATTS, M. JR.: Multiple myeloma; review of 40 cases. Arch. Surg., Chicago 39:807–823 (1939).

BAY, E.: Neurologische Störungen bei Blutkrankheiten. Z. ärztl. Fortbild. 55:879–887 (1966).

BAYRD, E. D. and HECK, F. J.: Multiple myeloma; review of 83 proved cases. J. amer. med. Ass. 133:147–157 (1947).

BECK: in Labauge et al.

BERLIN: In Ferrata and Storti, Le malattie del sangue, vol. II, p. 1529 (Fr. Vallardi, Milan 1958).

BERNARD, J.; INCEMAN, S.; ZARA, M. and CHRISTOL, D.: La dysglobulinémie maligne hémorragipare. Rev. Hémat. 7:264–295 (1952).

BETHLEM, J.; GOOL, VAN and HARTOG-JAGER, W. A. DEN: Progressive multifocal leukoencephalopathy associated with multiple myeloma. Acta. neuropath. 3:525–528 (1964).

BIANCHI, V.; GIAMPALMO, A. and MARMONT, A.: Contributo alla conoscenza della gelificazione plasmatica 'a frigore' e della plasmocitosi aleucemica con emogelificazione (gel-plasmocitomatosi). Minerva med. 40/II:101–136 (1949).

BIONDETTI, P.: Mieloma multiplo osteoplastico. Radiol. med. 38:1076 (1952).

BLODGETT, R. C. JR.; LIPSCOMB, P. R. and HILL, R. W.: Incidence of hematologic disease in patients with carpal tunnel syndrome. J. amer. med. Ass. 182:814–815 (1962).

BODECHTEL, G.; BORCHERS, H. G. and KOLLMANNSBERGER, A.: Enzephalopathie bei Blutkrankheiten. Dtsch. med. Wschr. 91:673–682 (1966).

BOLLINI, V. and FRASSINETI, A.: Un caso di plasmocitoma con aspetto osteomalacio. Radiol. med. 38:575–576 (1952).

BORCHERS, H. G. and MITTELBACH, F.: Neurologische Störungen bein Blutkrankheiten. Internist, Berl. 2:105–117 (1961).

BOUDIN, G.; PÉPIN, B. and BRION, S.: Neuropathie périphérique et myélome. Observation anatomo-clinique. Bull. Soc. méd. Hôp., Paris 77:490–500 (1961).

BOULET, P.; SERRE, H.; VEDEL, A.; VALLAT, G.; MIROUZE, J. and SALVAING, J.: Plasmocytome radiologiquement latent relevé par un syndrome de la queue de cheval. Montpellier méd. 33/34:372 (1948).

BOURDREAUX: in Labauge et al.

BROWDER, J. and VEER, A. DE: Lymphomatoid diseases involving spinal epidural space; pathologic and therapeutic consideration. Arch. Neurol., Chicago 41:328–347 (1939).

BROWNELL, E. G.: Multiple myeloma; review of 61 proved cases. Arch. intern. Med. 95:699–704 (1955).

CALVET, J.; CLAUX, J.; GAYRAL, L.; RASCOL, A. and CADENAT, H.: Syndrome de Garcin aigu par plasmocytome de la base du crâne. Rev. Oto-Neuro-Ophtal. 22:481–484 (1950).

CAPPELL, D. F. and MATHERS, R. P.: Plasmacytoma of petrous temporal bone and base of skull. J. Laryng. 50:340–349 (1935).

CARSON, C. P.; ACKERMAN, L. V. and MALTBY, J. D.: Plasma cell myeloma; clinical, pathologic and roentgenologic review of 90 cases. Amer. J. clin. Path. 25:849–888 (1955).

CHRISTOPHE AND DIVRY: in Olmer et al.

CLARKE, E.: a) Cranial and intracranial myelomas. Brain 77:61–81 (1954). b) Spinal cord involvement in multiple myelomatosis. Brain 79:332–348 (1956). c) Peripheral neuropathy associated with multiple myelomatosis. Neurology, Minneap. 6:146–151 (1956).

CLARKE, S. W.: Myelomatosis with meningitis and eye changes. Proc. roy. Soc. Med. 59: 423 (1966).

COSACESCO, A.: Le myélome chez les jeunes; forme vertébrale initiale. Lyon chir. 43:677–684 (1948).

COSTE *et al.* a): in Olmer et al.

COSTE, F.; DELBARRE, F. and LAPRESLE, J.: b) A propos du diagnostic clinique et radiologique de la maladie de Kahler. Bull. Soc. méd. Hôp., Paris 64:361–364 (1948).

CROW, R. S.: Peripheral neuritis in myelomatosis. Brit. med. J. ii: 802–804 (1956).

CUSHING: in Labauge et al.

DALRYMPLE, J.: On the microscopic character of 'mollities ossium'. Dublin Quart. J. Med. Sci. 2:85 (1848).

DANEO, V.: Mieloma e herpes zoster (un caso di mieloma associato ad herpes zoster generalizzato). Reumatismo 7:263 (1955).

DAVISON, C. and BALSER, B. H.: Myeloma and its neural complications. Arch. Surg., Chicago 35:913–936 (1937).

DEGENHARDT, D. P. and SHEEHAN, D.: Multiple myeloma; note on 8 cases. Brit. med. J. ii: 1016–1018 (1949).

DELANEY, W. V. JR. and LIARICOS, S. V.: Chorioretinal destruction in multiple myeloma. Amer. J. Ophthal. 66:52–55 (1968).

DELMAS-MARSALET, P.; PAULY; LÉGER; POUYANNE, H. and LÉMAN, P.: Troubles oculo-trigémellaires par myélome piétreux révélateurs d'une maladie de Kahler. Rev. Oto-Neuro-Ophtal. 23:411–415 (1951).

DENKER, D. G. and BROCK, S.: Generalized and vertebral forms of myeloma: their cerebral and spinal complications. Brain 57:291–306 (1934).

DOMMELEN VAN: in Wuhrmann.

DONNELLY, W. J. and GRAHN, E. P.: Extraosseous manifestations of multiple myeloma. Med. Clin. N. Amer. 49:229–240 (1965).

ELISABALDE and LAMBLIAS: in Labauge et al.

ERBSLÖH, F.: Das Zentralnervensystem bei Krankheiten des Blutes. In Lubarsch and

Henke, Handbuch der speziellen pathologischen Anatomie und Histologie, vol. XIII/2, pp. 1468–1525 (Springer, Berlin-Göttingen-Heidelberg 1958).

ESTES, H. R. and MILLIKAN, C. H.: Polyneuritis and radiculitis associated with multiple myeloma: report of case. Proc. Staff Meet. Mayo Clin. 29:453–455 (1954).

FRANTZEN, E.; HERTZ, H.; MATZKE, J. and VIDEBAEK, AA.: Protein studies on cerebrospinal fluid and neurological symptoms in myelomatosis. Acta neurol. scand. 45:1–17 (1969).

FRENCH, J. D.: Plasmacytoma of hypothalamus; clinical-pathological report of case. J. Neuropath. exp. Neurol. 6:265–270 (1947).

GESCHICKTER, C. F. and COPELAND, M. M.: Multiple myeloma. Arch. Surg., Chicago 16:807–863 (1928).

GILBERT-DREYFUS; MAMOU, H. and ATTAL, C.: Myélome ostéomalacique (myélomatose décalcifiante diffuse de Weissenbach et Lièvre). Bull. Soc. méd. Hôp., Paris 63:987–990 (1947).

GIOVANELLI, E.; POLETTI, T. and MASCARELLO, M.: Rilievi clinici su 24 casi di malattia plasmocitomatosa. Minerva med. 59:1188–1205 (1968).

GIRAUD, G.; LATOUR, H.; LÉVY, A.; PEUCH, P. and OLIVIER, G.: a) Syndrome de l'angle ponto-cérébelleux révélateur d'une maladie de Kahler. Montpellier méd. 53:624–627 (1958).

GIRAUD, G.; LATOUR, H.; DERMENGHEN, M.; OLIVIER, G.; NAVARRO, M. and SIMON, L.: b) Tétraplégie révélatrice d'une maladie de Kahler. Aspects anatomiques et mecanisme de production. Montpellier méd. 57:494–498 (1960).

GREENSTEIN, R. H. and CAHN, N. M.: Generalized herpes zoster: an unusual case associated with multiple myeloma. J. Albert Einstein med. Cent. 4:33 (1955).

GROKOEST, A. W. and DEMARTINI, F. E.: Systemic disease and carpal tunnel syndrome. J. amer. med. Ass. 155:635–637 (1954).

GROSGURIN, J. R.: Le myélome multiple. Sang 13:30–65 (1939).

GROSSMAN, L. A.; KAPLAN, H. J.; OWNBY, F. D. and GROSSMAN, M.: Carpal tunnel syndrome. Initial manifestation of systemic disease. J. amer. med. Ass. 176: 259–261 (1961).

GUGLIELMO, R. DI: I plasmocitomi (Abruzzini, Rome 1955).

GUPTA, S. P. and PRABHAKAR, B. R.: Peripheral neuropathy and solitary myeloma. Brit. med. J. ii: 1004 (1965).

HAGELSTAM, L.: Solitary vertebral plasmocytoma causing paraplegia; satisfactory results of roentgen treatment on paraplegia and serum globulins; case report, Acta chir. scand. 109:384–394 (1955).

HANSEN, P. F. and FABER, M.: Raynaud's syndrome originating from reversible precipitation of protein. Acta med. scand. 129:81–100 (1947).

JAMES, T. N.; MONTO, R. W. and REBUCK, J. W.: Thrombocytopenia and abnormal bleeding in multiple myeloma. Ann. intern. Med. 39:1281–1287 (1953).

KENNY, J. J. and MOLONEY, W. C.: Multiple myeloma: diagnosis and management in a series of 57 cases. Ann. intern. Med. 46:1079–1091 (1957).

Kirshbaum, J. D.: Metastatic plasma cell myeloma of testicles, with report of case. Urol. cutan. Rev. 51:456–459 (1947).

KISSEL, P.; HARTEMANN, P. and PERSON, H. C.: Le plasmocytome vertébral solitaire et ses manifestations nerveuses. Gaz. méd. France 64:1559–1561 (1957).

KRAMER, W.: Plasmocytoma of the brain in Kahler's disease (multiple myeloma). Acta neuropath. 2:438–450 (1963).

KURNICK, N. B. and YOHALEM, S. B.: Peripheral neuritis complicating multiple myeloma. Arch. Neurol., Chicago 59:378–384 (1948).

KYLE, R. A. and BAYRD, E. D.: 'Primary' systemic amyloidosis and myeloma. Discussion of relationship and review of 81 cases. Arch. intern. Med. 107:344–353 (1961).

LABAUGE, R.; IZARN, P. and CASTAN, P.: Les manifestations nerveuses des hémopathies. Rapport LXI Congr. Franç. de Psychiatrie et de Neurologie, Nancy 1963 (Masson, Paris 1963).

LAYANI, F.; ASCHKENASY, A. and NADAL, R.: Paraplégie, manifestation initiale d'un plasmocytome reconnu par ponction de l'apophyse épineuse. Guérison neurologique par radiothérapie. Bull. Soc. méd. Hôp., Paris 68:1186–1191 (1952).

LINDEBOOM, G. A. and MULDER, H. J.: Multiples Myelom mit leukämischem Blutbild und degenerativen Rückenmarksänderungen. Acta med. scand. 108:363–373 (1941).

LUGARESI, E.; TASSINARI, C. A. and GHEDINI, G.: Complicanze neurologiche in corso di emopatie a carattere iper-displastico. Minerva med. giuliana 3:88–90 (1963).

MAC INTYRE, W.: A case of mollities and fragilitas ossium, accompanied with urine strongly charged with animal matter. Trans. med. Soc. Lond. 33:211–232 (1850).

Madonick, M. and SOLOMON, S.: Total protein content of cerebrospinal fluid in multiple myeloma. Neurology, Minneap. 3:369–374 (1953).

MAGNUS-LEVY, A.: Multiple myelome. Acta med. scand. 95:217–280 (1938).

MAHOUDEAU, D.; LEBEAU, J. and DAUM, S.: Plasmocytome multiple à forme cérébrale. Bull. Soc. méd. Hôp., Paris 68:1150–1155 (1952).

McKISSOCK, W.; BLOOM, W. H. and CHYNN, K. Y.: Spinal cord compression caused by plasma cell tumors. J. Neurosurg. 18:68–73 (1961).

MEDOC, J.; RODRIGUEZ, B. and RODRIGUEZ JUANOTENA, J.: Meningeal myeloma. An. Fac. Med. Montev. 46:82–91 (1961).

MEIERS, H. G. and GEHRMANN, G.: 'Maligner Zoster' bei normproteinämischem Plasmozytom (Bence-Jones-Plasmozytom). Dtsch. med. Wschr. 93: 435–438 (1968).

MERIGAN, T. C. JR. and HAYES, R. E.: Treatment of hypercalcemia in multiple myeloma. Report of two patients. Arch. intern. Med. 107:389–394 (1961).

MICHON, P. and STREIFF, F.: Macroglobulinémie de Waldenström (Masson, Paris 1959).

MICHON, P.; LARCAN and STREIFF, F.: Etude clinique de la macroglobulinemie de Waldenström. Sang 31:369–386 (1960).

MILLIEZ, J. and MALLARMÉ, J.: Leucose à plasmocytes; confrontation avec la maladie de Kahler et la leucose leucoblastique. Sem. Hôp., Paris 25:763–769 (1949).

MOESCHLIN, S.: Klinische unde experimentelle Untersuchungen über den Wirkungsmechanismus des Urethans. Acta haemat., Basel 1:225–247 (1948).

MORIN, M.; GRAVELEAU, J.; PÉROL, R.; SHIMMEL, H. and TESTARD, R.: Les manifestations cérébrales du myélome plasmocytaire. Sem. Hôp., Paris 34:2663–2669 (1958).

MUNSAT, T. L. and POUSSAINT, A. F.: Clinical manifestations and diagnosis of amyloid polyneuropathy. Report of three cases. Neurology, Minneap. 12:413–422 (1962).

OJEA, M.; UCHA UDABE, R. and CARMENA, A.: Poliglobulia y polineuritis en el curso de un mieloma. Prensa méd. argent. 48:1457–1460 (1961).

OLMER, J.; MONGIN, M.; MURATORE, R. and DENIZET, D.: Myélomes, macroglobulinémies et dysglobulinémies voisines (Masson, Paris 1961).

PAGÈS, P.; BÉTOULIÈRES, P. and CAZABAN, R.: La forme isolée des plasmocytomes fronto-orbitaires. Ann. Oculist. 185:632–639 (1952).

PAILLAS, J.; SERRATRICE, G. and LEGRE, J.: Les tumeurs primitives du rachis (Masson, Paris 1963).

PENDE, G. and CHIARIONI, T.: Revisione critica degli aspetti anatomo-clinici della malattia plasmocitomatosa sulla base di 16 osservazioni personali. Medicina, Parma 3:669–728 (1953).

PÉTRIDÈS: in Labauge et al.

PINEY, A. and RIACH, J. S.: Multiple myeloma. Aleukaemic and leukaemic. Folia haemat., N.F. 46:37–58 (1931).

PINO, V.: Plasma cell myeloma of vertebrae with amyloid tumor, producing paraplegia; report of case. Surgery 36:804–807 (1954).

POLLI, E.: I comi metabolici. Relaz. LXVIII Congr. Soc. Ital. Med. Intern., Florence 1967 (Pozzi, Rome 1967).

RISER, M. and SOREL, R.: Contribution à l'étude des plasmocytomes. Plasmocytome intra-crânien avec paralysies unilaterales multiples. Ann. méd. 26:385–396 (1929).

RITTMEYER, K. and SCHLACHETZKI, J.: Paramiloidosi, macroglossia e sindrome del canale del carpo in un caso di plasmocitoma. Med. tedesc. 4:372–375 (1968).

ROHMER, F.; MENGUS, M. and BUCHHEIT, F.: Paraneoplastic neuropathy of the type of the Guillain-Barré syndrome in a patient with solitary myeloma. Rev. Oto-Neuro-Ophtal. 34:97–107 (1962).

ROSLUND, J.; SUNDBERG, K. and TOVI, D.: Plasma cell myeloma of thoracic vertebra with amyloid deposits. Acta path. microbiol. scand. 49:273–279 (1960).

ROVIT, R. L. and FAGER, C. A.: Solitary plasmocytoma of petrous bone. Report of a case with neurologic and radiographic remission following roentgen-ray therapy. J. Neurosurg. 17:929-933 (1960).

SCHEINKER, I.: Myelom und Nervensytsem. Dtsch. Z. Nervenheilk. 147:247–273 (1938).

SCHNEIDER, M. and MAZABRAUD, M.: Les signes révélateurs du myélome et leur fréquence relative. Rev. Rhum. 26:660–675 (1959).

SCHOTT, B.; COTTE, L.. and TOMMASI, M.: Ramollissement spinal postérieur en D7–D8 par myélome osseux plasmocytaire de D11–L1. Rev. neurol. 101:16–27 (1959).

SERRE, H.; SIMON, L. and BARJON, M. C.: Aspects du rachis myélomateux; à propos de 80 observations. Rev. Rhum. 29:635–645 (1962).

SHANBROM, E.; MILLER, S. and HAAR, H.: Herpes zoster in hematologic neoplasias: some unusual manifestations. Ann. intern. Med. 53:523–533 (1960).

SHENKIN, H. A.; HORN, R. C. JR. and GRANT, F. C.: Lesions of spinal epidural space producing cord compression. Arch. Surg., Chicago 51:125-146 (1945).

SILVERSTEIN, A. and DONIGER, D. E.: Neurologic complications of myelomatosis. Arch. intern. Med. 113:102–112 (1964).

SNAPPER, I.; TURNER, L. B. and MOSCOVITZ, H. L.: Multiple myeloma (Grune & Stratton, New York 1953).

SNAPPER, I. and KAHN, A.: Myelomatosis. Fundamentals and clinical features (University Park Press, Baltimore, 1971).

SNYDER, L. J. and WILHELM, S. K.: Multiple myeloma with spinal cord compression as initial finding. Ann. intern. Med. 28:1169–1177 (1948).

SOD, L. M. and WIENER, L. M.: Intradural extramedullary plasmacytoma; case report. J. Neurosurg. 16:107–109 (1959).

SPARLING, H. J.; ADAMS, R. D. and PARKER, F.: Involvement of nervous system by malignant lymphoma. Medicine, Balt. 26:285–332 (1947).

STANKIEWICZ, D. and DYMECKI, J.: Mental disorders in a case of multiple myeloma. Pol. Tyg. Lek. 15:553–555 (1960).

STEFANINI, M. and DAMESHEK, W.: Le malattie emorragiche (Italian translation by Dr. C. Buoni) (arti e Scienze, Rome 1965).

STRATEMEYER, J.: Solitary extramedullary plasmacytoma causing paraplegia. J. Phila. Gen. Hosp. 1:92 (1950).

SVIEN, H. J.; PRICE, R. D. and BAYRD, E. D.: Neurosurgical treatment of compression of spinal cord caused by myeloma. J. amer. med. Ass. 153:784–786 (1953).

SWINTON, N. W. JR.; ROSEN, B. J.; SHEFFER, A. L. and LEACH, R. E.: The carpal tunnel syndrome and multiple myeloma. Lahey Clin. Found. Bull. 19:49–53 (1970).

THIERS, H.; MOULIN, G. and GUIBAUD, P.: Zona et hémopathie maligne (à propos d'un zona généralisé révélateur d'un myélome). J. Méd., Lyon 47:1823–1834 (1966).

THOMAS et al.: in Labauge et al.

TOLOSA, A.; CANELAS, H. M.; TENUTO, R. A. and CRUZ, O. R.: Compressões medulares provocadas por mielomas vertebrais. Arg. Neuro-Psiquiat. 14:101–116 (1956).

TREMBLAY, E. C.; GILBRIN, E. and HOUDART, R.: Maladie de Kahler. Constatation anatomique 'in vivo' de la régression plasmocytome. Presse méd. 70:1452 (1962).

VERDA, D. J.: Malignant lymphomas of spinal epidural space. Surg. Clin. N. Amer. 24:1228–1244 (1944).

VICTOR, M.; BANKER, B. Q. and ADAMS, R. D.: The neuropathy of multiple myeloma. J. Neurol. Neurosurg. Psychiat. 21:73–88 (1958).

VORREITH, M.: Primary extramedullary plasmocytoma of the rectum with metastases to the central nervous system. Cas. Lek. ces. 99:421–426 (1960).

WILLIAMS, H. M.; DIAMOND, H. D.; CRAVER, L. F. and PARSONS, H.: Neurological complications of lymphomas and leukemias (C. Thomas, Springfield, Ill. 1959).

WUHRMANN, F.: Über das Coma paraproteinaemicum bei Myelomen und Makroglobulinämien. Schweiz. med. Wschr. 86:623–625 (1956).

Appendix. Cryoglobulinemia, Waldenström's disease

AARSETH, S.; OFSTAD, E. and TORVIK, A.: Maroglobulinaemia Waldenström. A case with haemolytic syndrome and involvement of the nervous system. Acta med. scand. 169:691–699 (1961).

ARSENI, C.; CHIMION, D. and GEORGIAN, M.: Hématome épidural spinal spontané conditionné par une dysimmunoglobulinémie maligne. Rev. roum. Neurol. 5:145–152 (1968).

ASCENZI, A.; FABIANI, F. and LUCENTINI, L.: Studio anatomopatologico di un caso di macroglobulinemia di Waldenström. Haematologica 42:153–178 (1957).

AZZENA D.; GHIGLIOTTI, G.; ASTENGO, F.; COSTA, U. and MOLINELLI, G.: Manifestazioni neurologiche in corso di "gammopatie monoclonali." Revista della letteratura e descrizione di 5 casi di mieloma multiplo e di z casi di macroglobulinemia di Waldenström con diverse compromissioni del sistema nervoso. Haematologica 52:999–1031 (1967).

BAYRD, E. D.: Continuous chlorambucil therapy in primary macroglobulinemia of Waldenström: report of four cases. Proc. Staff Meet. Mayo Clin. 36:135–147 (1961).

BICHEL, J.; BING, J. and HARBOE, N.: Another case of hyperglobulinemia and affection of central nervous system. Acta med. scand. 138:1–14 (1950).

BING, J. and NEEL, A. VAN: Two cases of hyperglobulinemia with affection of the central nervous system on a toxi-infectious basis (myelitis, polyradiculitis, spinal-fluid changes). Acta med. scand. 88:492–506 (1936).

BING, J.; FOG, M.and NEEL, A. VAN: Report of third case of hyperglobulinemia with affection of the central nervous system (radiculo-meningo-myelo-encephalitis) on a toxi-infectious basis, and some remarks on differential diagnosis. Acta med. scand. 91:409–427 (1937).

BODECHTEL, G.; BORCHERS, H. G. and KOLLMANNSBERGER, A.: Enzephalopathie bei Blutkrankheiten. Dtsch. med. Wschr. 91:673–682 (1966). 96.

BOUDIN, G.; BARBIZET, J. and DALLOZ, J. C.:Cryoglobulinémie et lymphoréticulosarcome: observation d'un cas avec purpure nécrotique, syndrome de Raynaud, parotidite et névrite multiple. Presse méd. 67:594–597 (1959).

BOUSSER, J. and BOIVIN, P.: Macroglobulinémie de Waldenström: à propos de deux nouvelles observations. Rev. Hémat. 12:100–115 (1957).

BUTTLER and PALMER: in Garcin et al[b].

CAGIANUT, B.: Le syndrome oculaire de la macroglobulinémie (syndrome de Waldenström). Ann. Oculist. 191:579–591 (1958).

CLATANOFF, D. V. and MEYER, O. O.: Response to chlorambucil in macroglobulinemia. J. amer. med. Ass. 183:40–44 (1963).

DANIS, P.; BRAUMAN, J. and COPPEZ, P.: Les lésions du fond d'oeil au cours de certaines hyperproteinémies (myélome à cryoglobuline, macroglobulinémie). Acta ophthal., Copenh. 33:33–51 (1955).

DARNLEY, J. D.: Polyneuropathy in Waldenström's macroglobulinemia. Case report and discussion. Neurology, Minneap. 12:617–623 (1962).

DINI, E.; VENTRUTO, V. and QUATTRIN, N.: Crioglobulinemie non macromolecolari. II Giornate Ematologiche, Naples 1968.

DOUMENC, J.; PROST, R. J.; SAMAMA, M. and BOUSSER, J.: Anomalie de l'agrégation plaquettaire au cours de la maladie de Waldenström (à propos de 3 cas). Nouv. Rev. franç. Hémat. 6:734–738 (1966).

EDGAR, R. and DUTCHER, T. F.: Histopathology of the Bing-Neel syndrome. Neurology, Minneap. 11:239–245 (1961).

FANKHAUSER, S.; ARNOLD, E.; SCHAUB, F. and LAPP, R.: Hämolytisches Syndrom und Makroglobulinämie Waldenström. Helv. med. Acta 23:645–648 (1956).

FIERE, H.: Contribution à l'étude de la macroglobulinémie de Waldenström (à propos de huit observations). Thèse Lyon (1957).

GARCIN, R.; MALLARMÉ, J.; HARTMAN, L. and RONDOT, P. a):Cryoglobulinémie et névrite multiple des membres inférieurs (presentation de malade). Bull. Soc. méd. Hôp., Paris 73:835–844 (1957).

GARCIN, R.; MALLARMÉ, J. and RONDOT, P. b): Forme névritique de la macroglobulinémia de Waldenström. Bull. Soc. méd. Hôp., Paris 74:562–573 (1958).

GARCIN, R.; MALLARMÉ, J.; RONDOT, P. and ENDTZ, L. c): Forme névritique de la macroglobulinémie de Waldenström (une nouvelle observation). Sang, 31:441–445 (1960).

GARCIN, R.; RONDOT, P. and GRUPPER, CH. d): Cryglobulinémie et périartérite noueuse à manifestations multinévritiques. Rev. neurol. 103:589–592 (1960).

GOTHAM, J. F.; WEIN, H. and MEYER, J. S.: Clinical studies of neuropathy due to macroglobulinemia (Waldenström's syndrome). Canad. med. Ass. J. 89:806–809 (1963).

GRIFONI, V.; BIGNOTTI, G.; TOGNELLA, S. and SCALTRINI, G.: Stato attuale della terapia del mieloma e della linforeticolosi macroglobulinemica di Waldenström. Recenti Progr. Med. 39:415–436 (1965).

GUGLIELMO, R. DI; MILIANI, A.; LOMBARDI, V.; ZINI, F. and ZILLI, A.: Effetti clinici e umorali indotti dalla terapia con prednisone a dosi elevate in alcune emopatie e altre situazioni morbose. Haematologica 46:309–352 (1961).

HAAS, W.; HOFMANN, H. and TEICHMANN, W.: Zur Nosologie der Makroglobulinämie Waldenström. Z. klin. Med. 154:252–273 (1956).

HAGEN, H.: Zur Differentialdiagnose der Makroglobulinaemie Waldenström. Ärztl. Forsch. 9:547–551 (1955).

HUTCHINSON, J. H. and HOWELL, R. A.: Cryoglobulinemia: report of a case associated with gangrene of digits. Ann. intern. Med. 39:350–357 (1953).

IZARN, P.; PALEIRAC, G. and ROBINET, M.: La fonction thromboplastique plaquettaire au cours des dysglobulinémies. Nouv. Rev. franç. Hémat. 6:729–733 (1966).

KAKULAS, B. A. and FINLAY-JONES, L. R.: A lymphoma with central nervous system involvement. Report of a case. Neurology, Minneap. 12:495–500 (1962).

KANZOW, U.: Die Makroglobulinämie Waldenström. Klin. Wschr. 32:154–159 (1954).

KAPPELER, R.; KREBS, A. and RIVA, G.: Klinik der Makroglobulinämie Waldenström. Beschreibung von 21 Fällen und Übersicht der Literatur. Helv. med. Acta 25:54–101 (1958).

KOLKER, A. E.: Ocular manifestations of hematologic disease. In Brown and Moore, Progress in hematology, pp. 354–389 (W. Heinemann Med. Books, London 1966).

KORSTEN, H. B. und BERNEAUD-KÖTZ, G.: Ein frühes Stadium des Fundus paraproteinaemicus bei einem Fall von Makroglobulinämie. Klin. Mbl. Augenheilk. 128:679–686 (1956).

LABAUGE, R.; IZARN, P. and CASTAN, P.: Les manifestations nerveuses des hémopathies. Rapport LXI Congr. Franç. de Psychiatrie et de Neurologie, Nancy 1963 (Masson, Paris 1963).

LAURELL, C. B.; LAURELL, H. and WALDENSTRÖM, J.: Glycoproteins in serum from patients with myeloma, macroglobulinemia and related conditions. Amer. J. Med. 22:24–36 (1957).

LAYANI, F.; ASCHKENASI, A. and BENGUI, A.: Macroglobulinémie avec lésions du squelette; dysplasie à la fois lymphoïde et plasmocytoïde de la moelle osseuse. Presse méd. 63:44–46 (1955).

LEVRAT; CREYSSEL, R.; MOREL, P.; THIVOLLET, J. and COSTOL: Un cas de macroglobulinémie de Waldenström. Lyon méd. 89:3–8 (1957).

LOGOTHETIS, J.; SILVERSTEIN, P. and COE, J. a): Neurologic aspects of Waldenström's macroglobulinemia. Report of a case. Arch. Neurol., Chicago 3:564–573 (1960).

LOGOTHETIS, J.; KENNEDY, W. R.; ELLINGTON, A. and WILLIAMS, R. C. b): Cryoglobulinemic neuropathy: incidence and clinical characteristics. Arch. Neurol., Chicago 19:389–397 (1968).

LONG, L. A.; RIOPELLE, J. L.; FRANCOEUR, M.; PARE, A.; POIRIER, P.; BEORGESCO, M. and COLPRON, G.: Macroglobulinaemia; effect of macroglobulins on prothrombin conversion accelerators. Canad. med. Ass. J. 73:726–733 (1955).

MACKAY, I. R.; ERIKSEN, N.; MOTULSKY, A. G. and VOLWILER, W.: Cryo- and macroglobulinemia; electrophoretic, ultracentrifugal and clinical studies. Amer. J. Med. 20:564–587 (1956).

MacKay, I. R.; Taft, L. I. and Woods, E. F.: Clinical features and pathogenesis of macroglobulinaemia. Brit. med. J. i: 561–563 (1957).

Mandema, E.: Macroglobulinemia (Waldenström) with report of 4 cases. Ned. T. Geneesk. 98:2109–2118 (1954).

Marshall, R. J. and Malone, R. G. S.: Cryoglobulinaemia with cerebral purpura. Brit. med. J. ii:279–280 (1954).

Melli, G. and Grifoni, V.: Terapia delle emoblastosi. Relaz. LXI Congr. Soc. Ital. Med. Intern., Naples 1960 (Pozzi, Rome 1960).

Michon, P. and Streiff, F.: Macroglobulinémie de Waldenström (Masson, Paris 1959).

Michon, P.; Larcan and Streiff. F.: Ètude clinique de la macroglobulinémie de Waldström. Sang 31:369–386 (1960).

Moulinier, J.; Servantie, X. and Mesnier, F.: Les effets thérapeutiques de la plasmapherèse dans la maladie de Waldenström. J. Méd., Bordeaux 144:1295–1300 (1967).

Olmer, J.; Mongin, M.; Muratore, R. and Denizet, D.; Myélomes, macroglobulinémies et dysglobulinémies voisines (Masson, Paris 1961).

Paufique, M. L. and Royer, J.: Manifestations oculaires au cours des macroglobulinémies. J. Méd., Lyon 39:525–530 (1958).

Quattrin, N.; Ventruto, V.; Dini E. and Cimino, R.: Stato attuale della diagnostica e nosologia delle paraproteinemie. Relaz. XIX Congr. Naz. Soc. Ital. Emat., Pavia 1963 (Tip. Viscontea, Pavia).

Rauber, G.; Martin, M. E. and Macinot, C.: La maladie de Waldenström. Étude particulière des manifestations viscérales. Ann. Anat. path. 8:159–194 (1963).

Revol, L.; Creyssel, R.; Morel, P. and Gauthier: Deux cas de macroglobulinémie de type Waldenström. Lyon méd. 196:533–552 (1956).

Ricci, C.; Arturi, F.; Carnevale, S.; Tizzani, P. L. and Blefari, D.: La sindrome de Waldenström. Studio clinico e biochimico di 6 casi. Haematologica 52:823–850 (1967).

Saric, R.; Moreau, F. and Tignol, J.: Neuropathie précédant de loin une maladie de Waldenström. Effet du traitement prolongé par le melphalan. J. Méd., Bordeaux 144:1301–1311 (1967).

Schaub, F.: Zum Krankheitsbild und zur Differentialdiagnose der Makroglobulinämie Waldenström. Schweiz. med. Wschr. 82:890–895 (1952). Gleichzeitiges Vorkommen von Makroglobulinämie Waldenström und von malignen Tumoren. Schweiz. med. Wschr. 83:1256–1257 (1953).

Schwab, P. J. and Fahey, J. L.: Treatment of Waldenström's macroglobulinemia by plasmapheresis. New Engl. J. Med. 263:574–579 (1960).

Stefanini, M. and Dameshek, W.: Le malattie emorragiche (Italian translation by Dr. C. Buoni) Artie Scienze, Rome, 1965).

Stirpe, M.: Il fondo oculare nelle anemie ed emoblastosi. Osservazioni sulla casistica esaminata nel Policlinico di Roma durante il decennio 1955–1964. Boll. Ocul. 44:577–591 (1965).

Tischendorff, W. and Hartmann, F.: Makroglobulinaemie (Waldenström) mit gleichzeitiger Hyperplasie der Gewebsmastzellen. Acta haemat. 4:374–383 (1950).

Vital, Cl.; Le Pennec, J. J. and Duvert, M.: Pathologie des neuropathies périphériques de la maladie de Waldenström. J. Méd., Bordeaux 144:1273–1281 (1967).

Waldenström, J.: Incipient myelomatosis or 'essential' hyperglobulinemia with fibrinogenopenia—a new syndrome? Acta med. scand. 117:216–247 (1944). Zwei interessante Syndrome mit Hyperglobulinämie (Purpura hyperglobulinaemica und Makroglobulinamie). Schweiz. med. Wschr. 78:927–928 (1948).

Wanebo, H. J. and Clarkson, B. D.: Essential macroglobulinemia. Report of a case including immunofluorescent and electron microscopic studies. Ann. intern. Med. 62:1025-1045 (1965).

Wanner, J. and Siebenmann, R.: Über eine subakut verlaufende osteolytische Form der Makroglobulinämie Waldenström mit Plasmazellenleukämie. Schweiz. med. Wschr. 87:1243–1246 (1957).

WUHRMANN, F.: a) Einige aktuelle klinische Probleme über die Serum-Gloubuline. Schweiz. med. Wschr. 82:937–940 (1952). b) Uber das Coma paraproteinaemicum bei Myelomen und Makroglobulinämien. Schweiz. med. Wschr. 86:623–625 (1956).

ZLOTNICK, A.: Macroglobulinemia of Waldenström. Amer. J. Med. 24:461–470 (1958).

ZOLLINGER, H. U.: Die pathologische Anatomie der Makroglobulinämie Waldenström. Helv. med. Acta 25:153–183 (1958).

Chapter XI

NEUROLOGICAL SYMPTOMS IN RETICULOSIS, RETICULUM CELL SARCOMA, FOLLICULAR LYMPHOMA, EOSINOPHILIC GRANULOMA, AND LIPOIDOSIS

The blood diseases dealt with in this chapter, together with Hodgkin's disease (Chapter VIII), sarcoidosis (Chapter IX), and multiple myeloma (Chapter X) form a large group of diseases of the reticuloendothelial system.

Their common characteristic is the proliferation of cells of the reticuloendothelial system, with a different anatomical and clinical expression in each disease. On occasions, however, there is a great similarity between one form and another, and eosinophilic granuloma has been known to progress to Hand-Schüller-Christian disease or to reticulosis.

The inclusion of Hodgkin's disease is debatable, since it is generally considered to be an immunopoietic cell tumor with a reagent allergy. According to some workers, it can be treated as a disease of the reticuloendothelial system; *Bufano*, for example, classes it as a malignant tumor of undifferentiated reticuloendothelial system cells progressing to granulation tissue, while *Rohr* suggests that it may be a tumor of lymphatic granulation tissue which might be called "postinflammatory granuloblastoma." *Moeschlin* treats the granulomatous tissue observed in Hodgkin's disease as a neoplastic proliferation of cells of the reticuloendothelial system, which constitutes the productive component of such tissue. The exudative component of the disease is, in his opinion, an aspecific intercurrent reaction or "reticulum allergy."

I. Nerve system involvement in reticulosis is rare (*Cazal*). Its picture is very similar to that of neuroleukemia, particularly when the blood picture is of the leukemic type.

A feature of reticulosis is its atypical proliferation of reticuloendothelial cells. Systemic diffusion takes place and skin localization may be

236

characteristic. Acute forms are by far the most common, though chronic forms are not unknown. A further distinction is made between the more frequent aleukemic and the leukemic forms. The latter usually run an acute or subacute course with reticulemia and are distinguished into histiocyte and monocyte leukemias, according to whether undifferentiated or differentiated cells are found in the circulating blood. The acute aleukemic forms include Letterer-Siwe disease (acute neonatal reticulosis). Similar to this form, though more reminiscent of Hand-Schüller-Christian disease with respect to its skeletal alterations, is a recently defined disease (*Sacrez et al.*) known as "neonatal malignant congenital histiocytopathy" (*Amato*) or "congenital Letterer-Siwe disease" (*Ahnquist and Holioke*).

Cazal has formed a larger nosological unit, histiomonocyte reticulosis, which includes Letterer-Siwe reticulosis, leukemic reticulosis (except the Naegeli and Marchal monocyte types, since these are held to be monocytoid paramyeloblastosis and lymphosis respectively), and some special forms of granulomatous reticulosis. The title "X reticulosis or histiocytosis" has been given by *Lichtenstein* to a nosological group including Letterer-Siwe disease, eosinophilic granuloma, and Hand-Schüller-Christian disease. The production of histiocyte granulomatous formations is a common feature of these diseases.

Nerve alterations in reticulosis may be attributable to specific infiltration, whether circumscribed or general (*Rubé et al.*), to osteoperiosteal or epidural neoplastic compression, or to hemorrhage or thrombosis. Anemia or toxic factors also may be responsible.

In a case reported by *Léger et al.*, necropsy following monocyte leukemia with a pseudotumoral neurological picture showed central nervous system (CNS) edema and widespread congestion. Microscopic examination revealed widespread glial reaction and histiomonocyte infiltration of the brain, bulb, and cerebellum. Numerous vessels were dilated and packed with histiomonocyte cells. Hemorrhagic suffusions were also observed.

The patient was a 62-year-old man who had presented five years earlier fever, intense anemia, and slight jaundice. Treatment with cortisone and repeated transfusions produced a rapid improvement followed by four years of good health. The ensuing neurological picture included mental confusion with disorientation in time and space, mistaken recognition and oneirophrenia. This lasted 48 hours and was accompanied by nocturnal urinary incontinence. Objective examination disclosed left brachial and very slight left facial paresis. Six days later the patient went into deep coma with left hemiplegia. Pauses in respiration were noted and swallowing ceased completely. There was rightward deviation of the head and eyes, and a bilateral Babinski's reflex was elicited. Examination of the fundus oculi showed extensive papillary edema. The patient appeared very anemic and there were signs of hemorrhagic diathesis. Arteriography showed a considerable shift of the anterior cerebral artery on to the median line. Following trepanation, a puncture was done for suspected hemorrhagic accumulation. Aspiration, however, produced a yellowish, streaky liquid, as seen in some gliomatous cysts. After a transient improvement, the patient died in hyperthermia and tachypnea caused by irreversible cardiorespiratory collapse.

In a case published by *Bamforth and Kendall* as megakaryocyte myelosis —but interpreted by *Cazal* as reticulosis—the terminal stage included paraplegia. This was shown to be caused by massive infiltration of the lumbar vertebrae, meninges, nerve roots, and cord at necropsy.

Peripheral compressions of nerve structures will give rise to localized and limited neurological manifestations. A patient observed by *Walther and Strocka* presented facial nerve paralysis caused by compression by a reticuloblastomatous skin nodule. The chin and lip anesthesia noted by *Cionini and Rotta* may be explained in the same way. The terminal stage here included signs of funicular myelosis, possibly secondary to anemia.

The clinical picture may cover a wide range: widespread brain involvement, with frequent alteration of consciousness and the appearance of neurological signs that are sometimes difficult to classify (*Di Guglielmo et al.; Duperrat et al.[a]; Basex et al.; etc.*); pseudotumoral conditions with coma, intracranial hypertension and focal signs. (*Leger et al.*); meningeal symptomatologies (*Leicher; Zimmermann; Bergouignan et al.*); cerebellar symptomatologies, with ataxia, tremor, dysmetria, dysarthria, nystagmus (*Cazal; Euzière et al.*); cord symptomatologies, with flaccid or spastic paraplegia (*Bamforth and Kendall; Chaptal et al.; Degos et al.; Lugaresi et al.*), or with funicular myelosis (*Cionini and Rotta; Litteral and Malamud*); peripheral involvement syndromes: quadriplegia (*Dupérié et al.*), polyneuritis (*Allison and Gordon; Aubertin et al.*), multineuritis (*Garcin; Basex et al.*), isolated mononeuritis (*Walther and Strocka*), simple sensitive type (*Cionini and Rotta*), or neuralgia (*Duperrat et al.[b]*).

In a case observed recently by *Bernard and Aguilar,* the clinical picture of the scintiscan and pneumoencephalographically demonstrated hypothalamic localization included diabetes insipidus, progressive obesity, hypogonadism and hypothyroidism, somnolence, and memory loss, together with symptoms suggesting intermittent intracranial hypertension. Necropsy confirmed the hypothalamic site and also showed fatty infiltration and cirrhosis of the liver and thyroiditis.

In a case of *Lindlar*, disseminated histiocytosis of the diencephalon and of the thoracic segment of the spinal cord caused impotence and disorders of the diencephalon and hypophysis.

Pathologic reticulohistiocytes may be observed in the cerebrospinal fluid (CSF) in reticulosis with meningeal involvement. The first observation in the literature is that of *Zimmermann* who reported two cases in 1961. In the first case the number of liquor cells was 400/mm³. These cells were pathologic with a large nucleus and nucleoli. Necropsy showed widespread reticulohistiocyte infiltration of the dura mater, the arachnoid membrane, and the perivasal sheaths of the brain and cerebellum.

Liquor pathologic cells were also reported in two cases by *Bergouignan et al.* Both of these patients presented signs of intracranial hypertension, the second with left choked disk and right optic atrophy. Chest X-ray revealed clinically silent miliary type lung damage in the first case and a mediastinal adenopathy in the second. Death occurred six months and four months, respectively, after the appearance of the first clinical signs.

In both cases, the CSF cytological picture was unusual. In the second case the number of cells was 220/mm³, with a slight increase in CSF protein content. Two types of cells could be distinguished; pathologic cells with tumoral features and accompanying cells without signs of malignancy. Polymorphism was very apparent in each type. Cells were usually observed in isolation and groupings were rare. The accompanying cells were about 30–40% of the total population and included lymphocytes, monocytes, plasma cells, polynucleates, or a few immature mycloid cells, small histiocytes, reticulum cells, and a great variety of meningeal cells. About one-third of the tumoral cells were of the histiocyte type with large protoplasm (diameters over 20–30 μ) and indistinct borders. The protoplasm contained inclusions, granulation, and vacuoles. The nucleus also was large, round or oval, and contained small blocks of chromatin. In some cases, one or two small nucleoli were observed. The same cell occasionally contained two or three nuclei recalling those of Langhans or Sternberg cells. The remaining tumoral cells showed the characteristics of reticulum cells or monocytes with dimensions varying from 15 to 30 μ. The relatively abundant basophile or polychromatophile protoplasm contained some azurophile granulations. The nucleus was large, round or oval, with clear and regular borders. Its position was more or less eccentric and the chromatin was very dense; nucleoli were not usually observed. Mitosis figures were also absent. Eccentric oval nuclei were found with their major diameter at right angles to the cell axis and with a paler protoplasmic area around the nucleus itself. In these cases, a plasma cell appearance was more or less marked. *Bergouignan et al.* stress the isolation of reticulohistiocytes and the high percentage of the accompanying cells as differential data:

in meningeal cancer, metastasis cells are usually found in groups with a small percentage of accompanying cells (1% according to *Kline*).

Neurological signs appear usually within a polyvisceral or hematologic reticulosis context, though they may be the first clinical expression of the underlying disease (*Chaptal et al.; Coquet;* case no. 2 of the series of *Bergouignan et al.*). In a case observed by *Garcin,* they were the only symptom of the disease.

On other occasions, the underlying picture may consist solely of skin symptoms (*Walther and Strocka; Duperrat et al.* [a,b] ; *Basex et al.; Aubertin et al.*).

In the first case observed by *Duperrat et al.*[a]; the initial picture was composed of skin signs which lasted for five years prior to rapid regression achieved with X-ray therapy. The later picture of consciousness disturbances, somnolence, sphincter disturbances, left facial paralysis, and left arm hypertonia was also dramatically improved by radiation. The patient died four months later, however. In their second case, a skin eruption on the back with beltwise pain as in herpes zoster was followed five years later by metamerically distributed left hemithorax hypersensitivity and pain, together with a skin eruption shown to be reticuloblastomatous on biopsy. In the case observed by *Walther and Strocka,* scalp neoformations and subcutaneous nodules were followed by left facial paralysis caused by compression of the nerve trunk by a skin nodule. At a much later date, visceral localization with leukemic episodes were observed. Necropsy showed widespread skin, lymph node, visceral, and meningeal infiltration.

The patient observed by *Basex et al.* presented an initial picture of erythematosquamous and a later picture of erythrodermic skin reticulosis which continued for four years without other manifestations. It was followed by depression, clouding of the senses, convergent squint resulting from paralysis of the 6th cranial nerves and terminal coma. The opening signs in the case reported by *Aubertin et al.* were erythematous and erythematosquamous manifestations on the face and neck, together with nonirritating reddish-violet right forearm nodules about the size of a pea. Later, erythematosquamous manifestations appeared on the left leg accompanied by considerable intractable local pain. Cutaneous reticulosis was diagnosed on biopsy. Nodules appeared later on the extensor surface of the left knee. About three months after the appearance of the first skin manifestations, the following neurological picture was observed: total paralysis of the right oculomotor nerve with ptosis, divergent squint, and paralytic mydriasis; right facial paresis; lower extremity paresis with loss of the Achilles reflex and right patellar reflex, though without Babinski's reflex. X-ray therapy produced a more or less total regression of the cranial nerve paralysis. The lower limb picture, however, was marked by increased pain and the appearance of sensory disturbances together with complete steppage gait of the left foot; while that of the upper limbs included hand pain and formication, loss of muscular force of the fist and thumb apposition, bilateral atrophy of the thenar eminence, and acrocyanosis. These manifestations gradually regressed, leaving only left foot steppage gait and slight thenar eminence atrophy.

In a case of reticulosis in a 27-year-old man studied by *Di Guglielmo et al.* the symptom picture consisted solely of nerve and skin signs, apart from intermittent and remittent fever and the presence of circulating pathologic histiocytes for a short period. The neurological signs were referable to disseminated brain sites, while the skin picture included nodules and hemorrhagic suffusion. Necropsy showed multiple brain hemorrhage sites. Histological examination indicated capillary, precapillary, venular and arteriolar endothelia, and adventitial reticular cell proliferation. These vasal changes were also found in the kidneys, testicles, and other organs, sometimes accompanied by aspecific lesions consisting of various degrees of hyalinosis with dissociation of the tunicae and regression of the elastic structures.

Herpes zoster in cases of monocyte leukemia has been reported by *Bluefarb* and *Cappelletti*. Trigeminally localized serious herpes zoster preceded fatal histioleukemia in a patient observed by *Panelli et al.*

The radiosensitivity of reticulosis is well known and very successful results are also obtained in neurological sites. Radioresistance, however, may be encountered in all localizations during the course of the disease, leaving antimetabolites and cortisones as the only means of treatment. In the case of meningeal forms, antimetabolites may be introduced intrathecally, accompanied by decompressive spinal puncture for the relief of intracranial hypertension.

Particularly serious reticulohistiocyte infiltration of the dura mater was observed in a personal case of acute aleukemic reticulosis in a 29-year-old man whose essentially febrile and neurological picture appeared one and a half months before death (*Gigante, D. and Levi*). The nerve symptoms consisted of violent headache, generalized hyperesthesia, peripheral right facial paralysis, abdominal and upper limb hyporeflexia, and absence of patellar and Achilles reflexes. Nuchal rigidity and Kernig's sign were absent. The CSF findings were normal. Later, confusion and delirium were followed by right hemiparesis and terminal coma. Necropsy showed involvement of the dura and cerebral edema.

II.   Reticulum cell sarcoma is the result of neoplastic proliferation of the reticuloendothelium and may be accompanied by neuralgia caused by compression of peripheral nerve trunks by infiltrated lymph nodes. Axillary involvement of the brachial plexus is typical. Invasion of the base of the cranium produces cranial nerve damage and exophthalmos may follow tumoral infiltration of the orbital cavity.

CNS involvement may form part of a generalized reticulum cell sarcoma picture. Diffusion may be attributed to metastasis from the lymph nodes or from primary sites or to multicentric proliferation.

A complex picture of damage to the nervous system was observed by *Galil-Ogly and Poroshin* in a 59-year-old woman with fever, anemia, dorsal radicular pain, facial paralysis, and deafness. The later signs included sensitivity disturbances, lower extremity paralysis, pelvic organ dysfunction, and sacral and gluteal skin dystrophy. Necropsy showed tumorous infiltration of the right paravertebral cellular tissue at D4 and D6, with nodules of about $1/2$ cm. in diameter in the right subpleural area and hilar adenopathies. Widespread CNS edema was also noted. Reticulum cells were observed in the CNS perivasal spaces and in the paravertebral and subpleural neoformations.

The same workers also observed lower limb edema and pain in a 72-year-old woman following fever diagnosed as influenza. Later, dark red irregular infiltration of the soft parts of the lower extremities was observed, together with a large, lympy swelling in the right breast. Marked right facial central type paralysis, right hemiparesis, and narrowing of the right pupil followed. Death was caused by pneumonia. The postmortem findings showed reticulum cells in the lower limb and breast swellings. The mesenteric lymph nodes and adrenal glands were completely replaced by pale gray tumor tissue. Softening was noted in the right subcortical area. In the nervous tissue, particularly in the site of the softening, the perivasal spaces were packed with reticulum cells.

Cord compression may be observed in the vertebral reticulosarcoma (*Rosendal*). In this connection it must be remembered that, like the lymph nodes, the bone marrow is a site of choice of reticulum cell proliferation.

Neurological signs indicating cord compression (anatomically demonstrated in two cases) were observed in three out of four spinal column reticulum cell sarcoma cases reported by *Drahozal et al.* Necropsy showed extensive myelomalacia. A further six cases have since been observed by *Goutelle et al.*

Cord compression may also be a result of the presence of a blastomatous mass of epidural origin. In a case of reticulum cell sarcoma observed by *Lugaresi et al.* a transverse medullary lesion was the first sign. Diagnosis was based on histological examination of a resected epidural neoformation.

Atrophic flaccid paraplegia was observed in a case reported by *Allison and Gordon*, together with paralysis of the 3rd and 7th cranial nerves and CSF albuminocytologic dissociation.

A left Horner's syndrome was noted by *Dell'Acqua* in a patient with left upper limb anesthesia and motor deficiency suggesting radicular paralysis. Necropsy showed a Pancoast's syndrome attributed to left lung reticulosarcomatous infiltration.

In a second case reported by the same author, systemic bone reticulosarcomatosis involving the skull cap was accompanied by a neurological picture with signs of 12th cranial nerve involvement, marked intracranial hypertension, and edema of the optic disk.

Thoracic herpes zoster followed by intractable neuralgia was observed by *Lugaresi et al.*

Three pathogenetic explanations were advanced by *Legeais et al.* to explain the neurological picture observed in a young man with a large reticulum cell sarcoma of the first left rib: paraneoplastic pathogenesis, metastatization, or simple concomitance of the neurological condition and the underlying disease.

The patient was a 14-year-old boy who, when first observed, presented a large swelling of three months' standing in the left clavicular area accompanied by severe pain in the left upper extremity, particularly the hand. The swelling extended from the upper border of the trapezius to the axilla. It was of a wooden consistency, with an irregular surface, indolent on palpation, and adherent to the costal plane. The neurological picture included considerable left upper extremity amyotrophy, particularly at the thenar and hypothenar eminences, the interosseal, and the flexor muscles. Muscular force was much reduced, though arm abduction, forearm flexion and extension, pronation and supination, and hand extension were all possible but flexion of the wrist and fingers was not. There was considerable hyporeflexia and, while sensibility was normal, the patient complained of violent piercing pain and formication at the fold of the elbow and in the hand. Electric irritability was normal in all four limbs. The electroencephalogram (EEG) showed left cerebral hemisphere irritation, without signs of localization. The chest X-ray suggested complete lysis of the first left rib, while biopsy of a subclavicular lymph node showed the reticulosarcomatous nature of the skeletal alteration.

Radiation and cortisone treatment, later replaced by cortisone and cyclophosphamide, produced marked regression of the left clavicular mass. At this stage the presence of calcareous deposits permitted radiographic visualization of the profile of the first rib, the anterior end of which had a roundish puffed appearance. Improvement of the neoplasia picture, however, was accompanied by further development of the neurologic symptomatology and the appearance of signs of intracranial hypertension. Frank bilateral Aran-Duchenne syndrome of the upper limbs, more marked on the left, was observed, with considerable amyotrophy and total areflexia. Lower extremity amyotrophy was present, though with unimpaired reflexes. Marked muscle galvanic and faradic hypoexcitability was noted, particularly in the left upper extremity. A degenerative electrical reaction could not be obtained. The ophthalmological data included convergent squint, suggesting involvement of the 6th cranial nerves, and considerable edema of the optic disk. There were EEG signs of more serious cerebral distress, particularly in the anterior regions, though without a precise localization. An increased CSF albumin content was noted (0.85 g%oo).

A paraneoplastic pathogenesis is suggested by *Blanchard* for a form of polyneuritis observed as the first manifestation of reticulum cell sarcoma in a 59-year-old woman whose presenting symptoms included hand and foot paresthesia and weakness in all four extremities. Paresthesia and pain in the left arm and hand had been noted some months before. The gait was hesitant and there was slight atrophy of the hand and foot muscles, with upper limb hyporeflexia and lower limb areflexia. A chest X-ray showed right pulmonary lesions and hilar and paratracheal adenopathies. Biopsy of a scalene muscle swelling showed a tumor with poorly differentiated cells. Following roentgen therapy of the chest and the administration of vitamin B12, the patient was discharged but was readmitted six weeks later upon progression of the neurological picture and died about three months from the date of first admission. Necropsy showed widespread reticulosarcomatosis with slight disseminated demyelinization of the spinal cord (permission to examine the brain was refused). There was no evidence of neoplastic invasion of the cord, the nerve roots, or the peripheral nerve trunks.

Waelbroeck et al. observed a "progressive multifocal leukoencephalopathy" in a case of reticulum cell sarcoma of the kidney. A picture of subacute multifocal leukoencephalopathy with progressive ataxia and dementia was noted in a case of reticulum cell sarcoma by *Martin and van Bogaert*. Anatomic examination of the CNS revealed striking degeneration of the cerebellar white matter, as well as multiple small demyelinative foci in the brain stem and at the corticomedullary junction of the cerebral hemispheres. Eosinophile inclusions, within the nuclei of neuroglia, neurons, and other cells, were conspicuous throughout the CNS.

III. Involvement of the nervous system is not common in follicular lymphoma (giant follicular lymphoblastoma, Brill-Symmers disease).

Only one example was found in a series of 229 cases of lymphoreticular disease studied by *Hutchinson et al.*

A case in a 34-year-old man with back pains irradiating beltwise from the right scapula was observed by *Borchers and Mittelbach.* Resection of an axillary lymph node enabled a diagnosis of follicular lymphoma to be established and radiation treatment led to the regression of the pain symptoms. One year later, however, an incomplete transverse spinal syndrome appeared. This yielded to combined radiation and triethylene melamine treatment, while a relapse was satisfactorily managed by radiation alone. Three months later, a typical herpes zoster was observed in the lumbar region and the CSF values showed inflammatory changes. Good results were obtained with cytostatics.

An anatomically demonstrated, aspecific peripheral neuropathy preceded the appearance of follicular lymphoma manifestations in a case observed by *Shafar.*

Herpes zoster involving the right gluteal region and the posterior surface of the right thigh was observed in a personal case diagnosed as follicular lymphoma two years earlier following the surgical removal and histological examination of the enlarged spleen. The patient—a 69-year-old man—also presented fever with maximum temperatures of about 38°C, a marked loss of general condition, and moderate anemia. Lymph node swellings were not observed.

IV.   Eosinophilic granuloma is more frequent in children and adolescents, than in adults and in males more than in females. Nerve manifestations are exceptional.

This disease is marked by the formation of a particular type of granulation tissue, of soft consistency and varying in color from brown to yellowish. Histological examination shows tissue formed of large round or oval histiocyte cells, with generous protoplasm and a roundish or kidney-shaped vesicular nucleus; large numbers of granulocytes or eosinophile myelocytes, sometimes in groups forming microabscesses; multinucleated giant cells (2–30 nuclei), sometimes with phagocytosis figures; macrophages and a variable number of plasma cells, lymphocytes and neutrophile granulocytes (*Green and Farber; etc.*). In most cases the course is that of a cicatricial sclerosis, with the disappearance of the eosinophiles.

The skeleton is the site of choice, usually in a single localization though multiple sites have been observed. All bones may be involved. The osteolytic effect of the granuloma leads to the formation of a usually cystic cavity, in which the pathological tissue is collected. The cortex, though usually unimpaired, suffers a considerable loss of thickness and acquires a parchment-like consistency, so that it can be cut readily with a knife.

Lymph node involvement may occur, usually limited to the stations corresponding to the diseased portion of the skeleton. Spleen enlargement is rare. Lung, skin, kidney, and gastroenteric alterations may be observed and these, like lymph node involvement, may offer the only sign of the underlying disease. Hepatomegaly has never been observed.

Granulomatosis of the cranium and vertebrae is the most frequent cause of neurological involvement which may present as paralysis of the cranial nerves or as ataxia (*Amato and Catalano*). Lower extremity paralysis and urine and stool incontinence were observed by *Oberman* in an adult patient with an osteolytic lesion of the 5th lumbar vertebra.

Diabetes insipidus indicating involvement of the diencephalon and hypophysis has been observed on several occasions (*Thoma; Engelbreth-Holm et al.; Versiani et al.; Ackermann; Kierland et al.; Ribuffo; Amato and Galloro; Cutillo et al.; Oberman*). Furthermore, there are cases with multiple localization and a frankly xanthomatous course that have progressed to Hand-Schüller-Christian disease, in which diabetes insipidus is a typical symptom.

Four adult cases of diabetes insipidus coupled with ulcers of the skin and mucosae, which were histologically referable to eosinophilic granuloma, have been reported by *Kierland et al.* In a case observed by *Amato and Galloro*, the clinical overture of large neck adenopathies was followed by osteolytic alterations of the cranium. About one and a half years after the first symptoms, when regression of the entire syndrome had begun, polydipsia and polyuria appeared. In a 1¹/₂-year-old child and a 43-year-old man observed by *Oberman*, diabetes insipidus appeared six months and 2¹/₂ years after the initial bone lesion respectively.

In some cases, diabetes insipidus shows no response to posthypophyseal antidiuretic hormone (*Amato and Galloro*). The reason for this is unknown.

Disturbances of body growth are also noted.

Exophthalmos is rare, though in a case reported by *Fasiani* it was the initial clinical sign.

Symptoms of general nervous distress, such as headache, nausea, and migraine, may be noted. These are not referable to the specific nerve location of the disease.

Eosinophilic granuloma is typically benign. Not only is it sensitive to radiation and medical (cortisones, antimetabolites and cytostatics) treatment, but also it tends to regress spontaneously. Surgical resection of the granuloma tissue may be done in the case of skeletal lesion. In the relatively rare instance of transformation into Hand-Schüller-Christian disease or Letterer-Siwe reticulosis the prognosis is less hopeful and the appearance of neurological complications may be fatal.

V.   Signs of neurological damage may also be noted in lipoidosis. This term is used to describe conditions such as Hand-Schüller-Christian, Gaucher's, and Niemann-Pick disease in which lipid substances are accumulated in reticuloendothelial cells. In the three diseases mentioned above these substances are cholesterol, kerasin, and sphingomyelin, and they are the source of the terms cholesterol, cerebroside, and sphingomyelin lipoidosis, respectively. The degree of proliferation of reticuloendothelial cells may vary in the different forms. It is not yet certain whether accumulation is attributable to a primary disturbance in lipid metabolism (overproduction, catabolic disturbances) or is a result of reticuloendothelial proliferation (*Müller and Orthner; etc.*), which is sometimes caused by infection. If the latter hypothesis is correct, the reticuloendothelial cells would subsequently take up the lipids or form them in an intracellular site. In the case of Hand-Schüller-Christian disease, however, many workers consider that reticuloendothelial proliferation—here typically granulomatous and similar to that of Hodgkin's disease (*Chester's* lipoidogranulomatosis)—precedes cholesterol ester accumulation. Recently it has been suggested that cell storage of lipids in Gaucher's disease may depend on a biochemical block at the reticuloendothelial level, caused by the lack of an enzyme (glycocerebrosidase) responsible for splitting cerebrosides into glucose and ceramide (*Berger*).

Hand-Schüller-Christian disease is not common. It usually occurs in early infancy and is found primarily in male subjects. Unlike the other forms of lipoidosis, it does not seem to be hereditary.

The anatomicopathological picture of the disease is marked by the formation of more or less voluminous histiocyte nodules or infiltrates of a yellowish or red-brown color. The typical histological finding is of foam cells (also called xanthomatous cells). These are large, polyhedric histiocytes with a foamy protoplasm and one or more nuclei at the circumference or in the center. In preparations not fixed with alcohol, cholesterol or cholesterol esters may be seen in the cells. Exudative cells (lymphocytes, plasma cells, eosinophile leukocytes, etc.) and connective cells may be observed also.

The clinical picture is marked by a typical triad: lacunar, osteolytic skeletal alterations (usually in the cranial bones) without signs of periosteal reaction; exophthalmos; and diencephalon and hypophyseal disturbances. Cranial bone alterations are typical of Hand-Schüller-Christian disease and usually seem to be secondary to granulomatous

infiltration of the dura mater or periosteum. Exophthalmos may be uni-
or bilateral and is usually a late manifestation. It may be caused by
granulomatous infiltration of the orbit or it may be secondary to collapse
of the walls of the orbit caused by infiltration from pathologic tissue. It
may be accompanied by optic nerve atrophy. Diencephalic and hypophyseal signs may be attributed to either direct compression by
granulomatous masses or infiltration of the sella turcica. Diabetes
insipidus, infantilism, and adiposogenital dystrophy are signs of this
type.

As long ago as 1893, *Hand* observed polyuria together with osteolytic
lacunae of the cranial bones and exophthalmos in a 3-year-old boy.
Necropsy showed grayish yellow granulomatous swellings in nearly
every organ and the picture was interpreted as tubercular. *Kay* (1905)
reported a case with cranial bone lacunae, exophthalmos, and polyuria,
and in 1915 *Schüller* observed three cases with cranial bone lacunae, two
of which presented exophthalmos in association with diabetes insipidus
and adiposogenital dystrophy, respectively.

It has been suggested that diabetes insipidus will be found in about
50% of all cases of Hand-Schüller-Christian disease (*Avery et al.;
Bluefarb*), though some writers claim an even higher frequency. Diabetes may be the initial and dominant sign or appear only months or
years after the onset of the underlying disease. Here its onset will be
insidious and will be revealed by increasing polyuria and polydipsia. In
some cases, urinary concentration capacity remains singularly unaffected (*Zöllner*). In the majority of cases, diabetes is responsive to
posthypophyseal antidiuretic hormone. *Roos et al.*, however, observed
hormone resistance in a 47-year-old man.

Strictly neurological symptoms attributable to true encephalomye-
lopathy are rare in Hand-Schüller-Christian disease and are observed
solely in adult subjects (*Guccione; Bossa; Fasanaro*). In *Bossa's* case, a
cerebellar symptomatology was accompanied by jacksonian epilepsy and
right hemiparesis. Data collected by *Giampalmo* show that nervous
system alterations may consist of granulomatous (glial-mesenchymal)
sites exclusively or of typical granulo-xanthomatosis sites with foam cells.

Müller and Orthner observed a progressive cerebellar and bulbar
symptomatology with diabetes insipidus and a meningitic symptomatology in a 47-year-old-man and a 57-year-old woman, respectively. In the
first case, necropsy showed numerous cerebral granulomas with diameters varying from 2 to 32 mm, in the left temporal lobe white matter, the
internal capsule, the hypothalamus and hypophysis region, the pons and
the cerebellum. The second case presented intraventricular granulomas.

Gradual onset of a neurological picture consisting of left hemiparesis,
left limp, slurring of speech, headache, loss of vision, left-sided ataxia,

right-sided weakness, and clumsiness in the use of both hands was observed recently by *Elian et al.* in a 41-year-old man. The later picture included severe spastic paraparesis, bilateral ataxia, and severe dysarthria, together with left-sided jacksonian fits, increasing in number and intensity, often to the point of generalized convulsion, and several psychotic episodes. Angiography showed leftward deviation of the distal segment of the anterior cerebral artery to the insertion of the falx cerebri, indicating the presence of a subdural (space-occupying) lesion in the parietal region. Craniotomy revealed a massive xanthoma. Necropsy showed widespread xanthomatosis and multiple, yellow lobulated nodules from 2 to 4 cm in diameter, bilaterally scattered over the inner surface of the dura, with corresponding cortical depression on the brain.

The natural history of Hand-Schüller-Christian disease is usually chronic but both spontaneous and therapeutic cures are known. Prognosis will be uncertain in all respects. Radiation therapy is the basic form of treatment.

Gaucher's disease is a familial congenital affection occurring most commonly in Jewish subjects. The disease runs a chronic course and patients may reach an advanced age. In the infantile forms, however, clinical signs are evident in the first six months of life and death occurs in less than two years or, at times, within the space of a few months (*Aballi and Kato; Amato; Meyer; Ullrich; etc.*).

The dominant feature of the clinical picture is splenomegaly, accompanied by hepatomegaly later in the course. The lymph nodes are usually unimpaired. Skeletal alterations, usually involving the head and neck of the femur, present a moth-eaten or widespread osteoporotic appearance on radiographic examination. The further course of the disease may be marked by a yellowish-brown or ochre color of the skin, while in the advanced stages, hemorrhage caused by thrombocytopenia is nearly always present.

Typical Gaucher cells are found in the bone marrow and diseased viscera. Infiltration is usually microscopic, but sometimes may be clearly apparent even on gross examination. Gaucher cells are usually of considerable size and may exceed $40\,\mu$ in diameter. Normal methods of tissue fixation dissolve the kerasin, leaving a "spider's web" or "creased tissue paper" residue of the protoplasm. The nucleus is shifted toward the perimeter and may be elongated, flat, or even pyknotic. Multinucleated cellls have been observed (*Pick* has counted 21 nuclei) and these are particularly large.

Neurological manifestations are more commonly seen in nurslings, while they arc rare in older subjects (only ten cases published up to 1962 according to *Mérab et al.*).

The usual picture in the nursling is one of retarded motor function development, widespread muscular hypertonia with hyperextension of the head, laryngospasm, squint, stupor, and pseudo-bulbar type symptoms (mastication, swallowing and phonation disturbances) (*Meyer; Portillo et al.; Banker et al.; Schettler and Kahlke*). The advanced stage of the disease in three cases reported by *Banker et al.* included hyperreflexia, tendon clonus, and Babinski's reflex, together with increasingly serious bulbar symptoms. Death was the result of intercurrent infection or lung inflammation caused by aspiration. Shortly before death, posture suggestions of decerebration were noted.

Anatomic and histologic study of the brain in these cases showed widespread nonuniform cell loss in layers 3 and 5 of the cortex and a predominance of microglia and Gaucher cells in this site. An equally serious nerve cell loss was observed in the thalamus, the other basic nuclei, the cerebral trunk, cerebellum, and spinal cord. Signs of neuronophagia and slight neuron cytoplasmatic storage of a glycolipid similar to Gaucher cell lipids were further outstanding features.

In the extremely rare cases of neurological complication in older subjects, hyperreflexia was observed by *Reiss and Kato* in three patients, and *Myers* observed involuntary movement of the eyes, mouth, face, and nucha in a splenectomized 8-year-old girl, whose irritability picture became more serious until death one year later with signs of bronchopneumonia and Gaucher cells in the sputum. Extrapyramidal symptomatologies were observed by *van Bogaert and Froehlich* in a 42-year-old man and by *Davison* in a 26-year-old patient. In the latter case, anatomicopathological examination of the brain showed lenticular and caudate nucleus cell degeneration and Alzheimer glial cells. An extrapyramidal symptomatology accompanied by dementia was observed by *Bird* in an 11-year-old patient. At necropsy (four years later), the neuron alterations proper to amaurotic familial idiocy were observed. Extrapyramidal involvement has also been observed by *Brain*. In a case reported by *Maloney and Cumings*, the neurological picture appeared at the age of five years and consisted of mental retardation and hyperreflexia followed by epileptic crises. Death from bronchopneumonia occurred at eight years, and histologic examination showed neuron storage of lipids.

In a case described by *Mérab et al.*, a Lebanese girl had presented increased abdominal volume at the age of four years as the first sign of the underlying disease. One year later, uncoordinated head and limb movements appeared, together with gait disturbances. When observed by the writers three years later, the patient presented marked hepatosplenomegaly accompanied by choreoathetoid head and limb movements and lower limb hypertonia and hyperreflexia. Widening of the basis of support was noted in the erect posture; walking was no longer automatic and normal swinging of the arms was absent; stiffness of the lower limbs was responsible for a slightly hesitant gait. Biopsy of the spleen, liver, and a laterocervical lymph node established a diagnosis of Gaucher's disease.

Peripheral nerve damage was observed by *Bischoff et al.* in a 43-year-old man with histologically demonstrated Gaucher's disease since infancy. Glycolipoids in the diseased nerve formations were shown ultramicroscopically.

A progressive deterioration of intellectual capacity was recently reported by *Balconi and Fornara* in a 13-year-old girl removed from school because of her inability to get into the third grade. The neurological picture included muscular hypotonia and hyporeflexia.

Treatment is symptomatic only. Splenectomy may lead to regression of hemorrhage caused by thrombocytopenia.

Niemann-Pick disease is also hereditary and appears in early infancy mainly in Jewish subjects. It usually runs a rapidly progressive course.

The picture is one of marked mental retardation, together with muscular rigidity and hyperreflexia. Involuntary muscle contractions, loss of coordination, athetosis, tremors, and seizures may be observed (*Schettler and Kahlke*), as well as opisthotonos and squint (*Fakatselli*). The mouth is often held open with the tongue protruding. Other manifestations of nerve involvement include vomiting, increased basal metabolism, and sweating (*Baumann et al.*). No particular abnormality will be observed in the electroencephalographic (EEG) data. The cranial nerves may be involved and deafness is a common symptom. Idiocy to the point of vegetation may be observed.

In 60% of cases, examination of the fundus oculi shows a cherry-red macular spot, reminiscent of that observed in Tay-Sachs disease, and the clinical picture of this disease may sometimes be similar to that of Niemann-Pick disease.

Considerable similarity undoubtedly exists between Tay-Sachs, Gaucher's, and Niemann-Pick disease. The first, in fact, is a form of lipoidosis in a cerebral and retinal site, with storage of gangliosides in the nerve cells. All three diseases may be described as neurodyslipidosis and some workers would include Hurler's disease as a further example of nerve tissue lipid storage. There is disagreement about the nature of the substance stored (*Tronconi*), however, and some workers (*Brante; Uzman; Dorfman and Lorincx*), consider Hurler's disease a familial metabolic systemic mesenchymopathy, in which the fundamental disturbance primarily concerns the mucopolysaccharides.

Other lipid storage diseases identified in recent years include:

sulfatide lipidosis, familial neurovisceral lipidosis (or generalized gangliosidosis), disseminated lipogranulomatosis, cephalin lipidosis, polyneuritiform ataxic heredopathy, etc. The respective neurological symptoms in each of these forms are: polyradiculitis followed by violent muscular pain and hyperesthesia; delayed mental and motor development; weak voice and nutrition and respiration difficulties; delayed mental development; polyneuritis with cerebellar ataxia and deafness. In cephalin lipidosis, reticuloendothelial cell lipid storage is responsible for massive spleen enlargement.

On gross examination, cerebral involvement in Niemann-Pick disease shows the white matter to be of a leathery consistency while the gray matter is rather soft. This is the reverse of the picture observed in Tay-Sachs disease (*Schettler and Kahlke*). Under the microscope, the large pyramidal cells are distended and swollen and sometimes have vacuoles instead of degenerated Nissl granules, and the nucleus is shifted toward the axon. There is a decrease in the total number of nerve cells and concomitant glial reaction. These alterations vary in intensity in different areas of the brain and biopsy may produce normal tissue, particularly in very young patients. Histological changes in the white matter are not observed. Increased sphingomyelin values are generally accompanied by increased concentrations of cholesterol and gangliosides, though Niemann-Pick cells are not observed since lipid storage involves the neurons only (*Schettler and Kahlke*).

Philippart et al. have recently observed a case in which normal brain sphingomyelin levels were accompanied by gray matter water accumulation and increased glycolipid values.

Fine cerebellar alterations were observed by *Wallace et al.* in a 13-month-old boy.

Histological changes similar to those described in the brain have been observed in the spinal cord.

Cerebral function damage in Niemann-Pick disease may vary considerably. As in Gaucher's disease, it is related to age and neurological abnormalities are both marked and frequent in patients up to the age of four or five years, since at this age lipid storage coincides with myelinization and general development.

Widespread brain alterations may be the cause of stupor or coma (*Plum and Posner*). This is thought to be caused by disturbances to nerve structure metabolism.

Appendix

Lastly, a word may be said concerning primary reticuloendothelial proliferation of the CNS. These forms are of unknown etiology and usually neoplastiform in nature (*Henschen*). They originate in nerve structure reticuloendothelial cells (adventitial histiocytes, fixed cells in the meningeal perivasal areas, microglia). Generally described as primary reticulosis of the nervous system, these proliferations have also been called peritheliomas or perithelial sarcomas (*Bailey; Hsü*), reticulosarcomas (*Yuile; Kinney and Adams; Fisher et al.*); microgliomas (*Russel et al.*), etc.

In the 40 or so cases reported in the literature, infiltration is primarily perivasal and is usually more abundant in paraventricular sites. The infiltrate cell picture may range from complete monomorphism, with relatively small cells and nuclei rich in chromatin, to polymorphism and the appearance of giant cells. Reticular fibers in the form of concentric rings around the vessels may also be noted.

The clinical picture often recalls that of cerebral tumor. The disease usually runs a rapid course of a few weeks or a few months; survival for more than a year is exceptional. In cases where no tumor is formed, two symptom patterns may be distinguished at the onset: aspecific psychological signs corresponding to progressive alteration to the point of mental confusion, and labyrinthine symptoms (static sense disturbances, nystagmus and sometimes kinetic cerebellar symptoms) (*Coste and Brion*). In this instance too, the disease runs a rapid course, with variable and nontypical accumulation of symptoms. Intracranial hypertension is nearly always observed.

In the first of two cases reported by *Marchiafava and Bignami* perivasal cell proliferation was present in all brain districts with the exception of the cerebral cortex and it was limited to the perivasal spaces, usually without invasion of nerve tissue. In the second case, however, the perivasal sleeves were fused together at the pons under the floor of the 4th ventricle.

The initial picture presented by the first patient, a 25-year-old man, included intense headache, localized at the temples, and cerebral type vomiting ten days before admission, accompanied by remittent fever with peaks of 38.5° C. An epilepsy episode, apparently originating in the left limbs, was observed on the morning preceding admission. The neurological picture included leftward fall in Romberg's position, slight nuchal rigidity, and a suggestion of Kernig's sign. Examination of the fundus oculi showed bilateral peripapillary edema. The CSF showed a cell value of $108/mm^3$ (90% mononucleates; 10% polynucleates); the Pandy test was slightly positive (±). The patient grew worse rapidly and progressively, with agitation followed by coma and death on the tenth day after admission. Necropsy showed wide meningeal and encephalic congestion, with infiltration around the white matter vessels in both hemispheres. Microscopic examination also revealed perivasal infiltrates in the basal nuclei, mesencephalon, pons, cerebellum, and bulb (the spinal cord was not studied). Medium and small caliber veins were primarily involved and infiltration was mainly confined to the Robin's spaces, though slight invasion of the surrounding nerve tissue was occasionally observed. The cells were of the reticuloendothelial type and were separated by fairly thick argyrophil fibers forming concentric rings around the vasal lumen.

The second patient was a 7-year-old boy who had presented leftward deviation of the eyes and mouth, accompanied by dribbling, and dysarthria two days before admission. He was unable to stand and vomited during fasting. On the following day, the deviation improved but right ptosis appeared. On admission, the patient was in a state of stupor, unresponsive to stimuli, and his eyes were closed. The neurological picture included, besides the ptosis mentioned above: bilateral internal squint, mydriasis with torpid reactions and loss of left corneal reflex, flattening of the right nasolabial plica, leftward displacement of the mouth slit, hypomobile soft palate, left limb hypotonia, upper extremity and abdominal areflexia, bilaternal patellar hyperreflexia, and bilateral Babinski and Oppenheim reflexes (more pronounced on the right). Craniography showed right occipital suture disjunction. Findings of right cerebral angiography were normal. The patient died two days later. Necropsy showed intense meningeal and encephalic congestion and an approximately 3 mm malacic patch in the pontine part of the 4th ventricle floor, surrounded by numerous petechiae. Histologic examination demonstrated that the malacic site was composed of primarily perivasal compact cell infiltration. Similar though more limited infiltration was observed in other parts of the brain.

In two cases of primary reticulosis of the nervous system studied by *Ederli and Merigliano,* reticuloendothelial infiltration had invaded the whole of the ventricular surface below the ependyma, the epithelium of which, though mostly free from infiltration, was in many places pushed into the ventricular cavity in the form of nodules of various shapes and sizes. The choroid plexuses, corpus callosum, transparent septum, caudate nucleus, and thalamus were invaded. In the first case, trigeminal neuralgia was followed by fulminant terminal coma. Increased CSF albumin and cell values were observed in both cases.

Primary hypothalamus and middle cerebellar peduncle localizations were noted by *Castaigne et al.* in a 62-year-old man with an 8-year history of diabetes insipidus. He presented postural disturbances and signs of intracranial hypertension and died of intercurrent pulmonary infection.

Clinical and anatomical evidence of a primary cerebellar localization was found by *White and Rothfleisch* in a 56-year-old man who presented blurred vision, vertigo, ataxia, papilledema, left central facial weakness, and bilateral Babinski's reflex. Pneumoencephalography suggested the presence of a left cerebellar mass. A short episode of headache, left earache and deafness, left cerebellar signs, and diminished sensation over all divisions of the left trigeminal nerve had been observed nearly two years earlier.

Granulomatous infiltration of the brain (*Wilke*'s granulomatous encephalitis) may be distinguished from the other mainly perivasal primary proliferations already mentioned by its outstanding cell polymorphism and its greater extension, combined with a notable tendency to form compact masses. *Wilke* considers this form of infiltration an inflammatory version of primary cerebral reticuloendotheliosis. This view is not shared by *Sigwald et al.* who observed multiple granuloma sites in the lungs, liver, and adrenal cortex as well as the CNS in a 50-year-old man. They regard the cerebral alterations as the expression of systematized nerve tissue proliferative reticulosis, with exceptional involvement of other organs.

Infectious mononucleosis is a virus-induced blood disease characterized by widespread benign reticuloendothelial cell hyperplasia. Occasionally neurological involvement is considerable and a so-called "nervous" variety of the disease has been recognized.

The first reports of neurological complications were made by *Epstein and Dameshek* and *Johansen* in 1931 and a series culled from the literature by *Leibowitz* in 1952 contained 83 cases.

Vasal congestion, edema, slight hemorrhage, mononuclear infiltration, and, in the more serious cases, various degrees of cell degeneration may be noted.

Neurological signs sometimes form the opening picture (*Giroire et al.*; *Münter, etc.*) or even the sole clinical expression (*Brogard et al.*) of the underlying disease. Frequencies of about 6% (*Prochazka and Kouba*) and from 1 to 9% (*Leibowitz*) have been noted. *Rentchnick* distinguishes meningeal, encephalitic, peripheral nervous, and ocular complications, and also neurological complications only demonstrated by electroencephalographs.

Meningeal involvement is the most common (*Gautier-Smith*) and may be accompanied by either normal or abnormal CSF values, the latter being the only clinical sign in some cases (*Klemola*). Increased albumin, positive Pandy reaction, and lymphocytosis are the usual findings. Encephalitic complications, with or without meningeal reaction, give rise to various degrees of psychological disturbance, including delirium and coma (*Amyot; Prochazka and Kouba; Brogard et al.*) (in an extremely serious, though successfully treated, case of meningoencephalitis observed by *Houtteville et al.* virtually complete flattening of the electroencephalographic trace lasted six hours). Convulsions and signs of local lesion may occur. Signs of cerebellar damage have also been reported, such as ataxia, asynergia, dysmetria, uneven or explosive speech, nystagmus, etc. (*Retif et al.; Dowling and van Slyck; etc.*). Peripheral complications include cranial (particularly the 3rd and 7th) and spinal nerve paralysis, Guillain-Barré syndrome, and Landry's paralysis.

Transverse myelitis has been observed by *Verliac et al., Cotton and Webb-Peploe,* and *Münter.*

Right central facial paralysis appeared a few days before the typical symptom picture in a personal case of infectious mononucleosis in a 2-year-old girl (*d'Eramo and Gualtieri*). This slowly regressed, as did the benign course of the underlying disease. Transient right arm paresis, lasting only a few hours, was observed during the disease. The CSF showed signs of hypertension and there was a slight increase in albumin level. The neurological picture was attributable presumably to focal cerebral cortex lesions. The brachial paresis was undoubtedly the expression of a rapidly resolved circulatory disturbance.

Ocular complications are less common than neurological ones. They include iridocyclitis or uveitis and retinopapillitis or signs of retinal detachment.

With the exception of the possibly fatal encephalitic forms and ascending polyradiculoneuritis, the prognosis is generally good; a 25% mortality in the presence of the latter complication is postulated by *Davie et al.,* in comparison to 0.5–1% mortality in uncomplicated cases. Persistent neuropsychiatric sequelae may result from encephalitic complications.

Treatment will make use of the remedies employed for the management of the underlying disease, and the efficacy of cortisones has been fully demonstrated (*Bender*). Rapid improvement was obtained with intrathecal steroids in a case of Guillain-Barré type syndrome with severe respiratory disturbances studied by *Erle.*

Finally, reference may be made to acute infectious lymphocytosis. This is probably caused by a virus and it has a typical blood picture. The symptomatology may occasionally include encephalitic syndrome (*Marinesco*) or signs of meningeal involvement (*Thelander and Shaw; Marinesco*). CSF lymphocytosis has also been reported (*Duncan*).

REFERENCES

Reticuloendotheliopathy in general

BUFANO, M.: Su le sarcomatosi sistemiche dei tessuti emopoietici. Boll. Soc. med. chir., Brescia 3 (1948).
MOESCHLIN, S.: Die Milzpunktion (Schwabe, Basel 1947).
ROHR: In Baserga, L'inquadramento attuale delle malattie del S.R.E. Fisiopatologia e clinica del sistema reticolo istiocitario (Atti delle Giornate Mediche Triestine), Trieste 1965, pp. 25–36 (Ediz. Scuola Med. Osped. Trieste, 1966).

Reticulosis

AHNQUIST, G. and HOLIOKE, J. B.: Congenital Letterer-Siwe disease (reticuloendotheliosis) in a term stillborn infant. J. Pediat. 57:897–904 (1960).
ALLISON, R. S. and GORDON, D. S.: Reticulosis of nervous system simulating acute infective polyneuritis. Lancet ii:120–122 (1955).
AMATO, M.: Istiocitopatia congenita maligna del neonato. Un nuovo aspetto della patologia infantile del sistema istiocitario. Haematologica 40:301–324 (1955).
AUBERTIN, E.; LAVIGNOLLE, A.; SUDRE, Y.; MOREAU, F. and BEYLOT, C.: Réticulose histiomonocytaire avec atteinte cutanée et neurologique. J. Méd., Bordeaux 141: 1693–1702 (1964).
BAMFORTH, J. and KENDALL, D.: Case of megakaryocytic myelosis with paraplegia. Acta med. scand. 99:494–509 (1939).
BASEX; DUPRÉ and PARANT: Réticulose à point de départ cutané ayant évolué pendant 4 ans. Terminaison rapide par un syndrome méningoencéphalitique. Bull. Soc. franç. Derm. Syph. 65:109–111 (1958).
BERGOUIGNAN, M.; LÉGER, H.; VITAL, CL. and COQUET, M.: Les formes méningées des réticulopathies malignes. J. Méd., Bordeaux 142:777–786 (1965).
BERNARD, J. D. and AGUILAR, M. J.: Localized hypothalamic histiocytosis X. Arch. Neurol., Chicago 20:368–372 (1969).
BLUEFARB, S. M.: Zona et leucémie monocytique. Arch. Derm. Syph., Paris 57:319–327 (1948).
CAPPELLETTI: in Panelli et al.
CAZAL, P.: La réticulose histiomonocytaire (Masson, Paris 1946).
CHAPTAL, J.; MOURUT, E. and CAZAL, P.: Réticulose histiomonocytaire subaiguë à forme hépato-splénique débutant par une paraplégie spasmodique. Sang 16:421–426 (1944).
CIONINI, A. and ROTTA, C.: Emoblastosi a decorso acuto con complessa sintomatologia nervosa. Linfogranuloma maligno o reticuloendoteliosi? Haematologica 15:593–631 (1934).
COQUET, M.: Contribution à l'étude des atteintes méningées au cours des réticulopathies malignes (à propos de deux cas de réticulose histiomonocytaire); Thèse Bordeaux (1963).
DEGOS, R.; DELORT, J.; OSSIPOWSKI, B.; CIVATTE, J. and TOURAINE, R.: Réticulose cutanée hyperplasique simple associée à un réticulosarcome ganglionnaire. Bull. Soc. franç. Derm. Syph. 64:11–12 (1957).
DUPÉRIÉ, R.; LACHAUD, R. DE and MONMAYOU, H.: Lymphadénie cutanée, épisode terminal de leucémie aiguë avec polynévrite et ictère. J. Méd., Bordeaux 23/24:397–405 (1943).
DUPERRAT, B.; GOLE and PEROT: a) Réticulomatose cutanée avec localisation cérébrale. Etat. précomateux. Effet spectaculaire de la radiothérapie. Bull. Soc. franc. Derm. Syph. 61:485–486 (1954).

DUPERRAT, B.; MEUNIER et BARBE, P.: b) Réticulose cutanée neurotrope. Bull. Soc. franç.
    Derm. Syph. 67:603–605 (1960).
EUZIÈRE, J.; GUIBERT, H. L.; FASSIO, E.; RODIER, J. and CAZAL, P.: Réticulose histio-
    monocytaire chronique à localisation nerveuse, du type 'réticulose syncytiale' de
    Dustin-Weill. Soc. Sc. méd. biol. Montpellier, meeting 9 January 1942.
GARCIN, R.: Sur le retentissement nerveux des réticulopathies et en particulier leurs
    modalités cliniques et leur mode de propagation. Bull. Acad. nat. Méd. 140:451–455
    (1956).
GIGANTE, D. and LEVI, M.: Su un caso di reticolo-endoteliosi acuta maligna a localizzazione
    meningea. Settim. med. 44:435–441 (1956).
GUGLIELMO, G. DI; FASANOTTI, A.; GIGANTE, D. and FERRARA, A.: Varietà nervosa della
    reticolo-endoteliosi acuta maligna. C.R. III Congr. Soc. Int. Européenne Hémat.,
    Rome 1951, pp. 380–382 (E.M.E.S., Rome 1952).
KLINE, T. S.: Cytological examination of the cerebrospinal fluid. Cancer, Philad. 15:591–
    597 (1962).
LÉGER, H.; ARNÉ, L.; MOULINIER, J.; SEILHAN, A. and SALLES, M.: Terminaison neurolo-
    gique d'une réticulopathie à forme de leucose à monocytes au long cours. Toulouse
    méd. 62:169–176 (1961).
LEICHER, F.: Zur Frage des Geschwulstcharakters der Reticulosen und ihrer Beziehungen
    zu den Leukämien. Z. klin. Med. 149:530–552 (1952).
LICHTENSTEIN, L.: Histiocytosis X: integration of eosinophilic granuloma of bone,
    'Letterer-Siwe disease' and 'Schüller-Christian disease' as related manifestations of
    single nosologic entity. Arch. Path. 56:84–102 (1953).
LINDLAR, F.: Histiozytose der Zentralnerversystems und der Lungen. Dtsch. med. Wschr.
    95:2075–2078 (1970).
LITTERAL and MALAMUD: In Revol, L.; Lacroix, P. R. and Croizat, P.: Contribution à
    l'étude des manifestations neurologiques au cours des leucémies. J. Méd., Lyon
    44:1007–1036 (1963).
LUGARESI, E.; TASSINARI, C. A. and GHEDINI, G.: Complicanze neurologiche in corso di
    emopatie a carattere iper-displastico. Minerva med. giuliana 3:88-90 (1963).
PANELLI, G.; MARIGO, S. and FERRERO, E.: Istioleucemia insorta in corso di grave herpes
    zooster disseminato. Haematologica 51:947–960 (1966).
RUBÉ, J.; DE LA PAVA, S. and PICKREN, J. W.: Histiocytosis X with involvement of brain.
    Cancer, Philad. 20:486–492 (1967).
SACREZ, R.; FRUHLING, L.; HEUMANN, G. and CAHN, R.: Réticulohistiocytose maligne à
    forme cutanée et hématologique chez un nouveau-né. Arch. franç. Pédiat. 11:141–
    150 (1954).
WALTHER, H. and STROCKA, G.: Akute leukämische Reticuloendotheliose unter dem Bilde
    einer 'Lymphosarcomatosis cutis'. Arch. franç. Derm. 166:699–710 (1932).
ZIMMERMANN, H.: Zum Problem der meningealen Leukämie und der meningealen
    Reticulose. Schweiz. med. Wschr. 91:1555–1561 (1961).

Reticulum cell sarcoma

ALLISON, R. S. and GORDON, D. S.: loc. cit.
BLANCHARD, B. M.: Peripheral neuropathy (non-invasive) associated with lymphoma. Ann.
    intern. Med. 56:774–778 (1962).
DELL'ACQUA, G.: Reticolosarcomi. C.R. III Congr. Soc. Int. Européenne Hémat., Rome
    1951, pp. 329–350 (E.M.E.S., Rome 1952).
DRAHOZAL, H.; FUSEK, I. and SVÁCINA, J.: Reticulum cell sarcoma of the spine with
    involvement of the cord. Rozhl. Chir. 40:707–712 (1961).
GALIL-OGLY, G.A. and POROSHIN, K. K.: On the problem of reticulosarcomatosis with
    disorders of the brain and spinal cord. Zhurn. Nevropat., Moskva 61:1655–1657
    (1961).

GOUTELLE, A.; LAPRAZ, CL; RAVON, R. and CHAPUIS, H.: Réticulosarcomes primitifs du rachis. À propos de six observations. J. méd., Lyon 51:937–963 (1970).

LEGEAIS, G.; BOINEAU, N.; BONNET, D. and PIOTROWSKI, J.: Syndrome d'Aran-Duchenne bilatéral au cours d'un réticulo-sarcome de la première côte. Pédiatrie, Lyon 16:727–730 (1961).

LUGARESI *et al.:* loc. cit.

MARTIN, J. B. and BOGAERT, L. VAN: Subacute multifocal leukoencephalopathy with widespread intranuclear inclusions. Arch. Neurol., Chicago 21:590–603 (1969).

ROSENDAL, T.: On reticulum cell sarcoma in bones. Acta radiol., Stockh. 26:210–221 (1945).

WAELBROECK, C.; SCHOUTENS, A.; GEPTS, W. and FLAMENT-DURAND, J.: A propos d'un cas de réticulosarcome du rein associé à une encéphalopathie multifocale progressive. Acta clin. belg. 20:300–310 (1965).

Follicular lymphoma

BORCHERS, H. G. and MITTELBACH, F.: Neurologische Störungen bei Blutkrankheiten. Internist, Berl. 2:105–117 (1961).

HUTCHINSON, E. C.; LEONARD, B. J.; MAUDSLEY, C. and YATES, P. O.: Neurologic complication of reticuloses. Brain 81:75–92 (1958).

SHAFAR, J.: Brill-Symmer's disease presenting as multiple symmetrical peripheral neuropathy. Lancet ii:470–471 (1965).

Eosinophilic granuloma

ACKERMANN, A. J.: Eosinophilic granuloma of bones associated with involvement of lungs and diaphragm. Amer. J. Roentgenol. 58:733–740 (1948).

AMATO, M. and GALLORO, V.: Granuloma eosinofilo con localizzazioni ossee e linfoghiandolari e diabete insipido. Haematologica 45:1181–1208 (1960).

AMATO, M. and CATALANO, D.: Istiocitopatie iperdisplastiche granuloxantomatose dell'infanzia (Ediz. Minerva Medica, Turin 1962).

CUTILLO, S.; CATALANO, D. and ESPOSITO, L.: Sulla evoluzione clinicoradiologica del granuloma eosinofilo. Pediatria 68:553–573 (1960).

ENGELBRETH-HOLM, J.; TEILUM, G. and CHRISTENSEN, E.: Eosinophilic granuloma of bone, Schüller-Christian's disease. Acta med. scand. 118:292–312 (1944).

FASIANI, G. M.: Granuloma eosinofilo dell'orbita. Minerva chir. 1:14–17 (1946).

GREEN, W. T. and FARBER, S.: 'Eosinophilic or solitary granuloma' of bone. J. Bone Jt. Surg. 24:499–526 (1942).

KIERLAND, R. R.; EPSTEIN, J. G. and WEBER, W. E.: Eosinophilic granuloma of skin and mucous membrane; association with diabetes insipidus. Arch. Derm., Chicago 75:45–54 (1957).

OBERMAN, H. A.: A clinicopathologic study of 40 cases and review of the literature on eosinophilic granuloma of bone, Hand-Schüller-Christian disease and Letterer-Siwe disease. Pediatrics 28:307–327 (1961).

RIBUFFO, A.: Granuloma eosinofilo della vulva; associazione con lesioni ossee e diabete insipido. Dermatologia 8:1 (1957).

THOMA, K. H.: Eosinophilic granuloma with report of one case involving first the mandible, later other bones, and being accompanied by diabetes insipidus. Amer. J. Orthod. 29:641–651 (1943).

VERSIANI, O.; FIGUEIRO, J. M. and JUNGUIERA, M. A.: Hand-Schüller-Christian's syndrome and 'eosinophilic or solitary granuloma of bone.' Amer. J. med. Sci. 207:161–166 (1944).

Lipoidosis

ABALLI, A. J. and KATO, K. J.: Gaucher's disease in early infancy; review of literature and report of case with neurological symptoms. J. Pediat. 13:364–380 (1938).

AMATO, M.: La tesaurismosi cerebrosidica (malattia di Gaucher) nella prima infanzia. Pediatria, Naples 55:31–51 (1947).

AVERY, M. E.; McAFFEE, J. G. and GUILD, H. G.: The course and prognosis of reticuloendotheliosis (eosinophilic granuloma, Schüller-Christian disease and Letter-Siwe disease); a study of forty cases. Amer. J. Med. 22:636–652 (1957).

BAFFI, V. and AURICCHIO, G.: Considerazioni sulla patogenesi dell' idiozia amaurotica familiare (a proposito di un caso di 'forma infantile' o 'malattia di Tay-Sachs'). Pediatria, Naples 59:527–538 (1951).

BALCONI, M. and FORNARA, P.: Considerazioni sulla forma giovanile della malattia di Gaucher e sulle sue manifestazioni neuro-psichiche. Minerva med. 60:4399–4415 (1969).

BANKER, B. Q.; MILLER, J. Q. and CROCKER, A. C.: The neurological disorder in infantile Gaucher's disease. Trans. amer. neurol. Ass. 86:43–48 (1961).

BAUMANN, T.; KLENK, E. and SCHEIDEGGER, S.: Die Niemann-Picksche Krankheit. Eine klinische, chemische und histopathologische Studie. Ergebn. allg. Path. path. Anat. 30:183–323 (1936).

BERGER, B.: Données nouvelles sur la maladie de Gaucher. Presse méd. 74:1127–1128 (1966).

BIRD, A.: Lipidoses and central nervous system. Brain 71:434–450 (1948).

BISCHOFF, A.; REUTTER, F. W. and WEGMANN, T.: Erkrankung des peripheren Nervensystems beim Morbus Gaucher. Neue Erkenntnisse auf Grund der Elektronenmikroskopie. Schweiz. med. Wschr. 97:1139–1146 (1967).

BLUEFARB, S. M.: Cutaneous manifestations of the reticuloendothelial granulomas (C. Thomas, Springfield, Ill. 1960).

BOGAERT, L. VAN and FROEHLICH, A.: Un cas de maladie de Gaucher de l'adulte avec syndrome de Raynaud, pigmentation, et rigidité du type extrapiramidal aux membres inférieurs. Ann. Méd. 45:57–70 (1939).

BOSSA, G.: Sul morbo di Schüller-Christian. R.C. Acad. Sci. med. chir. Soc. reale, Naples 91:58 (1937).

BRAIN, W. R.: Les affections dues à la thésaurismose de kérasine. Acta neurol. belg. 54: 597–605 (1954).

BRANTE, G.: Gargoylism-mucopolysaccharidosis. Scand. J. clin. Lab. Invest. 4:43–46 (1952).

CHESTER, W.: Über Lipoidgranulomatose. Virchows Arch. path. Anat. 279:561–602 (1930).

DAVISON, C.: Disturbances in lipoid metabolism and central nervous system. J. Mt. Sinaï Hosp. 9:389–406 (1942).

DORFMAN, A. and LORINCZ, A.E.: Occurrence of urinary acid mucopolysaccharides in Hurler's syndrome. Proc. nat. Acad. Sci., Wash. 43:443–446 (1957).

ELIAN, M.; BORNSTEIN, B.; MATZ, S.; ASKENASY, H. M. and SANBANK, U.: Neurological manifestations of general xanthomatosis (Hand-Schüller-Christian disease). Arch. Neurol., Chicago 21:115–120 (1969).

FAKATSELLI, N. M.: La maladie de Niemann-Pick. À propos de quatre observations personnelles. Méd. Hyg. 28:311–316 (1970).

FASANARO, G.: Encefalopatie dismetaboliche. Lavoro neuropsichiat. 74:109–190 (1954).

GIAMPALMO, A.: Le tesaurosi lipidiche. Atti Soc. ital. Pat. 2:29–230 (1951).

GUCCIONE, F.: Sulle alterazioni del sistema nervoso centrale nella malattia di Hand-Schüller-Christian. Arch. ital. Anat. Istol. pat. 7 (supplm.):427–470 (1937).

HAND, A.: Polyuria and tuberculosis. Arch. Pediat., N.Y. 10:673 (1893).

KAY, T.: Acquired hydrocephalus with atrophic bone changes, exophthalmos and polyuria. Penn. med. J. 9:320–321 (1905).

MALONEY, A. and CUMINGS, J.: A case of juvenile Gaucher's disease with intraneural lipid storage. J. Neurol. Neurosurg. Psychiat. 27:207–213 (1960).

MÉRAB, A.; TALEB, N.; NASSR, W. and HAKIMÉ, H.: Maladie de Gaucher avec manifestations neurologiques. À propos d'un cas chez un enfant de 8 ans. Sem. Hôp., Paris 39:366–371 (1963).

MEYER, R.: A proposito di un nuovo caso di malattia di Gaucher nel lattante. Riv. Pediat. 45:434–447 (1937).

MÜLLER, D. and ORTHNER, H.: Intracerebrale Lipoidgranulomatose. Bericht über zwei Fälle. Dtsch. Z. Nervenheilk. 187:608–636 (1965).

MYERS, B.: Gaucher's disease of lungs. Brit. med. J. ii:8–10 (1937).

PICK, L.: Classification of diseases of lipoid metabolism and Gaucher's disease (Dunham lecture). Amer. J. med. Sci. 185:453–469 (1933). Neimann-Pick's disease and other forms of so-called xanthomatosis (Dunham lecture). Amer. J. med. Sci. 185:601–616 (1933).

PHILIPPART, M.; MARTIN, L.; MARTIN, J. J. and MENKES, J. H.: Niemann-Pick disease. Morphologic and biochemical studies in the visceral form with late central nervous system involvement (Crocker's group C). Arch. Neurol., Chicago 20:227–238 (1969).

PLUM, F. and POSNER, J. B.: Diagnosis of stupor and coma. (Blackwell Scient. Publ., Oxford 1966).

PORTILLO, J. M.; MAÑE-GARZON, F.; BIDEGAIN, S. and LEGNAZZI, E.: Enfermedad de Gaucher de lactante y su sindromo neurologico. Arch. Pediat. Uruguay 31:653–659 (1960).

REISS, O. and KATO, K.: Gaucher's disease; clinical study, with special reference to roentgenography of bones. Amer. J. Dis. Child. 43:365–386 (1932).

ROOS et al.: in Amato and Catalano (loc. cit.)

SCHETTLER, G. and KAHLKE, W.: Gaucher's disease and Niemann-Pick disease; in Schettler Lipids and lipidoses, pp. 260-309 (Springer, Berlin-Heidelberg-New York 1967).

SCHÜLLER, A.: Ueber eigenartige Schädeldefekte im Jugendalter. Fortschr. Röntgenstr., vol. 23, pp. 12–18 (Hamburg 1915–1916).

TRONCONI, V.: Sindromi neurologiche da alterato metabolismo dei fosfoeglico-lipidi (neurodislipidosi). Asclepieo, Milano 3:121–125 (1957).

ULLRICH, O.: Die Pfaundler-Hurler'sche Krankheit. Ergebn. inn. Med. Kinderheilk. 62:929 (1943).

UZMAN, L. L.: Chemical nature of storage substance in gargoylism; Hurler-Pfaundler's disease. Arch. Path. 60:308–318 (1955).

WALLACE, B. J.; SCHNECK, L.; KAPLAN, H. and VOLK, B. W.: Fine structure of the cerebellum of children with lipidoses. Arch. Path. 80:466–486 (1965).

ZÖLLNER, N.: Schüller-Christiansche Krankheit. In Heilmeyer and Hittmair, Handbuch der gesamten Hämatologie, vol. V/1, pp. 202–209 (Urban & Schwarzenberg, Munich-Berlin 1964).

Appendix. Primary reticulosis of the nervous system

BAILEY, P.: Intracranial sarcomatous tumors of leptomeningeal origin. Arch. Surg. 18: 1359–1402 (1929).

CASTAIGNE, P.; CAMBIER, J.; ESCOUROLLE, R. and MASSON, M.: Réticulose cérébrale circonscrite à double localisation hypothalamique et protubérantielle (observation anatomo-clinique). Presse méd. 76:1213–1216 (1968).

COSTE, F. and BRION, S.: Étude anatomo-clinique d'un cas de périthélio-sarcome du système nerveux central. Sem. Hôp., Paris 82:3305–3312 (1952).

DELARUE, J.; SIGWALD, J.; BOUTTIER, D.; VEDRENNE, C. and CHOMETTE, G.: L'encéphalite réticulo-granulomateuse. Essai d'interprétation nosologique: les réticuloses proliféra-tives du névraxe. Ann. Anat. path. 6:429–455 (1961).

EDERLI, A. and MERIGLIANO, D.: Reticolosi primitive del sistèma nervoso. Riv. Neurol. 37:589–617 (1967).

FISHER, E. R.; DAVIS, E. R. and LEMMEN, L. J.: Reticulum cell sarcoma of brain (microglioma). Arch. Neurol., Chicago 81:591–598 (1959).
HENSCHEN, F.: In Lubarsch and Henke, Handbuch der speziellen pathologischen Anatomie und Histologie, vol. XIII/3, p. 641 (Springer, Berlin-Göttingen-Heidelberg 1955).
HSÜ, Y. K.: Primary intracranial sarcomas. Arch. Neurol., Chicago 43:901–924 (1940).
KINNEY, T. D. and ADAMS, R. D.: Reticulum cell sarcoma of brain. Arch. Neurol., Chicago 50:552–564 (1943).
MARCHIAFAVA, G. and BIGNAMI, A.: Reticulosi primitive del sistema nervoso centrale. Contributo anatomo-clinico. Osservazione di due casi. Arch. ital. Anat. Istol. pat. 29:511–532 (1955).
RUSSEL, D. S.; MARSHALL, A. H. E. and SMITH, F. B.: Microgliomatosis: a form of reticulosis affecting brain. Brain 71:1–15 (1948).
SIGWALD, J.; DELARUE, J.; BOUTTIER, D.; CHOMETTE, G. and VEDRENNE, C.: Ètude anatomo-clinique d'un cas d'encéphalite réticulo-granulomateuse. Les réticuloses prolifératives du névraxe. Rev. neurol. 105:526–528 (1961).
WHITE, B. E. and ROTHFLEISCH, S.: Primary cerebellar lymphoma. A case report. Neurology, Minneap. 18:582–586 (1968).
WILKE, G.: Uber primäre Reticuloendotheliosen des Gehirns. Mit besonderer Berücksichtigung bisher unbekannter eigenartiger granulomatöser Hirnprozesse. Dtsch. Z. Nervenheilk. 164:332–380 (1950).
YUILE, C. L.: Case of primary reticulum cell sarcoma of brain; relationship of microglia cells to histiocytes. Arch. Path. 26:1036–1044 (1938).

Infectious mononucleosis

AMYOT, R.: Les syndromes neuro-hématologiques. Union méd. Canada 90:1118–1126 (1961).
BENDER, C. E.: The value of corticosteroids in the treatment of infectious mononucleosis. J. amer. med. Ass. 199:529–531 (1967).
BROGARD, J. M.; CORET, F. and JAHN, H.: Encéphalo-méningite à forme comateuse révélatrice d'une mononucléose infectieuse. Strasbourg méd. 19:269–276 (1968).
COTTON, P. B. and WEBB-PEPLOE, M. M.: Acute transverse myelitis as a complication of glandular fever. Brit. med. J. i:654–655 (1966).
DAVIE, J. C.; CEBALLOS, R. and LITTLE, S. C.: Infectious mononucleosis with fatal neuronitis. Arch. Neurol., Chicago 9:265–272 (1963).
DOWLING, M. D. JR. and SLYCK, E. J.VAN: Cerebellar disease in infectious mononucleosis. Arch. Neurol., Chicago 15:270–274 (1966).
EPSTEIN, S. H. and DAMESHEK, W.: Involvement of central nervous system in case of glandular fever. New Engl. J. Med. 205:1238–1241 (1931).
ERAMO, N.D. and GUALTIERI, G.: Su un caso di mononucleosi infettiva con manifestazioni neurologiche. Gaz. int. Med. Chir. 73:209–212 (1968).
ERLE, G.: Sindrome di Guillain-Barré e mononucleosi infettiva. Descrizione di un caso trattato con corticosteroidi in rachide. Minerva med. 56:3626–3628 (1965).
GAUTIER-SMITH, P. C.: Neurological complications of glandular fever (infectious mononucleosis). Brain 88:323–334 (1965).
GIROIRE, H.; CHARBONNEL, A.; VERCELLETTO, P.; FÈVE, J. R. and BESANÇON, G.: Les manifestations neurologiques de la mononucléose infectieuse. J. Méd., Nantes 4:1–14 (1964).
HOUTTEVILLE, J. P.; GACHES, T.; GARREAU, T. and TREMAN, G.: Méningo-encéphalite gravissime avec silence. E.E.G. totale au cours d'une mononucléose infectieuse, Guérison. Bull. Soc. méd. Hôp. Paris 121:347–353 (1970).
JOHANSEN, A. H.: Serous meningitis and infectious mononucleosis. Acta med. scand. 76:269–272 (1931).

KLEMOLA, E.: Studies of infectious mononucleosis. Acta med. scand. 127:149–170 (1947).
LEIBOWITZ, S.: Infectious mononucleosis (Grune & Stratton, New York 1953).
MÜNTER, M. D.: Querschnitts myelitis bei infektiöser Mononukleose. Med. Klin. 64:1752–1755 (1969).
PROCHAZKA, J. and KOUBA, K.: Complicazioni nella mononucleosi infettiva. Minerva med. 52:3680–3684 (1961).
RENTCHNICK, P.: Les formes nerveuses de la mononucléose infectieuse. Presse méd. 64:473–478 (1956). Les formes nerveuses de la mononucléose infectieuse. Presse méd. 64:589–590 (1956).
RETIF, J.; BEGHIN, P. and BRIHAYE, J.: Ataxie cérébelleuse aiguë, forme neurologique de la mononucléose infecticuse. Acta neurol. belg. 62:884–899 (1962).
VERLIAC et al.: In Bulgarelli, La mononucleosi infettiva, p. 17 (Ediz. Minerva Medica, Turin 1968).

Acute infectious lymphocytosis

DUNCAN, P. A.: Acute infectious lymphocytosis in young adults. New Engl. J. Med. 233:177–179 (1945).
MARINESCO, G.: La lymphocytose infectieuse aiguë, (une nouvelle lymphoréticulite aiguë bénigne) (Masson, Paris 1965).
THELANDER, H.E. and SHAW, E.B.: Infectious mononucleosis, with special reference to cerebral complications. Amer. J. Dis. Child. 61:1131–1145 (1941).

Chapter XII

NEUROLOGICAL SYMPTOMS IN
MYELOSCLEROSIS

Neurological alterations have been reported in Albers-Schönberg disease (osteopetrosis or marble bones). This is a familiar condition of generalized bone sclerosis and extreme fragility, followed by marrow fibrosis and deficient hemopoiesis. Extramedullary hemopoiesis may take place in the spleen, liver, or even in the lymph nodes and other sites.

Osteosclerotic anemia (or osteomyelosclerosis) is a cryptogenic, acquired form of myelosclerosis. Secondary forms of myelosclerosis (toxic, leukemic, etc.) are also known. *Di Guglielmo* holds that osteomyelosclerosis is an expression of primary marrow sclerosis followed by metaplastic bone sclerosis, whereas *Bufano* considers it an example of "systemic-tending histiocyte sarcomatosis." In his view, the observed bone marrow, spleen, and other organ alterations are caused by histiocyte proliferation, with differences of course and manifestation in the various tissues affected.

Cranial bone alterations or narrowing of the basal foramina may lead to 2nd, 7th, 8th, and 12th cranial nerve lesions in Albers-Schönberg disease. *Keith* observed a picture of retinal atrophy and optic nerve damage (gliosis, reduced nerve fiber number, and degeneration) in a case in which neither optic canal stenosis or relevant bone compression was present.

Cerebrospinal fluid (CSF) hypertension is common and may be accompanied by intracranial hypertension. Hydrocephalus is rare. It may be the cause of serious optic nerve alterations (*Lorey and Reye*) and psychological disturbances, and is thought to be the result of occlusion of emissary vessels in the sclerotic cranial diploë.

Nerve compression may also be caused by tumor-like extramedullary hemopoietic masses (*Appleby et al.*). *Polliack and Rosenmann* noted such masses in the cranial dura mater of three patients at necropsy, following their *in vivo* clinical silence in pictures of myelofibrosis and terminal leukemia, thalassemia major, and chronic myeloid leukemia, respectively.

REFERENCES

APPLEBY, A.; BATSON, G. A.; LASSMAN, L. P. and SIMPSON, C. A.: Spinal cord compression by extramedullary hematopoiesis in myelosclerosis. J. Neurochem. Neurosurg. Psychiat. 27:313–316 (1964).

BUFANO, M.: L'inquadramento delle fibrosi e delle osteosclerosi criptogenetiche del midollo osseo tra le sarcomatosi poliblastiche del sistema delle cellule istiocitarie. Fisiopatologia e clinica del sistema reticolo istiocitario (Atti delle Giornate Mediche Triestine), Trieste 1965, pp. 101–112 (Ediz. Scuola Med. Osped. Trieste 1966).

GUGLIELMO, G. DI: Alterazioni acquisite concernenti l'ematopoiesi e la struttura ossea. V kongr. europ. Gesellschaft f. Hämat., Freiburg i Br. 1955, pp. 518–523 (Springer, Berlin-Göttingen-Heidelberg 1956). La malattia osteomielosclerotica. Progr. med., Naples 12:353–350 (1956).

KEITH, C. G.: Retinal atrophy in osteopetrosis. Arch. Ophthal., Chicago 79:234–242 (1968).

LOREY and REYE: Ueber Marmorknochen (Albers-Schönbergsohe Krankheit). Fortschr. Röntgenstr., vol. 30, pp. 35–43 (Hamburg 1922–1923).

POLLIACK, A. and ROSENMANN, E.: Extramedullary hematopoietic tumors of the cranial dura mater. Acta haemat., Basel 41:43–48 (1969).

Chapter XIII

NEUROLOGICAL SYMPTOMS IN HEMOCHROMATOSIS

Hemochromatosis is a metabolic disease caused by increased intestinal mucosa iron absorption (endogenous or idiopathic form). Deposits of iron in various tissues are responsible for the symptomatology (skin pigmentation, liver sclerosis, testicular atrophy, diabetes mellitus, and cardiac insufficiency). The exogenous form is the result of repeated blood tranfusions.

Neurological complications have been observed in the endogenous form only. They are of importance, however, even if only hypothetically, in questions of differential diagnosis relating to nerve signs in blood diseases treated with transfusions over a long period.

Their pathogenesis is a matter of controversy. With the exception of the case reported by *Ott* (hemosiderin deposits in the hypophysis and diencephalon), and the clinical data have never been confirmed on necropsy. Furthermore, hemosiderin deposits have no precise diagnostic value, since they have been observed in nerve formations of hemochromatosis patients with no signs of neurological involvement during life. The finding may come as a surprise at necropsy, in cases where no other clinical and anatomic signs of hemochromatosis are observed. It has therefore been suggested that metabolic disturbances are responsible for the nerve pictures observed in this disease (*Bergouignan et al.*).

Such pictures are, in any event, rare and, as stated, appear only in the endogenous form.

Weil has reported alternating depression and excitement in three cases and convulsions in one of a series of seven cases. *Raverdy et al.* observed an association of hemochromatosis and epilepsy in two families. *Ott's* patient, a 55-year-old man, had presented behavior disturbances for many years before the appearance of glycosuria, prostration, and terminal coma within the space of a few weeks.

Necropsy showed hepatic hemochromatosis accompanied by carcinoma, together with hemosiderin deposits in the myocardium as well as those in the hypophysis and diencephalon.

Depression and touches of delirium had been observed by *Boudin et al.* in a 55-year-old man some months before the sudden appearance of anxiety, slight confusion, dysarthria, an extrapyramidal syndrome, and, later, signs of pyramidal irritation. An increased CSF albumin value was noted. Following two convulsion episodes the neurological symptoms regressed, dysarthria being the most persistent. The patient's condition was satisfactory three years later.

Hemochromatosis appeared with diabetes some years earlier in a 43-year-old man observed by *Bergouignan et al.* and had been diagnosed from hepatomegaly, hemosiderin deposits in the liver biopsy specimen, testicular atrophy, and hyperferremia. The EEG picture was marked by generalized low voltage. Behavior disturbances (occupational instability, constant unpunctuality, jealousy, and threats of aggression toward his family) had been present for a long time. Later, episodes of somnolence and one of agitation with hallucinations were observed. Neurosurgical examination excluded the possibility of an expanding intracranial process. The CSF protein level was increased only slightly. When observed by *Bergouignan et al.* the patient presented a certain degree of agitation and jumbled speech. Persistent questioning resulted in answers indicative of a state of confusion. Neurological examination showed widespread hyperesthesia and lower extremity areflexia. The most important feature of the case was the occurrence of psychological changes from one moment to another. Death took place in a state of coma.

REFERENCES

BERGOUIGNAN, M.; MOUTON, L. and VITAL, CL.: Hémochromatose et manifestations neuro-psychiatriques. J. Méd., Bordeaux 142:743–749 (1965).

BOUDIN, G.; LAURAS, A. and ISMAIL, B.: Manifestations neuro-psychiques au cours d'une hémochromatose idiopatique. Rev. neurol. 109:564–568 (1963).

OTT, B.: Ueber psychische Veränderungen bei Hämochromatose. Nervenarzt 28:356–360 (1957).

RAVERDY, P.; CHRISTOPHE, M. and SIGWALD, J.: Épilepsie et hémochromatose. Deux observations familiales. Rev. neurol. 107:530–533 (1962).

WEIL, J. P.: Thèse Strasbourg (1954).

CONCLUSIONS

Our discussion of nerve damage in the course of diseases of the blood, itself sometimes without expression on the clinical level and detectable solely as a result of systematic investigation or during necropsy, has shown that a wide variety of clinical pictures, sometimes of notable complexity, may be encountered.

Classification of these clinical pictures, including, as they do, symptoms that are in no way specific in themselves, is not easy, though some of the more frequently observed patterns can be distinguished. In the case of the brain, one may point to vascular syndromes (malacia caused by ischemia, hemorrhage), pseudotumoral syndromes, multifocal syndromes, and some forms of infantile encephalopathy (noted in constitutional hemolytic jaundice and in the sequelae of sickle cell anemia, erythroblastosis fetalis, hemophilic intracranial hemorrhage, and hemorragic disease of the newborn). In the case of the spinal cord, there are cord compression and section sydromes as well as those affecting the posterior and lateral funiculi (funicular myelosis), while peripheral pictures include poly-, radiculo-, mono-, and multineuritis syndromes. Lastly, reference may be made to meningeal infiltration or hemorrhage syndromes and to signs of muscle involvement, particularly in cases of sarcoidosis.

There is usually a cause-and-effect relationship between the underlying blood disease and the nerve lesion. This may be direct, or indirect—as in degeneration and in the so-called paraneoplastic alterations of the nervous system sometimes observed in systemic blood diseases, though their relationship with the hemopathic process is no more than hypothetical. In some cases, a common etiology may be discerned. Thus vitamin B_{12} deficiency is the cause of both the blood disease and its accompanying neurological damage in pernicious anemia. The same is usually true of the albeit singular cause of Albers-Schönberg disease, namely bone sclerosis.

With respect to leukemia, some workers have suggested that a virus is responsible for the hemopoietic disturbances that are the essential features of the disease and is also active on the nervous system. In the case of paraneoplastic alterations, the suggestion has been made that a congenital or acquired systemic metabolic deficiency is the cause of both the blood disease and the neurological syndrome.

Chromosome abnormality has been seen as a common causal factor in both the hematological and the neurological manifestations observed in some deformity conditions (Fanconi's syndrome, etc.)

The appearance of nerve involvement is the source of difficulties in diagnosis when it is the initial, or more particularly, when it is the only clinical expression of the underlying blood disease (so-called simple neurologic forms).

Nerve system damage is a poor prognostic sign, particularly in systemic blood diseases. Even in these cases, however, medical, surgical, and radiation therapy may sometimes be followed by considerable improvement or even regression of neurological symptoms, while long periods of regression equivalent to cure are not unknown. It will be clear, therefore, that the early formulation of an exact diagnosis and the commencement of suitable treatment are matters of prime importance.

APPENDIX

RECENT REFERENCES NOT CITED IN TEXT

CHAPTER I

Perniciosiform anemia

BANERJI, N.K. and HURWITZ, L.J.: Nervous system manifestations after gastric surgery. Acta neurol. scand. 47:485–513 (1971).

Iron-deficiency anemia

KNIZLEY, H. JR. and NOYES, W.D.: Iron deficiency anemia, papilledema, thrombocytosis and transient hemiparesis. Arch. intern. Med. 129:483–486 (1972).

Hemolytic anemia

JOHNSON, R.V.; KAPLAN, S.R. and BLAILOCK, Z.R.: Cerebral venous thrombosis in paroxysmal nocturnal hemoglobinuria. Marchiafava-Micheli syndrome. Neurology. Minneap. 20:681–686 (1970).

CHAPTER IV

ALEMÀ, G.: Porfiria acuta intermittente. Atti Accad. Lancisiana, vol. XV, pp. 279–292 (Roma 1971).

RAMAN, P.T.; SAHADEVAN, M.G. and HOON, R.S.: Recurrent Landry-Guillain Barré syndrome in intermittent acute porphyria. J. Ass. Physicians India 17:267–268 (1969).

CHAPTER V

BERNARD, J. and DELOBEL, J.: Studio clinico, evolutivo e terapeutico di 341 casi di porpore trombopeniche idiopatiche. Minerva med. 63:1333–1344 (1972).

DINI, E. and ROSA, L. DE: La porpora trombocitopenica idiopatica. Consuntivo clinico e terapeutico di un dodicennio. Minerva med. 63:1345–1355 (1972).

LEHMANN, W.; FRITZSCHE, S. and SCHMECHTA, H.: Todliche intracranielle Blutung bei Thrombocytopenie. Mitteilung eines Falles. Psychiat. Neurol. med. Psychol., Lpz 22:262–265 (1970).

LÉVY, A. and STULA, D.: Neurochirurgische Aspekte bei Antikoagulantienblutungen in Zentralnervensystem. Dtsch. med. Wschr. 96:1043–1048 (1971).

MYLES, S.T.; HARRIS, C.E.C. and HANSEBOUT, R.R.: Epidural hematoma in hemophilia: successful treatment. Canad. med. Ass. J. 14:51–52 (1971).

CHAPTER VI

BALLARD, H.S. and MARCUS, A.J.: Hypercalcemia in chronic myelogenous leukemia. New Engl. J. Med. 282:663–665 (1970).

BAUTERS, F.; LERCHE, B. and GOUDEMAND, M.: Les méningites leucémiques. A' propos d'une statisque de 33 cas. Sem. Hôp., Paris 46:2516–2523 (1970).

BENOIT, P.; RAYMOND, R. and DROLET, Y.: Méningite leucémique chez l'enfant. Union méd. Canada 100:1100–1104 (1971).

BENVENISTI, D.S.; SHERWOOD, L.M. and HEINEMANN, H.O.: Hypercalcemic crisis in acute leukemia. Amer. J. Med. 46:976–984 (1969).

CLINE, M.J.: Cancer chemotherapy, pp. 128–130 (Saunders, Philadelphia and London 1971).

FERRARA, A.; LAGHI, V. and MANGO, G.: Compressione midollare e paraplegia da formazione neoplastiforme in corso di leucemia mieloide cronica in remissione. Progr. med., Roma 27:634–638 (1971).

FIERE, D.; BYRON, P.A.; DECHAVANNE, M. et al.: Evolution thérapeutique de 30 leucémies aiguës lymphoblastiques récentes. Lyon méd. 225:109–114 (1971).

GEILS, G. F.: Treatment of meningeal leukemia with pyrimethamine. Blood 38:131–138 (1971).

GUPTA, S.P.; AGARWAL, P.K. and PRATAP, V.B.: Proptosis. A manifestation of acute myelogenous leukaemia. Orient. Arch. Ophthal., New Delhi 8:94–97 (1970).

HURWITZ, B.S.; SUTHERLANDS, J.C. and WALKER, M.D.: Central nervous system chloromas preceding acute leukemia by one year. Neurology, Minneap. 20:771–775 (1970).

JHA, B. K. and LARUBA, P.A.: Proptosis as a manifestation of acute myeloid leukaemia. Brit. J. Ophthal. 55:844–847 (1971).

MAJ MELVIN, L. and BUTLER, M.C.: Hypercalcemia and leukemia. Proc. roy. Soc. Med. 63:591–592 (1970).

MANDELLI, F.: La polichemioterapia delle leucemie acute. Atti Accad. Lancisiana, vol. XIV, pp. 427–453 (Roma 1970).

MUSSA, G.C.; MADON, E. and MARTINI MAURI, M.: La scintigrafia cerebrale nella complicanza meningoencefalica durante la leucemia mieloblastica acuta infantile. Minerva pediat. 23:1017–1022 (1971).

OBERLING, F.; LANG, J.M.; HERDLY, J.; BUCHHEIT, F.; THIEBAUT, J.B. and WAITZ, R.: Syndrome aigu de la fosse postérieure au décours d'une poussée évolutive de leucémie lymphoblastique. Irradiation d'urgence. J. Méd. Strasbourg 3:47–49 (1972).

POUILLART, P.; SCHWARZENBERG, L.; SCHNEIDER, M.; AMIEL, J.L. and MATHÉ, G.: Méningites lymphoblastiques. Incidence, prévention et traitement. Nouv. Presse méd. 1:387–390 (1972).

RUBINSTEIN, M.A.: Carpal tunnel syndrome in lymphatic leukemia. J. amer. med. Ass. 213:1037 (1970).

STEIN, R.C.: Hypercalcemia in leukemia. J. Pediat. 78:861–864 (1971).

STORTI, E. and QUAGLINO, A.: Dysmetabolic and neurological complications in leukemia patients treated with L asparaginase. Recent Results Cancer Res., Berl. 33:344–349 (1970).

STORTI, E. and FONTANA, G.: Il punto sull'impiego della L-asparaginasi in terapia con particolare riguardo alla leucemia linfatica acuta. Minera med. 63:1445–1456 (1972).

CHAPTER VII

RAMAN, P.T.; SAHADEVAN, M.G. and HOON, R.S.: Landry-Guillain-Barré syndrome complicating lymphosarcoma. A case report. J. Ass. Physicians India 17:215–216 (1969).

CHAPTER VIII

CLINE, M.J.: Cancer chemotherapy, p. 161 (Saunders, Philadelphia and London 1971).

Le Gall, E.; Beley, G.; Mayer, G.; Guerci, O.; Thibaut, G. and Herbeuval, R.: Localisations cérébrales de lymphoréticulopathies. Ann. méd. Nancy 11:205–210 (1972).

Reagan, T.J. and Derby, B.M.: Intracerebral Hodgkin's disease. Dis. nerv. Syst. 32:843–847 (1971).

CHAPTER IX

Dickinson, E.S.: Sarcoid meningoencephalitis. Diagnostic difficulties encountered in two cases. Dis. nerv. Syst. 32:118–124 (1971).

Schubert, J.C.F.; Güllner, H.R.; Fischer, M. and Kropp, R.: Boecksches Sarkoid des Nervensystems. Dtsch. med. Wschr. 96:945–951 (1971).

CHAPTER X

David-Jones, G.A. and Esiri, M.M.: Neuropathy due to amyloid in myelomatosis. Brit. med. J. ii:444 (1971).

Djaidane, A.; Mayer, G.; Guerci, O.; Thibaut, G.; Andre, J.L. and Herbeuval, R.: Les encéphalopathies hypercalcémiques au cours du myélome multiple (sans insuffisance rénale). Ann. méd. Nancy 11:229–237 (1972).

Gordon, H.; Bandmann, M. and Sandbank, V.: Multiple myeloma associated with progressive multifocal leukoencephalopathy and Pneumocystis carinii pneumonia. Israel J. med. Sci. 7:581–588 (1971).

Gravano, L.; Schajowicz, F. and Menzani, A.: Mieloma multiplo de forma osteoblastica. Sindrome neurologico paraneoplasico. Prensa med. argent. 57:1659–1663 (1970).

Heesen, H.; Engelhardt, K. and Reiner, F.: Polyneuropathie als Leitsymptom eine gamma-G-Plasmocytoms. Z. ges. Neurol. Psychiat. 193:145–150 (1971).

Kollar, A.W.A.F.: Plasmozytome als Tumor spinalis. Wien. med. Wschr. 121:848–850 (1971).

Manigand, G.; Delarue, R.; Foulon, D. and Deparis, M. Hypercalcémie et anomalies électroencéphalographiques. A' propos d'une observation de maladie de Kahler avec hypercalcémie. Sem. Hôp., Paris 45:2026–2030 (1969).

Appendix. Cryoglobulinemia, Waldenström's disease

Abramsky, O.; Herishanu, Y. and Lavy, S.: Cryoglobulinemia and cerebrovascular accident. Confin. neurol. 33:291–296 (1972).

Huth, K.; Ehlers, G.; Knoth, W.; Kunze, K.; Loeffler, H.; Maehr, G. and Petzoldt, D.: Lichen myxoedematosis bei Makroglobulinämie Waldenström mit Polyneuropathie und carpal-tunnel Syndrom. Dtsch. med. Wschr. 97:152–159 (1972).

CHAPTER XI

Reticulum cell sarcoma

Bertelsen, K.: Primary cerebral reticulosarcoma. Path. Microbiol. 78/2 (sect. A): 209–214 (1970).

Mikol, J. Bousser, M.G. and Grellet, F.: Paraplégie au cours d'une lymphographie chez une malade atteinte d'un réticulosarcome ganglionnaire cervical. (Étude anatomo-clinique). Ann. Méd. intern. 121:355–362 (1970).

NEAULT, R.W.; SCOY, R.E. VAN; OKAZAKI, H. and MC CARTY, C.S.: Uveitis associated with isolated reticulum cell sarcoma of the brain. Amer. J. Ophthal. 73:431–436 (1972).

PLAFKER, J.; MARTINEZ, A.J. and ROSENBLUM, W.I.: A neoplasm of the reticuloendothelial system involving brain (microglioma) and viscera (reticulum cell sarcoma). Sth. med. J. 65:385–389 (1972).

POVLSEN, C.O.: Reticulum cell sarcoma in the cerebellum. Ugeskr. Laeg. 132:1724–1726 (1970).

Follicular lymphoma

CURRIE, S. and HENSON, R.A.: Neurological syndromes in the reticuloses. Brain 94:307–320 (1971).

Appendix. Infectious mononucleosis

KIFFER, A. and DUFOUR, P.: Paralysie laringée et pharingée unilatérale régressive complication d'une mononucléose infectieuse. A'propos de 2 cas. Rev. Oto-Neuro-Ophtal. 43:157–160 (1971).

LIEBERMAN, A.N. and SHATTUCK, C.: Seizures in infectious mononucleosis. Milit. Med. 135:569–570 (1970).

ROBERGE, C.; BOUCHE, B.; GIGUÈRE, R.; DROLET, M. and BÉLANGER, C.: L'encéphalite de la mononucléose infectieuse. Union méd. Canada 101:272–278 (1972).

SWORN, M.J. and URICH, H.: Acute encephalitis in infectious mononucleosis. J. Path. 100:201–205 (1970).

CHAPTER XII

HEFFNER, R.R. JR. and KOEHL, R.H.: Hemopoiesis in the spinal epidural space. Case report. J. Neurosurg. 32:485–490 (1970).

INDEX

INDEX

Abdominal symptoms, in porphyria, 69, 72
Afibrinogenemia, congenital, 87
Albers-Schönberg disease, 264
Amaurosis, in anemia from hemorrhage, 2
Amyloidosis, and carpal tunnel syndrome, 215
Anemia, 1–35
  from anticonvulsant drugs, 15
  aplastic, 2
  in benzolism, 26
  bothriocephalus, 15
  cold agglutinin, 24–26
  Cooley's, 23–24
  drepanocytic, 18
  erythroblastosis fetalis, 26–35
  in folic acid deficiency, 4–5, 15
  and geophagy, 22
  in hemoglobinuria, paroxysmal nocturnal, 24
  hemolytic, 17–35
    from autoantibodies, 24–26
  iron-deficiency, 16–17
  methemoglobinemia, 24
  osteosclerotic, 264
  ovalocytary, 23
  perniciosiform, 15
  pernicious, 2–15, 167
  postgastrectomy, 15
  in pregnancy, 15
  sickle-cell, 18–23
    treatment of, 23
Anticonvulsant drugs, anemia from, 15
Aphasia
  in polycythemia vera, 50
  in sickle-cell anemia, 21
  in thrombocythemia, hemorrhagic, 92
  in Waldenström's macroglobulinemia, 223

Apraxia, in polycythemia vera, 52
Arachnoid infiltrations, in leukemia, 102–103, 109
Arachnoiditis, in sarcoidosis, 183, 185
Astereognosis, in pernicious anemia, 9
Asthenia
  in leukemia, 124
  in porphyria, 70
  in Waldenström's macroglobulinemia, 224
Ataxia, in infectious mononucleosis, 256
Atherosclerosis, cerebral, in polycythemia vera, 48
Athetosis, in erythroblastosis fetalis, 30, 33
Auditory nerve, in pernicious anemia, 11

Babinski reflex
  in Gaucher's disease, 250
  in Moschcowitz disease, 95
  in pernicious anemia, 9
  in polycythemia vera, 51
  in porphyria, 71
  in Waldenström's macroglobulinemia, 222
Benzolism, anemia from, 26
Biermer's disease. *See* Anemia, pernicious
Bilirubin in brain, effects of, 26–27
Bing and Neel syndrome, 221
Bone marrow, in pernicious anemia, 12
Bothriocephalus anemias, 15
Brill-Symmers disease, 142, 143, 244–245
Brown-Séquard syndrome
  and Hodgkin's disease, 153, 155, 164
  and multiple myeloma, 211
Brudzinski sign, in leukemia, 109

funicular
in cold agglutinin disease, 25
in iron-deficiency anemia, 16
and multiple myeloma, 214
in pernicious anemia, 10, 12–13
postgastrectomy, 15
and reticulosis, 138
in sickle-cell anemia, 21
in sprue, 15
in thalassemia minor, 23
Myopathy
in leukemia, 123–124
in reticulum cell sarcoma, 244
in sarcoidosis, 193–194
in Waldenström's macroglobulinemia, 224

Nausea and vomiting
in anemia from hemorrhage, 1
in hemorrhagic disease of newborn,
86
in Hodgkin's disease, 160
in leukemia, 109, 124
in Moschcowitz disease, 94
in polycythemia vera, 46, 49, 54, 56
in porphyria, 69, 70
Neuritis and polyneuritis
in cryoglobulinemia, 220
in Hodgkin's disease, 158
in iron-deficiency anemia, 16
in leukemia, 123, 127
in lymphosarcoma, 142
in pernicious anemia, 11, 12
in polycythemia vera, 55
in porphyria, 70
in reticulosis, 238
in sarcoidosis, 192
in sickle-cell anemia, 22
in thrombocythemia, hemorrhagic,
93
Niemann-Pick's disease, 251–252
Nissl degeneration, in erythroblastosis
fetalis, 27
Nucha
in erythroblastosis fetalis, 28–29, 31
in hemorrhagic disease of newborn,
86
in leukemia, 109
Nystagmus
in erythroblastosis fetalis, 33

in hemorrhagic disease of newborn,
86
in mononucleosis, infectious, 256
in pernicious anemia, 11
in sarcoidosis, 190, 191

Ocular symptoms. *See* Eye signs
Oculogyric crisis, in erythroblastosis
fetalis, 33
Oculomotor paralysis
in Hodgkin's disease, 157, 158
in polycythemia vera, 54
Opisthotonos
in erythroblastosis fetalis, 31
in hemorrhagic disease of newborn,
86
in Niemann-Pick's disease, 251
Optic nerve atrophy, in anemia from
hemorrhage, 1–2
Osteomyelosclerosis, 264
Osteopetrosis, 264
Osteotendinous reflexes
in cold agglutinin disease, 25
in erythroblastosis fetalis, 29, 31
in porphyria, 70
Ovalocytary anemia, 23

Pain
in Hodgkin's disease, 152, 158
in multiple myeloma, 210
in polycythemia vera, 50
Pancoast syndrome, and Hodgkin's
disease, 159
Papilledema
in intracranial hypertension, 116
in leukemia, 116
in Moschcowitz disease, 94
in pernicious anemia, 11
in sarcoidosis, 183, 191
in Waldenström's macroglobulinemia, 225
Papillitis, in iron-deficiency anemia, 17
Paragranuloma, 146
Para-Hodgkin syndromes, 166–172
Paralysis. *See also* Hemiplegia; Paraplegia
in porphyria, 70
Paraplegia
in Burkitt's lymphoma, 143
in hemolytic icterus, 18
in Hodgkin's disease, 152